Essentials of Community Medicine
A Practical Approach

Essentials of Community Medicine

A Practical Approach

SECOND EDITION

Lalita D Hiremath MD
Professor
Department of Community Medicine
S Nijalingappa Medical College
Bagalkot, Karnataka, India

Dhananjaya A Hiremath MD
Professor
Department of Anesthesia
S Nijalingappa Medical College
Bagalkot, Karnataka, India

Foreword
SJ Nagalotimath

JAYPEE BROTHERS MEDICAL PUBLISHERS
The Health Sciences Publisher
New Delhi | London

Jaypee Brothers Medical Publishers (P) Ltd

Headquarters
EMCA House
23/23-B, Ansari Road, Daryaganj
New Delhi 110 002, India
Landline: +91-11-23272143,
+91-11-23272703
+91-11-23282021, +91-11-23245672
E-mail: jaypee@jaypeebrothers.com

Corporate Office
Jaypee Brothers Medical Publishers (P) Ltd.
4838/24, Ansari Road, Daryaganj
New Delhi 110 002, India
Phone: +91-11-43574357
Fax: +91-11-43574314
E-mail: jaypee@jaypeebrothers.com

Overseas Office
JP Medical Ltd.
83, Victoria Street, London
SW1H 0HW (UK)
Phone: +44-20 3170 8910
E-mail: info@jpmedpub.com

EU GPSR Authorised Representative
Logos Europe, 9 rue Nicolas Poussin
17000, La Rochelle, France
Phone: +33 (0) 6 67 93 73 78
E-mail: Contact@logoseurope.eu

Website: www.jaypeebrothers.com
Website: www.jaypeedigital.com

Inquiries for bulk sales may be solicited at: jaypee@jaypeebrothers.com

Essentials of Community Medicine—A Practical Approach

First Edition: 2004
Reprint: 2006
Second Edition: 2012, Reprint: **2026**

ISBN: 978-93-5025-044-0

Printed in India

Foreword

There was a time when medical students used to consider community medicine as a less important subject. The result sheet used to show passing percentage over 95 percent. But the subject has gained importance steadily. Today it is one of the important subjects. Not only the theory but the practicals are also important.

Students need a manual to complete the practicals. However, a useful practical manual was not available. This lacunae is being fulfilled herewith by Dr Dhananjaya A Hiremath and Dr Smt Lalita D Hiremath. This is a gift from the authors to all the students. They have covered in this book all topics required by the medical students. The explanation and descriptions are so detailed that even the postgraduates can refer.

The book is quite useful to dental, nursing and paramedical students and public health consultants.

I wish all the best to the authors and they should produce such useful books for the students in future.

SJ Nagalotimath MD
Medical Director
S Nijalingappa Medical College
Bagalkot, Karnataka, India

Preface to the Second Edition

The community medicine subject undergoes frequent changes according to the needs of the community and to match its dynamic growth, the updating of the subject is essential. It gives us a great pleasure to present this revised second edition. Considering mainly the interests of the postgraduate students, the following topics are updated, viz. Economics, Reproductive and Child Health, Contraceptive Methods, Immunization, Nutrition, and Hospital Waste Management.

Newer topics, viz. Integrated Disease Surveillance Project, Integrated Management of Neonatal and Childhood Illness, National Rural Health Mission, Community-based Rehabilitation, Indian Systems of Medicine, Hospital Statistics, and Social Security, are added.

Lalita D Hiremath
Dhananjaya A Hiremath

Preface to the First Edition

We are living in a world different from that of previous generation. The "information superhighway" is a reality and has become a tool for instant sharing of vast amounts of information. This book is written to serve both the undergraduates and postgraduates to face the practical and viva voce confidently and derive the maximum benefit from their honest endeavor.

It is generally observed that students face acute difficulties in accurately answering questions raised in viva voce. The practical portion has been written in a systemic and lucid manner so as to enable the students to grasp the subject easily and quickly answer any question to the complete satisfaction of the honorable examiners.

The book also serves the needs of the dental, nursing and paramedical students. It is a good tool for the personnel working in the department of health and family welfare services and public health administrators and consultants.

Dhananjaya A Hiremath
Lalita D Hiremath

Acknowledgments

We express our deep sense of gratitude to Dr Ashok S Mallapur, Principal, S Nijalingappa Medical College and HSK Hospital and Research Centre, Bagalkot, Karnataka, India, for his incessant inspiration and encouragement. We convey our sincere thanks to Dr TM Chandrashekhar, Dean, HSK Hospital, Bagalkot, Karnataka, India.

We are thankful to Shri Veeranna Charantimath, the Chairman of BVV Sangh, who is the visionary and founder of many educational institutions. We are also thankful to Shri Siddanna Shettar, Chairman, Governing Council of S Nijalingappa Medical College and HSK Hospital and Research Centre, Bagalkot, Karnataka, India, who is an eminent educationist and able administrator.

We convey our sincere thanks to Dr CH Ghattargi, Professor and Head, and all members of the Department of Community Medicine, S Nijalingappa Medical College, Bagalkot, Karnataka, India. We are grateful to all the students and teaching faculty, who have encouraged us to bring the revised second edition. We also express sincere thanks to Smt Kalpana Kulkarni, who contributed chapters on Biostatistics. The critical appraisal of the book by readers is always welcome. We are thankful to M/s Jaypee Brothers Medical Publishers (P) Ltd, New Delhi, India.

Contents

Introduction

COMMUNITY MEDICINE

Community medicine is comparatively a newcomer among academic disciplines of medicine. Previously it was taught to medical students as hygiene and public health. This name was later changed to preventive and social medicine when it was realized that the subject encompassed much more than merely the principles of hygiene and sanitation and public health engineering. The name preventive and social medicine emphasizes the role of: (a) disease prevention in general through immunization, adequate nutrition, etc. in addition to the routine hygiene measures and (b) social factors in health and disease. The modern day message is that the discipline variously labeled in the past as public health or preventive and social medicine cannot be divorced from health care, including clinical care of the community. It is in recognition of this wider role that the Medical Council of India has recently decided to label the discipline as Community Medicine in place of Preventive and Social Medicine.

CHALLENGES OF 21ST CENTURY

Challenges of 21st century are not only to combat diseases producing microbes but also to recognize that many of the causes of ill health are increasingly related to lifestyle, man-made changes in environment, and disparity and inequality in resources distribution within country and between the countries.

Developed world is facing *epidemiological transition* that is transition from infectious diseases as measles, diphtheria, and pneumonia to chronic diseases as heart diseases, cancer, stroke and diabetes, which consisted 9 out of 10 leading causes of deaths. This transition is mainly due to improved water supply, sewerage, and less crowded living environment, application of the preventive health services, such as immunization, preventive health check-ups, specific food interventions and use of highly developed curative technology.

Now, developing countries are experiencing the double burden of diseases, i.e. one which is caused by poverty, poor water supply and sanitation and low standard of livings and other which is due to adopting similar lifestyles as of developed world.

Another important concern is the world population that has increased three-fold in last century whereas India has increased almost five times in the same duration. The number of persons living in urban areas increased globally from 32 percent of world population in 1955 to 38 percent in 1975, and to 45 percent in 1995. It is expected to reach 54 percent by 2015 (World Health Report 1998).

In India, the urban population during 1911-1931 was 11-12 percent only and in 1951 was 17.3 percent only, however, in 1991 it reached to 25.7 percent and it is estimated 31 percent in 1996-97 and it was going to be 38 percent in 2006-07.

Chapter 1 Present Health Status

CHAPTER OUTLINE

- DISEASE BURDEN
- COMMUNICABLE DISEASES
- MATERNAL AND CHILD HEALTH
- REASONS FOR HIGH DISEASE BURDEN IN INDIA
- CHRONIC NONCOMMUNICABLE DISEASES AND CONDITIONS
- NOTIFIABLE DISEASES

DISEASE BURDEN

It has been estimated that the disease burden of the people of India is one of the highest in the world (Table 1.1). We have a triple burden of infectious diseases. Firstly, we have those infectious diseases that are prevalent worldwide and for which specific preventive measures are yet not available. Secondly, we have infectious diseases that are prevalent because of insufficient public health measures. Thirdly, we have infectious diseases perpetuated by the prevalence of vectors (hematophagous arthropods) as well as vertebrate fauna, the ecological determinants of which are given due to our geoclimatic features.

REASONS FOR HIGH DISEASE BURDEN

1. Poor economy of the country
2. Maldistribution of country resources
3. Poor governance and management to utilize resources appropriately
4. Poor people participation.

Table 1.1: Ten leading causes of burden of disease,world, 2004 and 2030

2004 Disease or injury	*As % of total DALYs*	*Rank*	*Rank*	*As % of total DALYs*	*2030 Disease or injury*
Lower respiratory infection	6.2	1	1	6.2	Unipolar depressive disorders
Diarrheal diseases	4.8	2	2	5.5	Ischemic heart disease
Unipolar depressive disorders	4.3	3	3	4.9	Road traffic accidents
Ischemic heart disease	4.1	4	4	4.3	Cerebrovascular disease
HIV/AIDS	3.8	5	5	3.8	COPD
Cerebrovascular disease	3.1	6	6	3.2	Lower respiratory infections
Prematurity and low birth weight	2.9	7	7	2.9	Hearing loss, adult onset
Birth asphyxia and birth trauma	2.7	8	8	2.7	Refractive errors
Road traffic accidents	2.7	9	9	2.5	HIV/AIDS
Neonatal infections and other*	2.7	10	10	2.3	Diabetes mellitus
COPD	2.0	13	11	1.9	Neonatal infections and other
Refractive errors	1.8	14	12	1.9	Prematurity and low birth weight
Hearing loss, adults onset	1.8	15	15	1.9	Birth asphyxia and birth trauma
Diabetes mellitus	1.3	19	18	1.6	Diarrheal diseases

COPD, chronic obstructive pulmonary disease

*This category also includes other noninfectious causes arising in the perinatal period apart from prematurity, low birth weight, birth trauma and asphyxia. These noninfectious causes are responsible for about 20% of DALYs shown in this category.

5. Poor level of literacy of the people
6. Geographical characteristics of the country for certain diseases like malaria, filaria, etc.
7. Poor political commitment
8. Poor policy
9. Poor scientific development
10. Religious belief system and cultural practices of the population.

COMMUNICABLE DISEASES

About 17 percent of all deaths and about 21 percent of all illnesses are due to communicable diseases. The major problems continue to be tuberculosis, filariasis, leprosy, malaria, diarrheal diseases and malnutrition.

Among viral diseases smallpox was eradicated in 1980. Measles continues to be rife frequency in occurrence, and so is viral hepatitis. Since 1973, the country has been experiencing large scale outbreaks of Japanese encephalitis. Dengue fever is also emerging as another health problem.

Among bacterial diseases meningococcal meningitis has shown a substantial increase. Cholera has significantly declined, but the other waterborne diseases (e.g. acute diarrheas, dysentery and enteric fever) have not abated. Half the world's tuberculosis patients are in India accounting for 14 million cases of which in the world, estimated to be 0.6 million. Tetanus and Diphtheria are not yet under control.

The country has one-third of leprosy cases. Among parasitic diseases, Malaria and Kala-azar have staged a comeback. During 1995, 3 million cases of malaria and 22,000 cases of Kala-azar were reported. About 420 million people are estimated to be living in known endemic areas of Filariasis.

Intestinal parasites such as *ascariasis,* hookworms, *giardiasis* and amoebiasis are widely prevalent. STDs are on the increase.

CHRONIC NONCOMMUNICABLE DISEASES AND CONDITIONS

Noncommunicable diseases such as hypertension, diabetes, cancer, road accidents, alcohol drug abuse and mental health problems are slowly emerging as health problems. One reason for this appears to be changes in lifestyle and growing stresses of urban life.

The Table 1.2 shows the percentage (approximately) of major causes of all deaths in developing countries.

Nutritional Deficiencies

Nutritional deficiencies are widespread and include protein energy malnutrition, vitamin deficiency, vitamin B complex deficiency, nutritional anemia and iodine-deficiency disorders. Undernutrition affects millions of people. In 1992, about 30 percent of babies were born with birth weight of less than 2.5 kg.

Table 1.2: The percentage (approximately) of major causes of all deaths in developing countries

Case	Years	
	1985	2000
Infections	35	25
Neoplasm	7	10
Circulatory diseases	20	30
Injuries	8	6

Recent trends with regard to nutritional status of women and children in India have been positive and modest. The improvement has been marked with respect to the prevalence of 'severe malnutrition'. Even with respect to moderate undernutrition modest improvements in anthropometry and birth weight have been noticeable even amongst the poor.

MATERNAL AND CHILD HEALTH

By virtue of the large group (Women 22% Children 38% together constitute 60%) of total population and also vulnerable or special risk group mother and children are the major consumer of health services.

Tables 1.3 and 1.4 show the poor status of MCH (Maternal and Child Health).

Burden of Occupational Diseases and Injuries

There are 100 million occupational injuries causing 0.1 million deaths in the world according to WHO (Leigh et al 1999). It is also estimated that in India 17 million occupational nonfatal injuries (17% of the world) and 45,000 fatal injuries (45% of the total deaths due to occupational injuries in world) occurs each year. Out of 11 million cases of occupational diseases in the world 1.9 million cases (17%) are contributed by India and out of 0.7 million deaths in the world 0.12 (17%) is contributed by India.

Table 1.3: Health facilities in India

	India
Population 2001 [Million]	1028.6[1]
Projected population 2010 [Million]	1176.7[1]
Health care infrastructure	
Community health centers	4276[2]
Primary health centers	23458[2]
Subcenters	146036[2]
Total FRUs	1813[2]

Contd...

Contd...

	India
CHCs owned building	3882[2]
PHCs owned building	19706[2]
SCs owned building	78803[2]
Manpower status	
Total allopathic doctors	725190[3]
Total allopathic doctors in Govt	84852[3]
Total dentist	73057[3]
Total dentist in govt sector	3233[3]
Total ayurvedic doctors	458418[3]
Total registered ANMs	549292[3]
Total ANMs in govt	153568[2]
Total registered GNMs	971574[3]
Total registered LHVs	51497[3]
Total specialist at CHCs	4279[2]
MBBs doctors at PHCs	24375[2]
Health care indicators	
Doctor population ratio [per 1000]	0.63[3]
Doctor nurse ratio	0.46[3]
Nurse population ratio [per 1000]	1.37[3]
Bed population ratio	0.87[4]
Population per subcenter ratio	7838[2]
Population per PHC	48799[2]

[1] Census of India [2]RHS-08 [3] NPH-08 [4]CBHI

Table 1.4: Health status in India

Infants mortality rate	53[2]
Maternal mortality ratio	254[2]
Total fertility rate	2.7[2]
Crude birth rate	22.8[2]
Crude death rate	7.4[2]
Life expectancy	66.9[1]
Under 5 mortality rate	74.3[3]
Total fertility rate	2.6[3]
ANC-3 check ups (%)	52[3]
I and FA Tab. received for 90 days %	23[3]
Two TT Inj. received in last preg %	72[3]
Birth in medical institutions (%)	49[3]
BCG (%)	78[3]
Polio 3 doses (%)	78[3]
DPT3 (%)	55[3]
Measles (%)	59[3]

[1] Census of India [2] NHP-08 [3] SRS-08

Clinical Diagnosis and Community Diagnosis (Table 1.5)

Table 1.5: Comparative model of clinical diagnosis and community diagnosis

Clinical diagnosis	*Community diagnosis*
• Sick patient	Sick community
• Patient decides to consult doctor	Community feels the need for consulting professionals
• Visits doctor	Professions and community interaction
• Doctor takes history and symptomology	Studies community history, hospital record, birth,death, notification analysis
• Provisional diagnosis	Community provisional diagnosis, (Identify community problems)
• Decides which system to examine and what type of investigations to be performed	Decides what type of exploration or studies to be conducted in the community
• Carry out clinical examination and investigations	Carry health surveys,screening for diseases surveillance
• Scrutiny, analysis and interpretation clinical examination and laboratory results	Scrutiny, analysis and interpretation of data
• Arrives at clinical diagnosis	Makes community diagnosis
• Decides treatment and advice	Decide on community treatment or community action on priorities.
• Administers the treatment and give advices	Plans and implements community service and program
• Monitor of follow-up of the patient (Symptomatic improvement, etc)	Monitor community change, reduction in morbidity, mortality, etc. (Evaluation)
• If no improvement change the treatment regimen	If no improvement, change or modify plan of action

NOTIFIABLE DISEASES

A disease that, by statutory requirements, must be reported to the public health authority in the pertinent jurisdiction when the diagnosis is made. Following are the notifiable diseases:

1. Lead poisoning or its sequelae.
2. Lead tetraethyl poisoning to its sequelae.
3. Phosphorus poisoning or its sequelae.
4. Mercury poisoning or its sequelae.
5. Manganese poisoning or its sequelae.
6. Arsenic poisoning or its sequelae.
7. Poisoning by nitrous fumes.
8. Carbon bisulfite poisoning.
9. Benzene and its derivatives poisoning or its sequelae.
10. Chrome ulceration or its sequelae.
11. Anthrax.
12. Silicosis.
13. Poisoning by halogens or its derivatives of hydrocarbons.
14. Pathological manifestation due to radium, radioactive substances, or X-rays.
15. Primary epitheliomatous cancer of the skin.

16. Toxic anemia.
17. Toxic jaundice due to poisonous substances.
18. Oil acne or dermatitis due to mineral oil or its derivatives in any form.
19. Byssinosis.
20. Asbestosis.
21. Occupational or contact dermatitis caused by direct contact with chemical or paints. It could be primary irritants or allergic sensitizers.
22. Noise induced hearing loss.
23. Beryllium poisoning.
24. Carbon monoxide.
25. Coal miner's pneumoconiosis.
26. Phosgene poisoning.
27. Occupational cancers.
28. Isocyanates poisoning.
29. Toxic nephritis.

Chapter 2 Family

CHAPTER OUTLINE

- FAMILY
- GENERAL INFORMATION FOR STUDENTS

FAMILY

Each student will be assigned families in the village. The objective of this program is to provide opportunities to the medical student to learn that the *family is the basic unit for epidemiological studies and obtain practical experience* in the health promotion, early diagnosis and treatment, disability limitation and rehabilitation.

Definition

Family is a group of individuals, who are related by blood or marriage, live under same shelter and share common kitchen.

Types of Family

There are four basic types of families:

Nuclear Family

When the family unit consists of husband, wife and children it is called nuclear family. Relationships of married couple in this type of family are more intimate than in other types of families. Nuclear family is mostly male dominated.

Polygamous type of nuclear family: It is made up of a husband, two or more co-wives and the children.

Polyandrous type: In some communities polyandrous type of families exists. This consists of wife, two or more co-husbands and the children. All family members either live in one house or each co-wife/co-husband occupies separate house. These houses (or huts) are usually within family compound or homestead. In most societies polygyny is socially permitted.

Extended Family

This type of family can be considered as a vertical extension of nuclear family. Thus, a small extended family consists of the old man, his wife, their sons, the son's wife and the son's children. Here the married son is a member of two nuclear families, his father's and his own. A large extended family, for example, may consist of, the old man, his wives, their unmarried children, married sons, son's wives (each son having one or more wives) along with their unmarried children.

Joint Family

This family can be considered as lateral extension of nuclear family. It consists of nuclear families of siblings (brothers in patrilocal system and sisters in matrilocal system), eldest brother/sister has the position of authority.

Three Generation Family

This is similar to joint family, but the reason for married son living with the parents is economical and not social.

Special Objectives

1. To study the family composition.
2. To study and observe environmental factors having their influence on the health and disease of the family members.
3. To study and observe social and economic factors associated with health and disease.
4. To observe the growth and development of the family.
5. To study the health status of the family members.
6. To study and follow—the morbidity encountered in the family and to learn the importance of observing the patient in his natural surroundings.
7. To learn the multiple factors associated with the cause of disease and in getting the treatment.
8. To study the mortality in the family.
9. To study the attitudes and practices of people towards health.

Method of Study

a. Observation
b. Questioning
c. Clinical examination
d. Investigation at field level.

Family—a Dynamic Unit

Family Cycle

Family is not a static unit. It is a dynamic unit. Four stages are described in family cycle.

Stage of formation: This stage begins with marriage.

Stage of growth: In this stage, the family grows due to procreation.

Stage of retraction: In this stage, there is reduction in the size of family. This is due to members leaving family due to marriage or due to death. It may also be due to married children forming a separate family.

Stage of disintegration: The original family looses its existence due to death of the couple which formed the original family.

All these stages may not follow the above sequence. Some may occur simultaneously. In joint and extended family the stage of retraction does not exist.

GENERAL INFORMATION FOR STUDENTS

1. In the family record, the details of the following done should be recorded namely immunization, environment, socioeconomic survey, diet survey, health check-up and annual family morbidity, etc.
2. In family record dead members (in last one year only) in household should also be recorded at the end with appropriate heading in the first column of living family members. The cause of death should be recorded in the "Remarks" Column. Any members dying during our care should be recorded.
3. A child under 1 year is not taken into account of while calculating for overcrowding, a child above 1 year but under 10 years is reckoned as a half unit.
4. Economic status should be enquired only when you have gained the confidence of the family.
5. In recording diet, note down seven days typical diet of the family. Weigh it and calculate the calories, proximate principles, vitamins and trace elements, etc.
6. Health knowledge should be assessed for common communicable diseases, diet, infant feeding, contraception, family planning, etc.
7. Past illness should be enquired for all infectious diseases.
8. While doing general physical examination look for the early signs of chronic diseases, common deficiency, skin infections, diseases prevalent in the family and treat them under the guidance of the staff.
9. For antenatal examination of the pregnant lady and examination of infants make an appointment in consultation with Public Health Nurse.
10. You will present your family study to the class, bringing out all the important features of environment, the growth and development of children in the family, common diseases in the family members, their problems and how you have helped them. The outlines for guidance are also provided.

Chapter 3

Economics

CHAPTER OUTLINE

- POVERTY LINE
- OVERCROWDING
- PER CAPITA INCOME

POVERTY LINE

Poverty line is generally defined in terms of minimum per capita consumption level of the people. As per the definition given by the Planning Commission, this level is the caloric intake of people. Thus, poverty line refers to the cut off point of income below which people are not able to purchase food sufficient to provide 2400 kcal per head per day. This income level has been fixed by the Planning Commission at Rs 356.35 per head in rural areas and Rs 538.60 (January 2010) in urban areas at 1987-88 prices.

Definitions and methodologies used for estimating poverty line differ from one source to other. According to the sixth five-year plan document, "A family having five members, whose annual income is less than Rs 3500 is said to be living below poverty line." This income limit was increased to Rs 6400 in the seventh plan. It was further raised to Rs 7200 as per the eighth plan document.

PER CAPITA INCOME

It is the per head income of the people of a country. It is calculated by dividing the national income of a country by its population.

Per capita income = National Income/Total population

Increase in the national income may not necessarily lead to an increase in the per capita income if there is a corresponding increase in population. The per capita income is the best indicator of measuring the standard of living of the people of a country. It provides an index of economic welfare.

Per capita income (1997-1998)	Rs. 13,193
Per capita income (2001-2002)	Rs. 15,746
Per capita income (2002-2003)	Rs. 16,123

OVERCROWDING

Degree of overcrowding can be best expressed as the number of persons per room, i.e.

$$= \frac{\text{Number of persons in household}}{\text{Number of rooms in the dwelling}}$$

Accepted Standards

1 Room	—	2 persons
2 Rooms	—	3 persons
3 Rooms	—	5 persons
4 Rooms	—	7 persons
5 Rooms or more	—	10 persons

(Additional 2 persons for each further room)

Floor Space Accepted Standard

110 sq ft	—	2 persons
90-100 sqft	—	1 ½ persons
70-90 sq ft	—	1 person
50-70 sq ft	—	½ person
Under 50 sq ft	—	Nil

(A baby under 12 months is not counted—children between 1-10 years counted as half a unit)

Sex Separation

Overcrowding is considered to exist if two persons over nine years of age, (not husband and wife) of opposite sexes are obliged to sleep in same room.

Housing

Housing Standards

Floor: The floors should be damp proof and free from cracks. The height of the plinth should be 2 to 3 feet.

Roof: The height of the roof should be minimum of 10 feet from the surface of floor.

Windows: Should be placed at a height of 3 feet above the ground level.
- Window area should be 1/5th of the floor area.
- Doors and windows combined should have 2/5th the floor area.

Lighting: The day light factor should exceed one percent of the floor area.

Cubic space: The height of the room should be such as to give an air space of at least 500 cft. per capita, preferably 1000 cft.

Living rooms: At least two rooms, one of which can be closed for security.

Social Classification

Methods of Social Classification

Prasad's method: This method is proposed by BG Prasad and is based on per capita income of family. It is useful for social classification of family and not for individuals. While using this classification it is necessary to update the value of rupee by applying appropriate correction factor.

Correction factor is obtained by multiplying AICPI by 4.93 percent (i.e. 0.0493) as suggested by Kumar[3]. This is preferred for rural areas. This is modified BG Prasad's social classification (Table 3.1).

= Per capita family monthly income of 1961 (as suggested by BG prasad) × correction factor (CF)

$$\text{Where, per capita monthly income} = \frac{\text{Total monthly income of the family}}{\text{Total members of the family}}$$

CF = Value AICPI, (Which is variable and it was Rs 741 in July 2009) multiplied by 0.0493, which is a finite number/multiplier (linking factor).

Therefore, CF during July 2009 was 741× 0.0493 = 36.53

Table 3.1: Assessment of socioeconomic status by modified BG Prasad's classification

BGP classification 1961 based on per capita monthly income × CF	*Modified BGP classification for the Year 2009 (July)*	*Socioeconomic class status*
Rs 100 and above × 36.53	Rs 3653 and below	I
Rs 99 to 50 × 36.53	Rs 3652 to 1826	II
Rs 49 to 30 × 36.53	Rs 1825 to 1096	III
Rs 29 to 15 × 36.53	Rs 1095 to 548	IV
Rs 14 and below	Rs 547 and below	V

Note:

i. Rs 100 during 1961 is equivalent to Rs 3653 during July 2009.

ii. Per capita family monthly income of today (as assessed by the above formula) has to be fitted in the second column and assessed accordingly.

iii. All India consumer's price Index (AICPI) is variable.

Thus, classification can be derived for any period by referring AICPI of that period.

Kuppuswamy's method: Kuppuswamy's socioeconomic status is an important tool in hospital and community based research in India. It was proposed in 1976.[1] This scale takes account of education, occupation and income of the family to classify study groups into high, middle and low socioeconomic status. As pointed out rightly by Mishra and Singh[2] from Rewa, "An income scale usually has relevance only for the period under study. Due to the steady inflation and consequent fall in the value of the rupee, the income criteria in the scale lose their relevance." Mishra, therefore, undertook important task of revision of family income per month (in Rs.) for 1976 when the price index was 296 according to base year 1960=100 (Table 3.2). He however revised it for 1998 using base year 1982=100. The base year has been changed from 2001."

Table 3.2: Reference index

Year	Reference index
1960	100 (base)
1976	296
1982	490 – 100 (new base)
1998	405
2001	458 – 100 (new base)
2007	April 128

We have attempted the same exercise using the new base year of 2001 for CPI-IW (All India average consumer price index for industrial workers).

Price index for 2001 by old base (1982=100) was 458. One needs to divide given years price index by price index of the base years. For example, Kuppuswamy's price index for 1976 was based on 1960 as 100. In other words means that any thing which cost Rs 100 in 1960 would cost Rs 296 in 1976. The criteria were, however, changed in 1982 to 100 (called as new base). As per criteria of 1960 (old base), the price index for 1982 was 490. Therefore, we get price index of 1976 converted to new base:

Price index by old base for 1982 = 490

Price index by new base for 1982=100

Price index by old base for 1976 was 296.

Conversion factor for 1976 by new base was calculated as follows: 100/490 × 296 = 60.04.

To know the price increase in 1998, price index by then new base (1982) was divided by conversion factor. Mishra, thus determined new income criteria for 1998 by multiplying old income ranges of 1976 by 6.745 (obtained by dividing price index of 1998 by 60.04 (405/60.04=6.745) on the basis of base year of 1982.

Now in view of new base for 2001 updating for current year is attempted hereby to help researchers in formulating their ranges of income for upcoming research. Conversion factor for 1982 base year has changed with considering 2001 as base year. To get updated conversion factor same exercise is adopted as follows:

Price index by old base for 2001=458

Price index by base for 2001 =100

Price index by old base for 1998 was 405

Price index by new base for 1998=100/458 × 405=88.42

To calculate conversion factor for the year 2007, we have to divide price index by 88.428. All-India average consumer price index numbers for industrial workers (Base 2001=100) shows general index as 128 on April 2007.

A conversion factor can be obtained by calculating from 1976 index also, and it comes as 9.764, which implies 9.764 times price increased as compared to 1976. Multiplying 1976 income by the factor of 9.764 would also provide scale for 2007.

Now the prices from 1982 levels have increased, and that increase can be obtained by multiplying prices of that time by the factor obtained as follows: 128/88.428 = 1.45.

Revised table (Table 3.3) for scales in 2007 to define socioeconomic status has thus obtained as follows (by multiplying 1998 income ranges by the factor 1.45): This revised prices scale for different socioeconomic status has shortcomings as educational and occupational factors also need to be revised by large scale survey. Another lacuna is also the same as were in modification for the year 1998.[2] However, this exercise will provide some clue for setting income group in researches as per current inflation rate.

Table 3.3: Kuppuswamy's socioeconomic status scale

A. Education score			
1. Profession or Honours			7
2. Graduate or postgraduate			6
3. Intermediate or post high school diploma			5
4. High school certificate			4
5. Middle school certificate			3
6. Primary school certificate			2
7. Illiterate			1
B. Occupation score			
1. Profession			10
2. Semi-profession			6
3. Clerical, Shop-owner, Farmer			5
4. Skilled worker			4
5. Semi-skilled worker			3
6. Unskilled worker			2
7. Unemployed			1
C. Family income per month (in Rs) original	**Score**	**Modified for 1982**	**Modified for 2007**
1. 2000	12	13500	19575
2. 1000-1999	10	6750-13499	9788-19574
3. 750-999	6	5050-6749	7323-9787
4. 500-749	4	3375-5049	4894-7322
5. 300-499	3	2025-3374	2936-4893
6. 101-299	2	676-2024	980-2935
7. 100	1	675	979
Total score	**Socioeconomic class**		
26-29	Upper (I)		
16-25	Upper middle (II)		
11-15	Middle lower middle (III)		
5-10	Lower upper lower (IV)		
<5	Lower (V)		

REFERENCES

1. Kuppuswamy B. Manual of socioeconomic status (Urban), Manasayan, Delhi, 1981.
2. Mishra D, Singh HP. Kuppuswamy's socioeconomic status scale— a revision. Indian J Pediatr 2003;70(3):273-74.
3. Kumar P. Indian Journal of Community Medicine 1993;18:2.

Chapter 4 Communicable Diseases

CHAPTER OUTLINE

COMMUNICABLE DISEASE

Definition

An illness due to a specific infectious agent or its toxic products capable of being directly or indirectly transmitted from man to man, animal to animal or from the environment (through air, dust, soil, water, food, etc.) to man or animal.

Definition of Infection

The entry and development or multiplication of an infectious agent in the body of man and animals.

Infectious disease: A clinically manifest disease of man or animal resulting from an infection.

Contamination: The presence of an infectious agent on a body surface; also on or in clothes, beddings, toys, surgical instruments or dressings or other inanimate articles.

Contagious disease: A disease that is transmitted through contact, e.g. scabies trachoma infestation.

Containment: The concept of regional eradication of communicable disease.

Infestation: For persons or animals the lodgment, development and reproduction of arthropods on the surface of the body or in the clothing, e.g. lice, itchmite.

Host: A person or other animal including birds and arthropods that affords subsistence or lodgment to an infectious agent under natural condition.

1. Obligate host — Means the only host
2. Definitive host — Parasite passes its sexual stage in host
3. Intermediate host — Parasite passes its a sexual stage in host
4. Transport host (carrier) — Organism remains alive but do not undergo development

Case

Case is defined as "a person in the population or study group identified as having the particular disease, health disorder or condition under investigation".

Primary case: Refers to the first case of communicable disease introduced into the population unit being studied.

Index case: Refers to the first case to come to the attention of the investigator.

Secondary case: Secondary case are those developing from contact with primary case.

Epidemic (*Epi—upon, demos—people*)

The "unusual" occurrence in a community or region, of disease, specific health-related behavior (e.g. smoking) or other health related events (e.g. traffic accidents) clearly in excess of " expected occurrence".

Endemic (*En—in, demos—people*)

It refers to the constant presence of a disease or infectious agent within a given geographic area or population group, without importation from outside may also refer to the "usual" or expected frequency of the disease within such area or population group.

Sporadic

The cases are so few and separated widely in space and time that they show little or no connection with each other, nor a recognizable common source of infection, e.g. polio, tetanus.

Pandemic

An epidemic usually affecting a large proportion of the population occuring over a wide geographic area such as a section of a nation, the entire nation, a continent or the world, e.g. influenza pandemics of 1918 and 1957.

Disease

Disease is a condition of the body or some part or organ of the body in which its functions are disrupted or deranged; in simple terms it is the physiological or psychological dysfunction.

Illness

Illness is a subjective state of the person who feels aware of not being well.

Sickness

Sickness is a state of social dysfunction, i.e. a role that the individual assumes when ill. It is quite difficult to assess the illness and sickness, however, disease can be measured directly or indirectly in terms of clinical state, disability, and death.

TUBERCULOSIS

It is a chronic bacterial infectious disease caused by *Mycobacterium tuberculosis* and is characterized by formation of granuloma in infected tissue and by cell-mediated hypersensitivity (Table 4.1). Dr Robert Koch discovered TB bacillus on 24th March 1882.

Sites Affected

Lungs, intestine, meninges, bones, lymph nodes and skin.

It has been reported as one of most important public health problem by all regions of WHO.

It affects the cream of population, i.e. adults in age group of 21 to 40 years.

Table 4.1: Important rates in relation to burden of tuberculosis

Prevalence of TB infection	30%
Incidence of TB infection (ARI)	1.4% in 0-4 years, 2.1% in 0-14 years, 1.7% is average ARI
Incidence of active TB	168/100,000/year
Incidence of sputum positive	075/100,000/year
Prevalence of sputum positive	0.4%
Primary drug resistance	3-13.3%
Primary resistance to INH	10.6-21.83%
Primary resistance to rifampicin	0-11.9%
Acquired resistance to INH	34.5%-76%
Acquired resistance to rifampicin	0.53.26%
Ethmbutol resistance	0-20.6%(0.5%)
Streptomycin resistance	0/35.8%(2.4%)
Any one drug resistance	(means 10.7%)
Multidrug resistant TB	3.5-42.3%
Resistance to 4 drugs	0%-14.1%
In new cases	(mean 1.0%)

(*Source:* Paramasivan, 1998, Jain, et al. 1992, Pablos-Mendez, et al. 1998, Espinal, et al. 2001, 2004; Negi, et al. 2003; WHO Report 2005).

Economic Burden of Tuberculosis

1. TB kills more people in India than HIV, STD, malaria, leprosy and tropical diseases combined.
2. Every year 30,000 children are forced to leave school because their parents have tuberculosis, and 1,00,000 women lose their status as mothers and wives because of social stigma.

3. Every year, more than 17 crores more days are lost to the National Economy on account of tuberculosis at a cost of Rs 700 crore.

Epidemiological Indices

1. Prevalence of infection
2. Prevalence of disease or case rate
3. Incidence of infection
4. Incidence of new cases
5. Prevalence of suspected cases
6. Prevalence of drug resistance cases
7. Mortality rate.

Epidemiology

Agent: Mycobacterium tuberculosis which is commonly known as "Koch" bacillus or tubercle bacilli or acid fast bacillus (AFB).

Sources

1. Human:
   a. Rapid multiplier
   b. Slow multiplier
2. Bovine—Infected milk
3. Atypical *Mycobacterium.*

Communicability

Patients are infective as long as they remain untreated.

Host Factors

- *Age:* Prevalence increases with age up to the age of 45 to 54 in males.
- *Sex:* In female the peak of tuberculosis prevalence is below 35 years.
- *One percent prevalence:* In under 5 years of age.
- *Thirty percent prevalence:* At the age of 15 years.
- *Common in elderly.*

Environmental Factors

Housing factors

1. Darkness
2. Illventilated
3. Overcrowded.

Social factors

1. Poor quality of life
2. Poor housing
3. Overcrowding.

4. Population explosion
5. Under nutrition
6. Lack of education
7. Large families
8. Early marriages
9. Lack of awareness regarding cause of illness
10. Poor sanitation
11. Air pollution
12. Spitting indiscriminately
13. Sharing of *Hukka* and smoke
14. *Purdha* system.

Incubation period: Three to six weeks

Mode of transmissions

1. Inhalation
2. Ingestion
3. Surface implantation.

Case Finding

Based on four cardinal symptoms:

1. Continuous, irregular, intermittent and low grade fever for more than two weeks
2. Cough with expectoration for more than two weeks
3. Chest pain (plural involvement)
4. Hemoptysis.

Definitions

(According to WHO)

Case: Patient whose sputum is positive for tubercular bacilli.

Suspected case: Patient whose sputum is negative for tubercular bacilli and X-ray suggestive of shadow.

Case Finding Tools (Table 4.2 to 4.7)

1. Sputum examination.
2. Mass miniature radiography (MMR)
3. Tuberculin test.
4. Other tests:
   a. Polymarase chain reaction (PCR)
   b. CT scan
   c. Magnetic resonance imaging (MRI).

Sputum Examination

Two samples are to be collected:

1. Over night sputum
2. Spot sputum.

Chemoprophylaxis

Primary

When drug is given to person not infected so far (Tuberculin negative) and who has been exposed to open case.

Secondary

INH is given to person already infected (Tuberculin positive) in order to prevent development of disease.

Treatment

Drug Regimens Currently used in India

- Standard regimens/Conventional regimens (Table 4.2)
- Short-course chemotherapy regimens (Table 4.3).

Conventional Regimens

Two types:
1. Daily regimens
2. Bi-weekly regimens.

Table 4.2: Standard regimens/conventional regimens

Regimen code	*Regimen with drugs and dosage*	*Duration (Months)*	*Mode and rhythm of administration*	*Instructions*
R_1	2 STH/10TH a. Intensive phase (2 months) S = 0.75 g H = 300 mg T = 150 mg b. Continuation phase (10 months) H = 300 mg T = 150 mg	12	Inj. S (IM) administered daily. Other two drugs orally daily in a single dose, self-administered at home	Inj. administered DTC/PHI/other health facilities Oral drugs issued on monthly basis by DTC/PHI
R_2	12TH H = 300 mg T = 150 mg	12	Both drugs orally daily at home in a single dose	Issued on monthly basis by DTC/PHI

Table 4.3: Short-course chemotherapy regimens (SCC)

Regimen code	*Regimen with drugs and dosage*	*Duration (Months)*	*Mode and rhythm of administration*	*Instructions*
R_A	2 EHRZ/6TH a. Intensive phase (2 months) E = 800 mg, H = 300 mg R = 450 mg, Z = 1.5 gm b. Continuation phase (6 months) H = 300 mg, T = 150 mg	8	All drugs daily at the same time, self-administered at home Both drugs orally daily, self-administered at home	Issued on fortnightly basis Issued on monthly basis by DTC/PHI
R_B	2 SHRZ/4 $S_2H_2R_2$ a. Intensive phase (2 months) S = 0.75g, H = 300 mg R = 450 mg, Z = 1.5 g b. Continuation phase (4 months) S = 0.75 g, H = 600 mg R = 600 mg	6	Inj. S (IM) administered daily. Other 3 drugs orally daily in a single dose, under supervision Twice weekly; all drugs together	All drugs administered under supervision at DTC/PHI All drugs administered under supervision at DTC/PHI

S = Streptomycin, R = Rifampicin, T = Thioacetazone, H = Isoniazid
Z = Pyrazinamide, E = Ethambutol

Table 4.4: Category of patients for treatment

Regimen code	*Category*
R_1	a. Smear negative patients with extensive radiological evidence of disease/cavity/toxemia b. New smear positive cases where SCC is not available or a patient is unable to continue SCC c. Extra- pulmonary patients in general (e.g. tubercular lymphadenitis) d. Cases, sputum positive after treatment completion with RA who are unable to attend DTC or other specialized centers on referral for further treatment
R_2	a. Smear negative patients with X-ray evidence of tuberculosis other than those in (R_1 a) b. Lost patients, smear negative on reporting back, irrespective of previous history of treatment c. Highly irregular patients (e.g. with cumulative default of more than a month in the intensive phase of any of the regimens or in continuation phase of RB) irrespective of the smear result
R_A	New cases a. All smear positive cases newly indexed under DTP, irrespective of age and previous treatment outside the program b. Serious forms of extrapulmonary tuberculosis (e.g. meningeal, spinal)
R_B	Retreatment cases a. Patients remaining smear positive on completion of treatment with R_1, R_2 and R_A or on return after lost b. Cured patients returning with smear positive result

Note: Patients requiring retreatment should be referred to DTC for initiation of treatment and sent back to the concerned PHIs for continuation of prescribed regimen.

Table 4.5: Doses of antitubercular drugs for adult and children

Medication	Adult		Children	
	Dose thrice a week	Number of pills in combipack	Daily dose	Thrice a week
Isoniazid	600 mg	2	5 mg/kg	10-15 mg/kg
Rifampicin	450 mg*	1	10 mg/kg	10 mg/kg
Pyrazinamide	1500 mg	3	25 mg/kg	35 mg/kg
Streptomycin**	0.75 mg	–	15 mg/kg	15 mg/kg
Ethambutol#	1200 mg	3	15 mg/kg	30 mg/kg

* Patient who weigh 60 kg or more are given an extra 150 mg dose.
** Patient over 50 years of age are given 0.5 gm of streptomycin.
# Ethambutol should not be given in children below 6 years of age.

Table 4.6: Important regimens in relation to burden of tuberculosis

Medication	Drug action	Daily dose regimen	Adult		Children	
			Dose thrice a week	No.of pills in combipack	Daily dose	Thrice a week
Isoniazid	Bactericidal	300 mg	600 mg	2	5 mg/Kg	10-15 mg/Kg
Rifampicin	Bactericidal	450-600 mg	450 mg*	1	10 mg/Kg	10 mg/Kg
Pyrazinamide	Bactericidal	1-1.5 gm	1.5 gm	2-3	25 mg/Kg	35 mg/Kg
Streptomycin**	Bactericidal	0.75-0.5 gm	0.75 gm	–	15 mg/Kg	15 mg?Kg
Ethambutol#	Bacteriostatic	800 mg	1200 mg	2-3	2.5 mg/Kg	30 mg/Kg
Thiacetazone	Bacteriostatic	150 mg	Not applied	–		Not applied
Ofloxacine/Cipro	Bactericidal	200/400 mg				
Kanamycine	Bactericidal	1 g m				
Ethionamide	Bactericidal	250-1 gm				
Cycloserine	Bacteriostatic	250 mg				

* Patient who weigh 60 kg. or more are given an extra 150 mg. dose
** Patient over 50 years of age are given 0.5 gm of streptomycin
# Ethambutol should not be given in children below 6 years of age

Important Definitions

Smear +ve TB

At least 2 initial sputum smear +ve for AFB or 1AFB +ve smear and 1+ve culture.

Smear –ve TB

At least 3 –ve smears, but tuberculosis suggestive symptoms and X-ray. Abnormalities or +ve culture (Fig. 4.1).

Adherence

Persons take appropriate drug regimen for required time (also known as compliance).

New Cases

A Patient with sputum +ve pulmonary tuberculosis who have never had treatment for TB or has taken anti-TB drugs for less than four weeks.

Table 4.7: Classification of categories, types of patients, regimens adopted under RNTCP

Category	*Type of patient*	*Regimens' in months*	*Duration*	*Color of the box*
Category I	New sputum smear Positive seriously ill sputum negative Seriously ill extra-pulmonary**	$2(HRZE)_3$@$4(HR)_3$	6	Red
Category II	Sputum positive relapse*** Sputum positive failure*** Sputum positive treatment after default	$2(HRZES)_3$ $1(HRZE)_3$# $5(HRE)_3$	8	Blue
Category III	Sputum negative extrapulmonary not seriously ill	$2(HRZ)_3$ $4(HR)_3$	6	Green
Category IV	MDR-TB cases##	[6(9)Km Ofx eto Cs ZE/18 Ofx eto Cs E]	24-27	

All the drugs are administered thrice weekly. The number before the letters refers to the number of months of treatment. The abbreviations are as follow: R-Rifampicin, E-Ethambutol, H-INH, S-Streptomycin, and Z-Pyrazinamide, K-Kanamycin, O-Oflaxacin, Et-Ethionamide, C-Cycloserine.

**Examples of seriously ill extrapulmonary TB cases are meningitis, disseminated TB, TB pericarditis,Tuberculous peritonitis, bilateral or extensive pleurisy, spinal involvement with neurological complications; smear negative pulmonary TB with extensive parenchymal involvement and intestinal and genitourinary TB.

If sputum smear is positive after two months of the start of treatment then same treatment regimen (Intensive phase) should be continued for another one month. Thereafter continuation phase should be started irrespective of sputum report at three months. If patient is sputum positive at five months also then he/she should be labeled as "failure" and category II treatment should be started from the beginning.

***In rare and exceptional cases, patients who are sputum smear-negative or who have extrapulmonary disease can have relapse or failure. This diagnosis in all such cases should always be made by a medical officer and should be supported by culture or histological evidence of current active tuberculosis. In these cases, the patient should be categorized "other" and given category II treatment.

If the Sputum smear is positive even after three months of the start of treatment in category II patients then four drugs (HRZE), excluding streptomycin, should be extended for one more month.

Smear examination should be conducted monthly during intensive phase and at least quarterly during continuous phase. Culture examination should be done at least at 4,6,12,18 and 24 months of treatment.

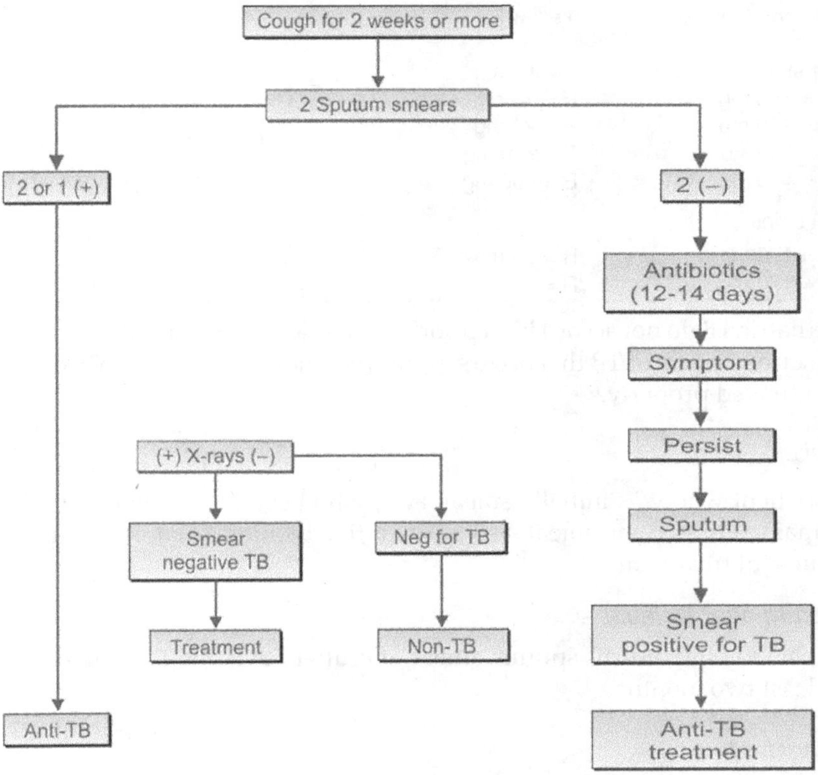

Fig. 4.1: Diagnosis of tuberculosis

Relapse

A patient who returns smear +ve having previously been treated for TB and declared cured after the completion of his treatment.

PEDIATRIC TUBERCULOSIS

Tuberculosis is a major cause of childhood morbidity and mortality. It is estimated that about six to eight percent of all new TB cases are in the pediatric age group and majority is in one to four years. Childhood TB is a reflection of the prevalence of sputum positive pulmonary tuberculosis in the community and the extent of transmission of infection in the community. Children suffer from severe forms of TB because of their poor immunity.

Pediatrics DOTS

Weight	*Box color*	*Regimen*
11-17 kg	1 Orange	$2(HRZE)_3 4\ (HR)_3$
6-10 kg	1 Yellow	$2(HRZE)_3 4\ (HR)_3$
18-25 kg	1 Orange + 1 Yellow	$2(HRZE)_3 4\ (HR)_3$
26-30 kg	2 Orange	$2(HRZE)_3 4\ (HR)_3$

Orange box	Yellow
24 strips H = 150 mg R = 150 mg Z = 500 mg E = 400 mg	24 strips H = 75 mg R = 75 mg Z = 250 mg E = 200 mg
18 strips	
H = 150 mg R = 150 mg	H = 75 mg R = 75

Pediatric TB do not accord high priority as it is less infectious. But because of serious forms of TB that occurs in children they are more likely to die if not treated properly.

Failure Case

A patient who was initially smear +ve , who began treatment and who remained or became smear +ve again at five months or later during the course of treatment.

Return after Default

A patient who returns sputum smear +ve, after having left treatment for at least two months.

Transfer In

A patient recorded in another administrative area register and transferred into another area to continue the treatment.

Transfer Out

A patient who has been transferred to another area register.

Cured

Initially smear +ve patient who completed treatment and had –ve smear result on at least two occasions (one at treatment completion).

Treatment Completed

Initially smear –ve patient who received full course of treatment, or smear +ve who completed treatment with –ve smear at the end of initial phase, but no or only one –ve smear during continuation phase and none at the end of the treatment.

Died

Patient who died during treatment regardless of cause.

Directly Observed Therapy Short-course (DOTS)

- 1993—DOT Pilots
- 1998—DOTS scale-up begins
- 2000—More than 30 percent of country covered by DOTS.

Principles

1. Case detection primarily by microscopic examination of sputum of patient presenting to health facilities.
2. Adequate drug supply.
3. Short-course chemotherapy given under direct observation.
4. Systematic monitoring and accountability for every patient diagnosed.
5. Political will.

Follow-up

Response to treatment

- Symptomatic and general well being usually within 10 to 15 days.
- Fever subsides by two weeks , occasionally may take up to one month
- Respiratory symptoms decrease by second month and may subside by third or fourth month.

Sputum Examination

In category I and III—Repeat sputum smear examination at the end of 2nd, 4th , and 6th month (Flow chart 4.1).

Flow chart 4.1: Category—I and III

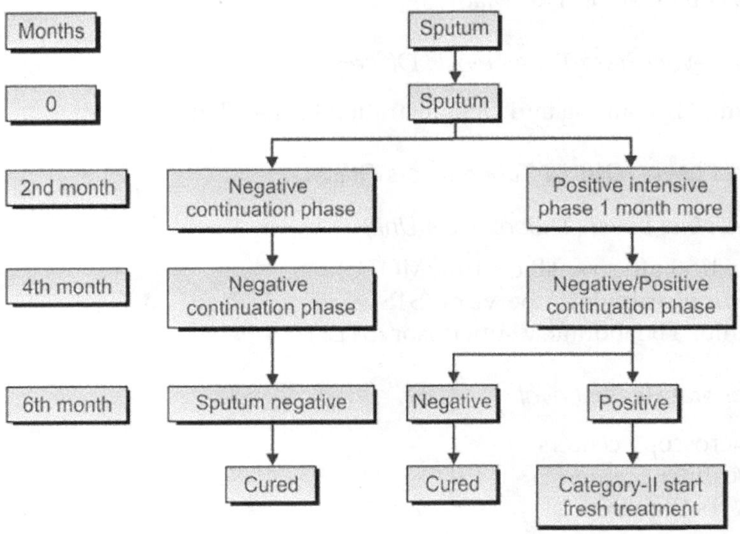

In category II—Repeat sputum smear examination at the end of 3rd, 5th and 8th month (Flow chart 4.2).

Flow chart 4.2: Category—II

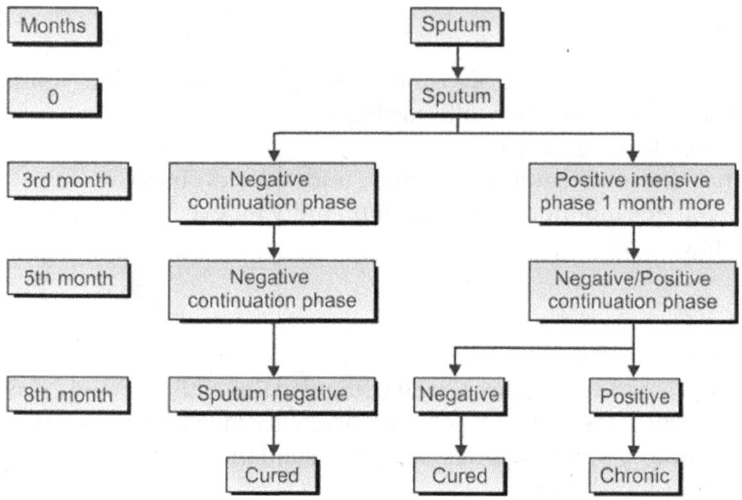

Structure of the RNTCP

National Level (Deputy Director General—TB)

- National Institutes
  (NTI Bangalore, TRC Madras)

State Level (State Tuberculosis Officer)

- State TB Training and Demonstration Center (Director)

District Level (District Tuberculosis Officer)

Sub-district Level (Tuberculosis Unit)

- Medical officer—TB control (MOTC)
- Senior treatment supervisor (STS)
- Senior TB laboratory supervisor (STLS).

Peripheral Health Level

- Microscopy centers
- Treatment centers
- DOTs Providers.

Difference in National Tuberculosis Program and Revised NTCP (Table 4.8)

Table 4.8: Difference in National Tuberculosis Program and Revised NTCP

	NTP	*RNTCP*
Objective	Early diagnosis and treatment	Breaking the chain of transmission
Operational	1. Not defined	1. Cure rate 85% 2. Case finding 70% of estimated cases
Strategy	1. Short-course chemotherapy (SCC) unsupervised 2. Conventional	1. DOTs (Directly observed treatment short-course) 2. Uninterrupted drug supply
Diagnosis	1. More emphasis on X-ray 2. Two sputum smears 3. One sputum +ve is considered a case	1. Mainly sputum microscopy 2. Three sputum smears 3. One +ve is not a case

Reasons for Dropout of the Treatment

1. Long distance from PHI/DTC
2. Transport facilities to PHI/DTC
3. Costing time
4. Affordability (economic status for travelling)
5. Unpleasant side effects
6. Uncooperative staff
7. Communication gap
8. Personal inconvenience
9. Discontinuous/improper treatment
10. Demoralization
11. Stigma
12. Ignorance
13. Sex bias
14. Views expressed by doctor, uncooperative staff, shortage of staff, shortage of drug
15. Interest in hospital admission
16. Belief in other systems of medicines.

National TB Control Program

Program has been in operation since 1962 in India.
Its objectives are:
1. Long-term
2. Short-term.

Objectives of NTCP (1962)

Long-term Objectives

To reduce tuberculosis in the community to that level when it ceases to be a public health problem, i.e.

a. One case infects less than one new person annually.
b. The prevalence of infection in age group below 14 years is brought down to less than 1 percent, against about 30 percent, as at present.

Short-term Objectives

a. To detect maximum number of TB cases among the outpatient attending any health institution with symptoms suggestive of TB and treat them effectively.
b. To vaccinate newborns and infants with BCG.
c. To undertake the above objectives in an integrated manner through all the existing health institutions in the country.

Disinfection of Sputum

1. Cheap handkerchiefs, cotton tissue towels and paper box, etc. used to receive the sputum and nasal discharge of the patient, should be burnt.
2. Sputum cups containing 50 percent carbolic lotion.
3. Disposal of sputum should be done by burying.
4. Safe, cheap and practical method is to receive sputum in small tin can and put boiling water in it, within a minute bacilli will be killed.
5. Cups and utensils should be disinfected by boiling.
6. Beds and beddings should be exposed to sunlight.
7. Wet mopping of floors.
8. Fly sitting on sputum and other discharges should be prevented.

DOTS-Plus Strategy

DOTS-Plus for MDR-TB is a comprehensive management initiative under development that is built upon the five elements of the DOTS strategy DOTS-Plus takes into account specific issues, such as the use of second-line anti-TB drugs, that need to be addressed in areas where there are significant levels of MDR-TB. The goal of DOTS-Plus is to prevent the further development and spread of MDR-TB. DOTS-Plus is not intended as a universal option and is not required in all settings. DOTS-Plus should be implemented in selected areas in order to combat an emerging epidemic. The underlying principle is that proper implementation of DOTS will prevent the emergence of drug resistance and should be the first step in fighting MDR-TB. It is not possible to conduct DOTS-Plus in an area without having an effective DOTS-based TB control program in place. The Working Group has identified access to second-line anti-TB drugs as one of the major obstacles to the implementation of DOTS Plus pilot projects. While access to second-line anti-TB drugs must increase, these drugs should only be used in DOTS-Plus pilot projects that meet the standards set forth by the Scientific Panel of the Working Group in the *Guidelines for the Establishment of DOTS-Plus Pilot Projects for the Management of MDR-TB* (the Guidelines). Adherence to the Guidelines results in proper management of existing cases of MDR-TB while preventing the rapid development of resistance to second-line anti-TB drugs. The Guidelines are based on the recommendations of the Scientific Panel of the Working Group and will be further developed based on evidence provided by DOTS-Plus pilot projects. In addition to explaining the DOTS-Plus concept, the Guidelines define the minimum requirements necessary to establish and maintain DOTS-Plus pilot projects. Sample protocols are available to design standardized or individualized treatment regimens with second-line anti-TB drugs to be used in DOTS-Plus pilot projects.

Components

DOTS-Plus refers to DOTS programs that add components for MDR-TB diagnosis, management and treatment. The DOTS-Plus strategy promotes full integration of DOTS and DOTS-Plus activities under the RNTCP, so that patients with MDR- TB are both correctly identified properly managed DOTS Plus is having five components:

1. Sustained government commitment.
2. Accurate, timely diagnosis through quality assured culture and drug susceptibility assured culture and drug susceptibility testing (DST).
3. Appropriate treatment utilizing second-line drugs under strict supervision.
4. Uninterrupted supply of quality assured anti-TB drugs: and
5. Standardized recoding and reporting system.

Strategy and Focus

1. DOTS reveals the emergence of drug-resistant TB and MDR-TB by ensuring that patient to the full course of treatment.
2. DOTS-Plus is designed to cure MDR-TB using second line anti-TB drugs.
3. DOTS-Plus is needed in areas where MDR-TB has emerged due to previous inadequate programs.
4. DOTS-Plus pilot project are only recommended in setting where the DOTS strategy place to protect against the creation of further drug resistance.
5. It is vital that DOTS-Plus pilot project are implemented following the recommendation. Stop TB working group on MDR-TB in order to minimize the risk of creating resistant second line anti-TB drugs.
6. Before launching DOTS-Plus pilot project, WHO member states are strongly recommended to consult WHO.

7. With the coordination of the working group on DOTS-Plus for MDR-TB and a partnership industry, the price of second line anti-TB drugs have fallen considerable, making these more accessible to the poor.

Green Light Committee Initiative

Component two of the stop TB strategy calls for the control and prevention of multidrug-resistant tuberculosis (MDR-TB) through: (i) increased access to quality-assured second-line anti-TB drugs; and (ii) prevention of development of resistance to anti-TB drugs.

The Green Light Committee (GLC) initiative, together with the working group on MDR-TB, promotes implementation of this strategy in accordance with the global plan to stop TB (2006–2015) and the global MDR/XDR-TB response plan (2007–2008).

Established in 2000, the GLC initiative is the mechanism that enables access to affordable, high-quality, second-line anti-TB drugs for the treatment of MDR-TB. Its objectives are:

- Ensuring effective treatment of patients with MDR-TB in accordance with guidelines published by the World Health Organization (WHO) on the programmatic management of MDR-TB;
- Increasing access to technical assistance to facilitate rapid scale-up of MDR-TB management;
- Increasing access to high-quality, low-cost, second-line anti-TB drugs for the treatment of MDR-TB among well-performing programs; preventing the development of resistance to second-line anti-TB drugs by ensuring rational drug use;
- Advising WHO on policy-related matters to effectively prevent and control MDR-TB based on the best available scientific evidence.

The GLC initiative therefore contributes to reducing transmission of TB, preventing further drug resistance and ultimately reducing the global burden of TB. The initiative is coordinated by the GLC Secretariat, which is hosted and administered by WHO. The Global Drug Facility (GDF), an arm of the stop TB partnership, which is also hosted and administered by WHO, carries out drug procurement for GLC-approved programs. Technical assistance to MDR-TB program is coordinated and delivered by WHO and its technical partners.

HIV Infection and Risk of Tuberculosis

HIV increases the susceptibility to infection with *M. tuberculosis*. In a person infected with *Mycobacterium tuberculosis*, HIV is a potent cause of progression of tuberculosis infection to disease. Compared to an individual who is not infected with HIV, an individual infected with HIV has a 10 times increased risk of developing tuberculosis.

As HIV infection progresses, CD4 lymphocytes decline in number and function. The immune system is less able to prevent the growth and local spread of *M.tuberculosis*. The duration of TB in HIV infected persons is more difficult on account of more non-TB respiratory diseases, more smear negative, disseminated and extrapulmonary TB and X-rays being less specific. Fortunately more than 90 percent of surviving HIV infected TB can be cured provided complete treatment is taken regularly.

LEPROSY

Leprosy continues to be a social and public health problem but the situation is gradually improving.

History

Milestones

1955	National Leprosy Control Program
1983	National Leprosy Eradication Program (MDT started)
1991	World Health Assembly resolution to eradicate leprosy by 2000 AD
1993	World Bank supported the MDT program Phase I
1997	Mid-term appraisal
1997-2002	Ninth Five Years Plan
2000	NLEP Project Phase II

It is a disease of antiquity. The causative organism, *Mycobacterium lepreae* was discovered in 1873 by Hanson Norway.

Sulphon drugs were introduced for treatment of leprosy in 1943.

Burden of Leprosy

World

There are around 1.3 million cases of leprosy in the world (1996). Leprosy remains a public health problem in 55 countries, but 16 countries account for 91 percent of the total number of registered cases and five of them (Brazil, India, Indonesia, Myanmar, and Nigeria) account for about 82 percent. Globally 60 percent of the estimated cases are contributed by India.

India

- Prevalence rate (PR) is 3.74/10,000 population (March 2001) which was 57/10,000 in 1981.
- Elimination level (<1/10,000) achieved in 13 states—Nagaland, Haryana, Punjab, Mizoram,Tripura, Himachal Pradesh, Meghalaya, Sikkim, Jammu and Kashmir, Rajasthan, Manipur, Assam, and Kerala.
- States close to achieve elimination—Gujarat, Arunachal Pradesh, Daman and Diu.

- Leprosy is endemic mainly in states of Bihar, Jharkhand, Chhattisgarh, UP, West Bengal, Orissa and MP where 64 percent are found.
- Bihar has 24 percent of recorded leprosy cases in India.
- A total of 5.59 lakh cases were detected in India by 2000-2001 due to intensification of the program, the highest number of cases detected in any year.
- Annual new cases detected were 4 to 7.8 lakh. Out of the total 18.5 percent were children.
- Deformity cases (Grade II and above) among new cases were 2.7 percent.
- MB cases among new cases were 34 percent.

Essential Indicators for Leprosy

An indicator is a calculation, which is used to measure different aspects of leprosy control. Indicators can give different information:

a. They can tell how big or how serious is the problem of leprosy in the area. It can help one to analyze the situation regarding leprosy in the area.
b. They can help to assess how well the leprosy control program is functioning. This will help to plan and run program more efficiently. The following indicators are mainly used.

Prevalence Rate (Point Prevalence Rate)

Prevalence indicates the quantum of morbidity due to leprosy in the community. Prevalence rate is calculated by using the following formula.

$$PR = \frac{\text{No. of Regd cases in the project are at a point of time}}{\text{Estimated mid-year population}} \times 10{,}000$$

A reduction in prevalence rate from year to year indicates a favorable impact of the measures taken.

New Case Detection Rate

NCDR or annual case detection rate ACDR. It is calculated as follows:

$$NCDR = \frac{\text{No. of new cases detected in the new year}}{\text{Mid-year population}} \times 10{,}000$$

New case detection roughly indicates the quantum of transmission. A reduction in new case detection rate indicates a reduction in transmission.

Disability Rate Among New Detection

It can be calculated as follows:

$$= \frac{\text{No. of new cases having disability grade '2'}}{\text{No. of new cases detected during the year}} \times 100$$

It indicates the efficiency in early detection of cases.

Proportion of Children among New Detection

It can be calculated as follows:

$$= \frac{\text{No. of children (0-14 year) cases among new cases}}{\text{Total new cases detected during the year}} \times 100$$

Reduction of this rate in the later years indicates favorable impact on disease transmission.

Multibacillary (MB) Rate

It can be calculated as follows:

$$= \frac{\text{No. of MB cases among new cases}}{\text{Total new cases detected during the year}} \times 100$$

Proportion of Single Skin Lesion (SSL) Case Rate

It can be calculated as follows:

$$= \frac{\text{No. of SSL cases detected during the year}}{\text{Total no. of new cases detected during the year}} \times 100$$

Cohort Cure Rate MB/PB

a. The No.of MB/PB cases put under treatment during the year.
b. The No.of those patients of the Cohort group who have completed full course of treatment during the next one and half years.

$$\text{Cohort cure rate} = \frac{b}{a} \times 100$$

Epidemiology

Agent (Mycobacterium leprae)

1. *Sources of infection:* Lepromatous and borderline lepromatous cases in the family or among close contacts.
2. *Mode of transmission:*
   a. Droplet infection
   b. Contact transmission.
3. *Period of communicability:* Lepromatous and borderline cases become noninfectious within two weeks of treatment with rifampicin or three months of treatment with dapsone.

4. *Incubation period:* Long, usually three to five years, shorter incubation in tuberculoid leprosy.
5. *Secondary attack rate:* Five to twelve percent.

Host

1. *Age*: Occurs at all ages, with maximum incidence during 10 to 20 years
2. *Sex*: More in males, M:F is 3:2 in all types of leprosy and 3:1 in lepromatous type of leprosy.

Environmental and Social Factors

1. Physical environment
2. Social environment
3. Biological environment.

Physical environment: The factors are:

a. Large family size
b. Over crowding
c. Poor ventilation
d. Urban slum.

M. leprae can remain viable in dried nasal secretions for 9 days and in moist soil for 46 days.

Social environment: Deep rooted prejudices lead to social ostracism of patients with leprosy, Thus, there is delay in seeking treatment, thereby increasing the possibility of transmission.

Biological environment: Wild armadillos in limited area of USA have been found to be infected.

a. Genetic factor-HLA linked gene
b. Migration

Mode of Transmission

1. Droplet infection
2. Contact transmission
3. Other routes
   a. Breast milk
   b. Insect vector
   c. Tattooing needles.

Clinical Features

Presentation depends upon cell mediated immunity of the patient (Tables 4.9 and 4.10).

Table 4.9: Classification of leprosy

NLEP	Ridely and Jopling	Indian	International (Madrid)
Paucibacillary	Indeterminate	Indeterminate	Indeterminate
	TT	Tuberculoid	Tuberculoid
	BT	Pure neuritic	
Multibacillary	BB	Borderline	Borderline
	BL	Lepromatous	
	LL	Lepromatous	Lepromatous

Table 4.10: Immunological status and type of leprosy

Immunological status	*Type of disease*
1. Poor immunity	Lepromatous (LL) leprosy
2. Intermediate immunity	Borderline leprosy (BB, BL, BT)
3. Good immunity	Tuberculoid (TT) leprosy

Lepromatous Leprosy

Early manifestations commonly missed by patients include:

1. Nasal symptoms:
   a. Stuffiness
   b. Crust formation
   c. Blood stained discharged from nose.
2. Edema of legs and ankles:
   a. Bilateral and symmetrical
   b. More marked in the evening.

Other overt manifestations include:

1. Skin lesions:
   a. Macules (more common, papules and nodules.
   b. Bilateral symmetrical and large.
   c. Sites: Face, arms, buttocks, legs and trunk.
   d. Hypopigmented.
2. Leonine facies:
   a. Thickening of skin of forehead, causes deepening of the natural lines.
   b. Ear lobes are thickened.
   c. Eyebrows are lost (madarosis).
   d. Nasal bridge may collapse.
3. Superficial nerves:
   a. Thickened
   b. Glove and stocking anesthesia.
4. Testicular atrophy leading to:
   a. Sterility
   b. Impotence
   c. Gynecomastia.

5. Bone:
   a. Periostitis
   b. Disuse osteoporosis.
6. Eye:
   a. Superficial punctate keratitis.

Diagnosis

1. Clinical examination
2. Bacteriological examination
3. Foot-pad culture
4. Histamine test
5. Biopsy
6. Immunological tests.

Clinical Examination

Diagnosis is fairly easy in lepromatous and non-lepromatous cases if the disease is just kept in mind. Simple diagnostic guidelines have been outlined by WHO. Difficulty may arise in the indeterminate type. It should be confirmed by bacteriological examination of the material obtained by the routine 'slit-and-scrape' method from the edge of the lesion or from the lobule of the ear. Nasal smear may also be used. Skin and nerve biopsy may be performed in non-lepromatous cases.

Early detection of subclinical cases is obviously of great importance in control of leprosy.

The following three are helpful in this:

i. Enlargement of great auricular nerve.
ii. Search for AFB in ear lobes of contacts of leprosy patients.
iii. Immunological test aimed at assessing cell mediated or humoral immunity. The most commonly used test for cell mediated immunity is the lepromin test, using either the Mitsuda or Dharmendra lepromin preparation. There is evidence that the tests for humoral immunoresponse, such as FLA-ABS, may be much more sensitive than lepromin test alone.

The government has brought out a simple guide for medical officers to help them to diagnose and manage leprosy patients. Some practical guidelines for diagnosis are given below.

What are the principles of skin examination? How does one examine the skin?

1. Choose a spot where good light is available.
2. As far as possible, choose a spot where there is privacy.
3. Always examine the whole skin from head to toe.
4. Use the same order of examination always so that you do not forget to examine any part of the body.
5. Compare both sides of the body.

What should one look for in the skin?

The following features must be noted when examining a patch on the skin:

- *Site:* This is useful for follow-up.
- *Number:* The number of lesions indicates the severity of the disease. This is useful for classification and follow-up.
- *Color:* May be hypopigmented (lighter in color than the rest of the skin), or erythematous (red). Lesions of leprosy are never depigmented. Erythematous color can be used to identify disease activity or a reactional state (Active lesions or those in reaction are often red).
- *Sensory loss:* This is useful both for diagnosis and classification of leprosy. Loss of sensation is a cardinal sign of leprosy.
- *Tenderness on gentle tapping:* This is seen in reactional states.
- *Presence of infiltration:* This term refers to skin which is thickened, shiny and erythematous. All three features must be present in the same area. This may be seen in severe forms of leprosy.

How should One Test for Sensation?

Remember the cardinal sign: Hypopigmented or reddish skin lesion(s) with definite loss of sensation.

It is very important to pick up the skill of eliciting sensory loss in skin patch.

- You will need a ball point pen/pin, etc.
- Explain to the person what you are going to do and demonstrate it.
- Touch the skin with the pen/pin. Ask the person to count aloud each time he feels the pen/pin. Alternatively, ask the individual to point to the spot touched with his finger.
- Repeat this procedure a few times until the patient is familiar and comfortable with the procedure.
- Now ask the patient to close his eyes and repeat over the area to be tested. Alternatively, the person should be blindfolded or some barrier should be used to prevent his or her from watching the procedure.

Remember

1. Do not keep asking the patient whether he feels the pen/pin or not. You may get misleading results.
2. When testing for sensation, touch the skin lightly with the pen/pin. Do not stroke.
3. Proceed from the normal skin to the abnormal.
4. Give only one stimulus at a time.
5. Vary the pace of testing.

What are the General Principles of Nerve Palpation?

Examination of nerves in all the patients is very important for prevention of deformity. This involves two aspects:

- Palpation of the nerves for thickening, tenderness and consistency.
- Assessment of nerve function.
  1. When palpating the nerves, you should look for three things: Thickening, tenderness and consistency.
  2. When palpating the nerve, the patient should be properly positioned. The examiner should also be positioned correctly.
  3. Always compare both sides to assess thickness and consistency.
  4. Look at the patient's face while palpating the nerve to elicit tenderness.
  5. Always palpate across the course of the nerve.
  6. Feel along the nerve as far as possible in both directions.
  7. Palpate gently with the pulp of the finger, not the tip.

How should We assess Nerve Function?

Nerve function assessment includes both motor and sensory function, i.e. Voluntary Muscle Test (VMT) and Sensory Test (ST). Both VMT and ST should be done for:

a. All patients with nerve thickening.
b. All patients with multibacillary leprosy.

How is Voluntary Muscle Testing done?

Voluntary muscle testing is done by first checking the range of movement to see whether movement is normal, reduced or absent due to paralysis. If movement is normal, a test for resistance is then done (Fig. 4.2). Press gently in the opposite direction while asking the patient to maintain position, resisting pressure as strongly as possible. Then gradually press more firmly and judge whether resistance is normal, reduced or absent. Always compare the right side with the left. The grading of the result can be done as follows:

- S (Strong)—Able to perform the movement against full resistance.
- W (Weak)—Able to perform the movement but not against full resistance.
- P (Paralysed)—Not able to perform the movement at all.

Bacteriological Examination

- Skin smear
- Nasal smear
- Nasal scraping.

Bacterial Index (BI)

Bacterial Index (BI) is the only objective way of monitoring the benefit of treatment. The WHO grading of smears for BI is as follows:

Negative	:	No bacilli found in 100 fields
One plus (+)	:	One or less than one bacillus in each microscopic field

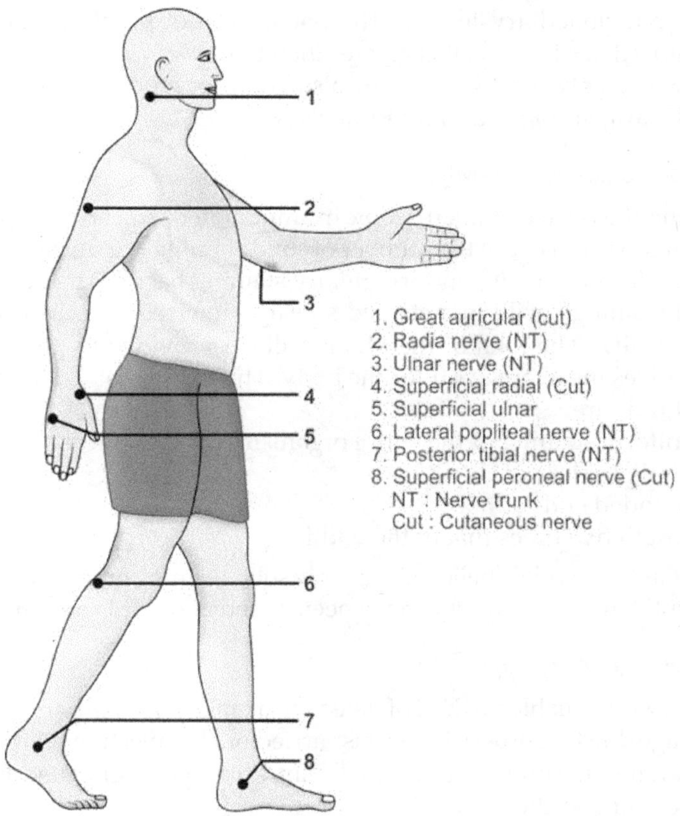

Fig. 4.2: Diagram of the human body showing nerves commonly invoiced in leprosy

Two plus (+ +)	:	Bacilli found in all fields
Three plus (+ + +)	:	Many bacilli found in all fields
		Add G to the entry if globi are present

Bacterial index is calculated by totalling the number of + given to each smear and dividing this number by the smears collected. A minimum of seven sites should be examined; smears from four skin lesions, one nasal swab, and smears from both ear lobes, e.g.

Right ear	+++
Left ear	+++
Nasal smear	+++
First skin lesion	+++
Second skin lesion	++
Third skin lesion	+++
Fourth skin lesion	++

$$\text{Bacterial index (BI)} = \frac{19}{\text{7 sites of examination}}$$

In paucibacillary leprosy the bacterial index is less than two; in multibacillary leprosy, it is greater than two.

Two other types of grading are also in use for reporting bacterial index, e.g. Dharmendra's scale and Ridley's scale.

Morphological Index (MI)

During the course of microscopic examination of smears, it is possible to distinguish and count the number of solid staining organisms (organisms that stain completely) and irregularly staining bacilli. The percentage of solid staining bacilli in a stained smear is referred to as Morphological Index (MI). The total of the MIs for all sites divided by the number of sites gives the average MI for the body. The criteria for calling the bacilli solid rods are:

a. Uniform staining of the entire organism
b. Parallel sides
c. Rounded ends
d. Length five times that of the width.

It has been widely believed that only solid-staining organisms are viable. Recently, however, doubts have been raised about this notion.

Histamine Test (Table 4.11)

This is very reliable method of detecting at an early stage peripheral nerve damage due to leprosy. The test is carried out by injecting 0.1 ml of 1:1000 histamine phosphate intradermally into the hypopigmented patches or in areas of anesthesia.

Table 4.11: Histamine test—result and interpretation

Result	*Interpretation*
Bright flare (triple response)	Normal skin
Delayed and feeble flare	Indeterminate
Flare absent	(BB)
	Tuberculoid (TT)

Sweat Test (Table 4.12)

This test is recommended when difficulty is experienced in the diagnosis, as for example, indeterminate leprosy.

0.2 ml of 1:1000 solution of pilocarpine is injected intra-dermally. Paint with iodine and dust with starch powder.

Table 4.12: Sweat test—result and interpretation

Result	*Interpretation*
Blue discoloration	Normal skin
No color	Leprosy

Lepromin Test

It is used to classify the type of lesion.

0.1 ml of antigen is injected intradermally. The reaction is read at 48 hours and 21 days.

Early reaction (Fernadez reaction): An inflammatory response develops within 24 to 48 hours and this tends to disappear after 3 to 4 days. It is evidenced by redness and induration at the site of inoculation. If the diameter of the red area is more than 10 mm at the end of 48 hours, the test is considered positive. The early positive reaction indicates whether or not a person has been previously sensitized by exposure to and infection by the leprosy bacilli. The early reaction is induced by soluble constituents of the leprosy bacilli. The reaction corresponds to Mantoux reaction in TB.

Late reaction (Mitsuda reaction): The test is read at 21 days. If there is a nodule more than 5 mm in diameter at the site of inoculation, the reaction is said to be positive. The late reaction is induced by the bacillary component of the antigen. It indicates cell mediated immunity.

Value of the lepromin test: Lepromin test is not a diagnostic test. It evaluates the immmune status of leprosy patients. It helps in classification of leprosy.

This test also helps in assessing the prognosis in cases of leprosy of all types.

Utility of lepromin test: In classifying the types of leprosy (Table 4.13).

Table 4.13: Classifying the types of leprosy

Test	*Type of leprosy*
+++	TT
++	BT
–ve	BB, BL, LL

Lepromin positive individuals either escape the clinical disease (the majority) or develop paucibacillary disease.

Lepromin negative individuals are at a higher risk of developing progressive multibacillary leprosy.

Deformities Occurring in Leprosy (Table 4.14)

Table 4.14: Deformities occurring in leprosy

Face	Mask face, facies leonina, sagging face, lagophthalmos, loss of eye-brows (superciliary madarosis) and eyelashes (ciliary madarosis), corneal ulcers and opacities, perforated nose, depressed nose, ear deformities, e.g. nodules on the ear and elongated lobules
Hands	Claw hand, wrist-drop, ulcers, absorption of digits, thumb-web contracture, hollowing of the interosseous spaces and swollen hand
Feet	Plantar ulcers, foot-drop, inversion of the foot, clawing of the toes, absorption of the toes, collapsed foot, swollen foot and callosities
Other deformities	Gynecomastia and perforation of the palate

Features of Lepra Reactions (Reversal Reaction) (Table 4.15)

Table 4.15: Features of lepra reactions (reversal reaction)

Features	*Type 1 (Reversal reaction)*	*Type 2 (Erythema nodosum leprosum reaction)*
Skin	Existing lesions suddenly become red, swollen warm, and tender. New lesions may appear	Red, painful, tender, subcutaneous (deep) nodules (ENL) appear commonly on face and arms and legs. They appear in groups and subside within a few days
Nerves	Lesions when subsiding may show scales on the surface. Nerves close to the skin may become enlarged, tender and painful (neuritis) with loss of nerve function	Nerves may be affected but not as commonly as in type 1
Other organs	Not affected	Other organs like eye, joints, bones, testes, kidney may be affected
General	Not common	Fever, joint pains, fatigue *symptoms*

Clinical Difference between Reversal Reaction and Relapse (Table 4.16)

Table 4.16: Clinical difference between reversal reaction and relapse

	Reversal reaction	*Relapse*
Time interval	Generally occurs during chemotherapy or within 6 months of stopping treatment	Usually occurs only when chemotherapy has been discontinued, after an interval of usually more than 6 months
Onset	Abrupt and sudden	Slow and insidious
Old lesions	Existing lesions become edematous, erythematous or tender	Lesions may show erythema and infiltration, but no tenderness
New lesions	Several new lesions appear	New lesions are few
Ulceration	Lesions may ulcerate	Ulceration does not occur
Nerve involvement	Multiple nerve involvement common, painful and tender	Nerve involvement may occur only in a single nerve; usually no pain, tenderness
General condition	May have fever, joint pains, malaise	Not usually affected
Response to steroid treatment	Rapid	Nil

Treatment of Reversal Reaction

During reversal reaction (multidrug therapy) MDT should be contained without interruption along with antireaction treatment.

Antileprosy Drugs and their Characteristics (Table 4.17)

Table 4.17: Antileprosy drugs and their characteristics

Drug	Dose (mg)	Bactericidal activity
Dapsone	100	+
Rifampicin	600	+++
Ethionamide	375	++
Prothionamide	375	++
Clofazimine	100	+

Patient Grouping for MDT (Table 4.18)

Table 4.18: Patient grouping for MDT

Group criteria	PB single skin lesion (patch) PB-SSL	PB (Paucibacillary) leprosy	MB (Multibacillary) leprosy
Skin lesions	1 skin lesions	2-5 lesions asymmetrically distributed	6 and above Symmetrically distributed
Nerve involvement	No nerve involvement	No nerve involvement/ only one nerve trunk	More than one nerve trunk involvement
Skin smear	Negative at all sites	Negative at all sites	Positive at all sites

Dosage Schedule for MDT (Table 4.19)

Table 4.19: Dosage schedule for MDT

	Drugs used	Dosage (adults)	Frequency of administration	Criteria for cure
MB leprosy	Rifampicin Dapsone Clofazimine	600 mg 100 mg 300 mg 50 mg	Once monthly Daily Once monthly Daily	Completion of 12 monthly. Pulses within 18 months
PB leprosy	Rifampicin Dapsone	600 mg 100 mg	Once monthly Daily	Completion of 6 monthly. Pulses within 9 months
Single skin lesion leprosy	Rifampicin Ofloxacin Minocycline	600 mg 400 mg 100 mg	Single dose Single dose Single dose	Administration of single dose treatment (ROM)

If there is no nerve involvement-rest and analgesics only are used. If there is nerve involvement-corticosteroids (Prednisolone) are given in addition to rest and analgesics.

A suggested course of prednisolone for an adult patient is as follows:

- 40 mg once a day for the first 2 weeks then
- 30 mg once a day for 3 and 4 weeks
- 20 mg once a day for 5 and 6 weeks
- 15 mg once a day for 7 and 8 weeks
- 10 mg once a day for 9 and 10 weeks
- 5 mg once a day for 11 and 12 weeks.

The daily dose of prednisolone should not exceed 1 mg/kg body weight.

Treatment of ENL Reaction

ENL reaction occurs only in MB cases.

- For mild reactions, bed rest, aspirin or paracetamol are sufficient.
- In case of nerve involvement, treatment with prednisolone should be started immediately during ENL reaction. MDT should be continued without interruption along with antibiotic treatment.

Completion of Treatment and Cure

- Any SSL patient who has taken one dose of ROM should be considered as cured.
- Any PB patient who has taken six months of PB-MDT within 9 months should be considered as cured.
- Any MB patient who has taken 12 months of MB-MDT within 18 months should be considered as cured
- All such patients should be told about the early signs of reactions and relapse and asked to report any such events promptly to the center. If the individual has sequelae due to the disease, such as disabilities he/she should be encouraged and helped to use the available facilities at the health centre or at an appropriate referral center.

It is important to remember that a leprosy patient who has completed a full course of treatment should no longer be regarded as a case of leprosy even if some sequelae of leprosy remain.

Side Effects of Anti-leprosy Drugs (Table 4.20)

Table 4.20: Side effects of anti-leprosy drugs

Common side effects	*Signs and symptoms*	*What to do if side effects occur*
Dapsone		
Anemia	Paleness inside the lower eyelids, tongue and finger nail Tiredness, edema of feet and breathlessness	Give anti-worm treatment and iron tablets. Continue dapsone
Severe skin complication (Exfoliative dermatitis)	Extensive scaling, itching, ulcers in the mouth, the eyes, jaundice and reduced urine output	Stop dapsone. Refer to hospital immediately. Never restart
Abdominal symptoms	Abdominal pain, nausea, and vomiting on high doses	Symptomatic treatment. Reassure the patient
Liver damage (Hepatitis)	Jaundice (Yellow color of skin, eyeballs and urine), loss of appetite and vomiting	Stop dapsone. Refer to hospital, restart after the jaundice subsides.
Kidney damage (Nephritis)	Edema of face and feet Reduced urine output	Stop dapsone. Refer to hospital

Contd....

Contd....

Rifampicin		
No significance	Reddish coloration of urine, saliva and sweat	Reassure the patient
Hepatitis (liver damage)	Jaundice (yellow color of skin, eyeballs and urine)	Stop Rifampicin. Refer to hospital restart after the jaundice subsides
Flu-like illness	Fever,malaise and body ache	Symptomatic treatment
Allergy	Skin rash	Stop rifampicin
Clofazimine		
No significance	Brownish-red discoloration of skin, urine, and body fluids	Reassure the patient, it will go after completion of treatment
Ichthyosis	Dryness and thickening of the skin, itching	Apply oil to the skin Reassure the patient
Eye	Conjuctival dryness	Moistening eye drops
Abdominal symptoms	Abdominal pain, nausea and vomiting on high doses	Symptomatic treatment Reassure the patient
Ofloxacin*		
Abdominal symptoms	Abdominal pain, nausea and vomiting on high doses	Symptomatic treatment Reassure the patient
Central nervous system complaints	Sleeplessness, headaches, dizziness, nervousness, hallucinations	Symptomatic treatment Reassure the patient
Dizziness	—	Reassure the patient
Discoloration of the teeth in children	—	Reassure the patient
Pigmentation of the mucous membranes	—	Reassure the patient
Abdominal symptoms	Abdominal pain, nausea and vomiting on high dose	Symptomatic treatment Reassure the patient

* With a single dose regimen (ROM) complications are rare. However, this drug is also not recommended for use in pregnant women and children below five years of age.

- Any patient showing a positive skin smear, irrespective of the clinical classification, should be treated with the MDT regimen for MB leprosy.
- When classification is in doubt, the patient should be treated with the MDT for MB leprosy.

LEPROSY CONTROL

Leprosy Control Programs

1. Medical measures
   a. Estimation of the problem
   b. Early case detection

c. Multidrug therapy
d. Surveillance
e. Immunoprophylaxis
f. Chemoprophylaxis
g. Rehabilitation
h. Health education
i. Others

2. Social support
3. Program management
4. Evaluation.

Candidate Vaccines

In view of the variable protective effect of BCG vaccine against leprosy, several alternative vaccine preparations are under development. They should more appropriately be called " Candidate Vaccines" (Table 4.21).

Table 4.21: Candidate vaccines

Category I (based on M. leprae)	*Category II (based on cultivable mycobacteria)*
Killed *M. leprae*	BCG
Killed *M. leprae* + BCG	BCG + *M. vaccae*
Acetoacetylated *M. leprae*	Killed ICRC bacillus

Health Education

Leprosy Educational Messages

1. Leprosy is the least communicable of all infectious diseases.
2. Four out of five leprosy cases in India are of the noninfectious kind.
3. The treatment available today renders infectious cases noninfectious in as little as five or six weeks with the help of MDT.
4. Leprosy does not strike overnight. It can take years to manifest itself. A very prolonged exposure to untreated, infectious cases is necessary for the signs of the disease to become manifest.
5. Leprosy is neither hereditary nor a curse. It is caused by a germ.
6. Leprosy is completely curable.
7. Leprosy need not result in deformities at all. If detected and treated early, it leaves no physical scars.
8. The nerve and limb complications that lead to deformity are not inevitable; they are the result of neglect.
9. Leprosy can be cured even at an advanced stage, though it may not be possible to correct all the deformities.
10. Leprosy is not a poor man's disease. It can occur in any social or economic class, even among the affluent.
11. Leprosy is not only an adult's disease: 20 percent of all newly detected cases are children.

12. Leprosy is more than just a medical problem and, for the disease to be fully treated, community support is as important as medical help.
13. The leprosy patients can stay at home without any risk and continue to work because, once the treatment is started, the disease is contained.
14. The first signs of leprosy are:
    a. A pale or red patch which could be oily, smooth or dry. The patch is neither painful nor itchy.
    b. Loss of hair and lack of sweating in the discolored area.
    c. Numbness in the patch.
    d. A tingling or "ant-crawling" sensation along the affected nerve.
15. Leprosy is curable. All it needs is:
    a. Early detection
    b. Early intervention
    c. Sustained treatment
    d. Community support throughout.
16. Treatment of leprosy is absolutely free.

Rehabilitation

All cured cases should be provided suitable jobs through government or private agencies. Modern plastic and orthopedic surgery and physiotherapy should be used to treat disfiguration and deformities and to restore appearance and function. Burnt out cases with marked deformities may be kept in special rehabilitation centers.

Leprosy Organizations in India

There are many voluntary organizations working in the field of leprosy in India. These include:

1. *Leprosy Mission:* This was the first voluntary organization for leprosy work in India. It was started in 1874 by Bailey in Chamba, Himachal Pradesh. Its headquarter is presently in Purulia, West Bengal.
2. *Hind Kushth Nivaran Sangh:* This pioneer organization was established in India in 1947 as a branch of the British Empire Leprosy Relief Association founded in London in 1925.
3. Gandhi Memorial Leprosy Foundation, Sevagram, Wardha.
4. Belgium Leprosy Center (Polambakkam, Chennai).
5. Danish Save the Children Fund.
6. Bharat Sewashram Sangh, Jamshedpur, Bihar.
7. Kashi Kushth Seva Sangh ,Varanasi, UP.
8. Tapovan, Amravati, Maharashtra.
9. Hindu Mission, Chennai, Tamil Nadu.

Two other important organizations active in the field of leprosy are the Jalma Central Institute of Leprosy (taken over by ICMR in 1975) and the Central Leprosy Teaching and Research Institute, Chingleput, Tamil Nadu.

National Leprosy Eradication Program (NLEP)

This program was started in 1983.

Strategies

The program has the following four strategies:

1. Provide domiciliary treatment (MDT) in endemic districts through staff trained in leprosy.
2. Provide services through mobile leprosy treatment units with the help of primary health care staff in moderate and low endemic districts.
3. Organize health education to patients, their families and the community to increase awareness and to remove stigma.
4. To Provide deformity and ulcer care and medical rehabilitation services to the needy patients.

Infrastructure

It is shown in Table 4.22.

The term elimination refers to the reduction in the prevalence of leprosy to below one case per 10,000 population. There will be drastic reduction in the prevalence of a disease to the extent that it no longer remains a public health problems.

Eradication refers to the complete stopping of transmission as a result of total disappearance of the diseases causing organism. The aim is to reduce case load to 1 or less than 1 per 10,000 population.

Modified Leprosy Elimination Campaigns

The Modified Leprosy Elimination Campaigns (MLEC) approach is actually organizing camps for one or two weeks duration in which services like cases detection, treatment and referral to reconstruction facilities are available. A wide level information about camps services and about disease disseminated through radio, TV, newspapers, loudspeaker, etc.

Table 4.22: Infrastructure

Unit	*Scale*	*No existing*	*Remarks*
Leprosy control unit (LCU) or modified LCU	One per 4.5 lakh population	778	In endemic rural areas headed by a Medical Officer
Urban leprosy center (ULC)	One for 50,000 population	907	Manned by one paramedical worker responsible to the MO of a dispensary or hospital
Survey education and treatment center (SET)	One per 25,000 population	5744	In low endemic areas, attached to a PHC or hospital manned by a paramedical worker under guidance of MO, PHC

Contd...

Contd....

Mobile leprosy treatment units (MLTU)	350	In non-endemic districts headed by a Medical Officer.
Temporary hospitalization ward (THW)	290	
Reconstructive surgery units (RSU)	75	
Samples survey cum assessment unit (SSAU)	40	

MLEC has proved quite effective for case finding and has been employed during phase II. Two rounds of MLEC will be held during phase II; the specific MLEC strategy is varied according to the endemicity of different regions:

Action Plan of MLEC (Table 4.23)

Table 4.23: Action plan of MLEC

Endemicity	*1 MLEC year 1*	*2 MLEC year 2*	*Year 3*
High endemic states	Active search statewise in UP, Bihar, West Bengal, mix of active search and VRCs in Orissa and Madhya Pradesh	Mixed approach active search and VRCs depending upon endemicity of individual districts/ pockets	Special action projects for the elimination of leprosy (SAPEL) and LECs in tribal areas. In Bihar, voluntary reporting centers (VRCs)
Moderate/low endemic states	VRCs for 2 days with training and IEC support	VRCs for 2 days with training and support	For 2 days
Very low endemic states	IEC activity, passive reporting	IEC activity, passive reporting	

Special Action Projects for the Elimination of Leprosy

Special Action Projects for the Elimination of Leprosy (SAPEL) is an initiative aimed at providing MDT services to patients living in special difficult to access areas or situation or to those belonging to neglected population groups. The most important thing is for the elimination program to reach everyone who needs MDT services. Innovative and practical strategies involving mainly operation solutions are be used in order to provide MDT to these patients.

Global Leprosy Elimination Program

Revised Intensified Strategy 2000-2005 (Modified Leprosy Elimination Campaign and SAPELS).

Elements of the Intensified Program

1. Identification of endemic districts
2. Integration of MDT services with general health services
3. Monitoring elimination at district level
4. Promoting community action
5. Social marketing/advocacy
6. Re-motivating the research community
7. Prevention of disability and rehabilitation.

FILARIASIS

Filariasis is a global problem. (More than 1.1 billion people live in areas where there is a risk of infection.) It is estimated that globally 751 million population is exposed to the risk of filariasis. Half of these cases are in India.

Burden of Disease

Lymphatic filaria is prevalent in 18 states and union territories. Bancroftian filariasis is widely distributed while brugian filariasis caused by Brugia malaya is restricted to 6 sates—Uttar Pradesh, Bihar, Andhra Pradesh, Orissa, Tamil Nadu, Kerala, and Gujarat. The WHO has estimated that 600 million people are at risk of infection in South-East Asia and 60 million are actually infected in the region (WHO-SEARO 1999). There are about 454 million people (75.6%) at the risk of infection with 48 million (80%) infected with parasite are contributed only by India.

Epidemiology

Human Filarial Infections

Agents

1. *Wuchereria bancrofti*
2. *Brugia malayi*
3. *Brugia timori*
4. *Onchocerca volvulus*
5. *Loa loa*
   T. perstans
   T. streptocerca
6. *Mansonella ozzardi*

Vectors

1. Culex mosquitoes
2. Mansonia mosquitoes
3. Anopheles mosquitoes
4. Simulum flies

5. Chrysopes flies
6. Culicoides.

Host

Man is the definitive host and mosquito is the intermediate host of Bancroftian filariasis.

- Age — All age group
- Sex — Higher in males
- Social factors — Urbanization, industrialization, poverty, illiteracy

Environmental Factors

Climate: It influences the breeding of mosquitoes.

- Temp 22 to 38°C
- Humidity—70 percent
- Town planning—this disease is associated with bad drainage.Vectors breed profusely in polluted water.
- Incubation period = 8 to 16 months.

Clinical Manifestations

I. Lymphatic filariasis
II. Occult filariasis

Lymphatic Filariasis

a. Asymptomatic amicrofilaremia
b. Asymptomatic microfilaremia
c. Stage of acute manifestation
d. Stage of chronic obstructive lesions—elephantiasis of leg, scrotum, arms, penis, vulva and breasts.

Survey

1. Mass blood survey
   a. The thick film
   b. Membrane filter concentration
   c. DEC provocation test
   (DEC—100 mg—administered orally, microfilaria begin to reach peak in 15 minutes and begin to decrease 2 hours later, the blood may be examined one hour after administration of DEC).
2. Clinical survey
3. Serological test
4. Xenodiagnosis
5. Entomalogical survey.

Control Measures

1. Chemotherapy
2. Vector control.

Chemotherapy

For the individual case treatment: Diethylcarbamazine (DEC) is given for Bancrofti filariasis in the dose of 6 mg/kg body weight orally daily for 12 days in divided doses after meal (a total of 72 mg per kg of DEC). For the Brugian filariasis, DEC is given 3 to 6 mg/kg body weight per day up to total dose of 18 to 72 mg per kg.

Mass treatment: Every member of the community irrespective of infection are treated with DEC. This mode of control has been tried in many areas. In some areas selective cases of microfilaria positive are treated with DEC.

Revised strategy: Single dose mass treatment of diethylcarbamazine (DEC) alone or combined with Ivermectine, repeated at six months or one year, is claimed to bring down the microfilaria rate by over 80 percent. DEC-fortified table salt brings the microfilaria rate to a negligible level within eight months of its introduction.

Vector Control

1. Antilarval measures
2. Antiadult measures
3. Personal prophylaxis.

National Filaria Control Program

It was launched in 1955. In June 1978, the operational component of the National Filaria Control Program (NFCP) was merged with urban malaria scheme. The program has been extended to rural areas since, 1994.

1. Delimitation of the problem in the hitherto unsurveyed areas.
2. Control in urban areas through recurrent anti-larval measures and antiparasitic measures.
3. Filaria clinic were established at the rate of one clinic for 50,000 population. Work involves collection of night blood samples by home visiting. Each unit is expected to cover the alloted population in 2 to 2.5 years. Cases are treated with 72 mg DEC.

National Health Policy

"Elimination of lymphatic filariasis by 2015".

DIARRHEA AND DYSENTERY

Diarrhea is one of the most common causes of death in under-five children. Almost 99 percent of death can be prevented by treating with ORS solution.

Definition

Diarrhea is defined as the passage of loose liquid watery stools. The liquid stools are usually passed more than three times a day. The recent change in consistency and character of stools rather than frequency that is more important.

Acute diarrhea — Lasts for three to seven days
Chronic diarrhea — Lasts for three weeks or more

What is Not Diarrhea?

- Passage of frequent formed stools
- Passage of pasty stools in a breastfed child
- Passage of stools during or immediately after feeding
- Passage of frequent loose greenish yellow stool in the 3rd and 4th day of life (Transitional diarrhea).

Dysentery

If blood is visible in stools the condition is called dysentery.

Gastroenteritis

The term gastroenteritis is used to describe acute diarrhea.

Problem of Diarrheal Disease

The median diarrheal incidence rate ranges from 1.0 to 4.7 episodes per year. In slum areas of major cities an incidence as high as 10.5 episodes per child per year was also reported. About 3 million deaths globally are associated with diarrhea. India alone account for one-third of these deaths. Around 65 percent of deaths are due to dehydration, 20 to 35 percent due to persistent diarrhea and remaining 15 percent due to dysentery. Beside this there is problem of re-emergence of new strains of Cholera, Escherichia and Shigella that need to be tackeld properly otherwise nation may face the severe epidemics.

Upto one-third of total pediatric admissions are due to diarrhea disease and up to 17 percent of all deaths in indoor pediatric patients are diarrhea related.

Causes of Diarrhea (Table 4.24)

Table 4.24: Causes of diarrhea

Pathogen		*% of cases*
Virus	Rotavirus	15-25
Bacterial	*Escherichia coli*	10-20
	Shigella	5-15
	Campylobacter jejuni	10-15
	Vibrio cholerae	5-10
	Salmonella	1-5
Protozoans	Cryptosporidium	5-15
No pathogen found		20-30

Diarrhea Control Program

Components of diarrhea disease control program—started in 1978. Since 1985 to 86 Nation has started oral rehydration therapy.

Short-term

1. Appropriate clinical management
2. Appropriate feeding
3. Chemotherapy.

Long-term

1. Better MCH care practices
   a. Maternal nutrition
   b. Child nutrition :
      i. Promotion of breastfeeding
      ii. Appropriate weaning practices
      iii. Supplementary feedings.
2. Preventive strategies
   a. Sanitation
   b. Health education
   c. Immunization
   d. Antifly measures
3. Preventing diarrhea epidemics.

CHOLERA

Cholera is a notifiable disease all over India as well as to WHO. Being a disease of poor sanitation, poor water, and food hygiene, it occurs as endemic, sporadic and pandamic.

Typical cases are characterized by the sudden onset of profuse, effortless, watery diarrhea followed by vomiting, rapid dehydration, muscular cramps and suppression of urine formation.

Case fatality rate is 30 to 40 percent varies from 10 to 80 percent.

Epidemiology, clinical features, complication and investigation.

Epidemiology

Agent

Vibrio cholerae: There are two types of *vibrio cholerae*:

1. Classical *vibrio cholerae*
2. ELT or *vibrio cholerae*

   There are two serotypes:
   a. Ogawa
   b. Inaba

Source of infection: Contaminated food and water.

Period of communicability: The patient is infective during the later part of incubation period and during the periods of disease and convalescence which lasts for 7 to 10 days.

Mode of transmission: Feco-oral route

Incubation period: One to five days , usually 12 hours to 2 days.

Clinical Features

Stage of evacuation

1. Profuse vomiting.
2. Frequent loose motions, watery, copious, with flakes of mucus (Rice water stool).

Stage of collapse

1. Hypovolemic shock, due to massive diarrhea and vomiting.
2. Tachycardia and tachypnea.
3. Oliguria.
4. Cold and clammy skin.

Stage of recovery

1. Vomiting and loose motions decrease.
2. Hydration improves.
3. Normal temperature returns.

Atypical Presentation

Cholera sicca: It is a fatal variety, in which there is very little or no diarrhea or vomiting, and patient develops collapse very rapidly with overt manifestations.

Complications

1. Hypovolemic shock
2. Acute renal failure
3. Electrolyte disturbances (hypokalemia)
4. Enteritis
5. Cholecystitis
6. Stroke in the elderly patient.

Investigations

1. Leucocytosis with polymorphonuclear predominance.
2. Stool swab, for demonstrating darting motility, of *V. cholerae*
3. Stool culture for *V. cholerae*
4. Slide agglutination using polyvalent anti-cholera, dignostic serum.

Control of Cholera

1. Verification of the diagnoses
2. Notification
3. Early case finding
4. Establishment of treatment centers
5. Rehydration therapy
6. Adjuncts to therapy
7. Epidemiological investigation
8. Sanitation measures
9. Chemoprophylaxis
10. Vaccination
11. Health education.

Rehydration Therapy

Oral rehydration: The introduction of oral rehydration, by WHO in 1971, has greatly simplified the treatment of cholera and other acute diarrhea diseases. The aim of oral fluid therapy is to prevent dehydration and reduce mortality (Tables 4.25 and 4.26).

Table 4.25: Composition of ORS—bicarbonate

Ingredient	*Quantity*
Sodium chloride	3.5 g
Sodium bicarbonate	2.5 g
Potassium chloride	1.5 g
Glucose (dextrose)	20.0 g
Potable water	1 liter

Table 4.26: Composition of ORS—citrate

Ingredient	*Quantity*
Sodium chloride	3.5 g
Trisodium citrate dehydrate	2.9 g
Potassium chloride	1.5 g
Glucose	20.0 g
Potable water	1 liter

Assessment of Dehydration (Table. 4.27)

Table. 4.27: How to assess your patient

		FOR DEHYDRATION			FOR OTHER PROBLEMS	
		A	B	C		
1. Ask about:	Diarrhea	Less than 4 liquid stools per day	4 to 10 liquid stools per day	More than 10 liquid stools per day	Longer than 14 days duration. Blood in the stool	
	Vomiting	None or a small amount	Some	Very frequent		
	Thirst	Normal	Greater than normal	Unable to drink		
	Urine	Normal	A small amount, dark	No urine for 6 hours		
2. Look at:	Condition	Well, alert	Unwell, sleepy or irritable	Very sleepy, unconscious floppy or having fits	Severe undernutrition	
	Tears	Present	Absent	Absent		
	Eyes	Normal	Sunken	Very dry and sunken		
	Mouth and Tongue	Wet	Dry	Very dry		
	Breathing	Normal	Faster than normal	Very fast and deep		
3. Feel:	Skin	A pinch goes back quickly	A pinch goes back slowly	A pinch goes back very slowly		
	Pulse	Normal	Faster than normal	Very fast, weak or you cannot feel it		
	Fontanelle (in infants)	Normal	Sunken	Very sunken		
4. Take temperature					Fever-38°C (or 101°F) or greater	
5. Weigh if possible		Loss of less than 25 grams for each kilogram of weight	Loss of 25-100 grams for each kilogram of weight	Loss of more than 100 grams for each kilogram of weight		
6. Decide		The patient has no signs of dehydration	If the patient has 2 or more of these signs, he has some dehydration	If the patient has 2 or more of these danger signs, he has severe dehydration	If your patient has:	Then:
					Blood in the stool and diarrhea for less than 14 days	Treat with an appropriate oral antibiotic for shigella dysentery If this child is also – Dehydrated – Severely undernourished or – Less than 1 year of age, reassess the child's progress in 24-48 hours. For the severely undernourished child, also refer for treatment of severe undernutrition
					Diarrhea for longer than 14 days with or without blood	Continue feeding and refer for treatment
					Severe undernutrition	Show the mother how to cool the child with a wet cloth and fanning.
					Fever - 38 °C (or 101°F) or greater	Look for and treat other causes (for example, pneumonia, malaria).

Treatment of Mild Dehydration (Table 4.28)

1. Amount of ORS solution to give in first four to six hours
2. If the mother can remain at the health center
   - Show her how much solution to give her child.
   - Show her how to give it—a spoonful every one to two minutes.
   - Check from time to time to see if she has problems.

Table. 4.28: Amount of ORS solution

Patient's age[1]	2 4 6 8 10 12 18 months → ← 2 3 4 6 8 15 years → adult						
Patient's weight in kilograms	Wt in kg	Under 5	5-7.9	8-10.9	11-15.9	16-29.9	30 or over
ORS solution (ml)	200-400	400-600	600-800	800-1000	1000-2000	2000-4000	

[1] Use the patient's age only when you do not know the weight.

Note: Encourage the mother to continue breastfeeding.

If the patient wants more ORS, give more.

If the eyelids become puffy, stop ORS and give other fluids. If diarrhea continues, use ORS again when the puffiness is gone.

If the child vomits, wait 10 minutes and then continue giving ORS, but more slowly.

Treatment of Severe Dehydration (Flow chart 4.3)

Flow chart 4.3: Treatment of severe dehydration

Follow the arrows. If the answer to the question is 'yes', go across. If it is 'no', go down.

Can the child drink? — Yes → 1. Start treatment with ORS solution, as in Treatment Plan B 2. Send the child for IV treatment

↓ No

Are you trained to use a nasogastric tube for rehydration? — Yes → 1. Start rehydration using the tube 2. If IV treatment is available nearby, send the child for immediate IV treatment

↓ No

URGENT: Send the child for IV treatment

Note: If the child is above two years of age and cholera is known to be currently occurring in your area, suspect cholera and give an appropriate oral antibiotic once the child is alert.

Intravenous Rehydration

The recommended dose of the IV fluid to be given is 100 ml/kg divided as follows (Table 4.29).

Table 4.29: Treatment plan for rehydration therapy

Age	*First give 30 ml/kg in*	*Then give 70 ml/kg in*
Infants (under 12 months)	1 hour	5 hours
Older	30 minutes	2½ hours

Maintenance Therapy (Table 4.30)

Table 4.30: Maintenance therapy

Amount of diarrhea	*Amount of oral fluid*
Mild diarrhea (not more than one stool every 2 hours or longer or less than 5 ml stool per kg per hour)	100 ml/kg body weight per day until diarrhea stops
Severe diarrhea (more than one stool every 2 hours, or more than 5 ml of stool per kg per hour)	Replace stool losses volume for volume; if not measurable, give 10-15 ml/kg body weight per hour

For more than 25 years WHO and UNICEF have recommended a single formulation of glucose based Oral Rehydration Salts (ORS) to prevent or treat dehydration from diarrhea irrespective of the cause or age group affected. This product, which provides a solution containing 90 mEq/l of sodium with a total osmolarity of 311 mOsm/l, has proved effective and without apparent adverse effects in worldwide use. It has contributed substantially to the dramatic global reduction in mortality from diarrheal diseases during the period.

For the past 20 years, numerous studies have been undertaken to develop an " improved" ORS. The goal was a product that would be at least as safe and effective as standard ORS for preventing or treating dehydration from all types of diarrhea but which, in addition, would reduce stool output or have other important clinical benefits. One approach has consisted in reducing the osmolarity of ORS solution to avoid possible adverse effects of hypertonicity on net fluid absorption. This was done by reducing the solution super glucose and salt (NaCl) concentrations.

Oral rehydration therapy is now preventing about one million dehydration deaths (Table 4.31).

Table 4.31: Oral rehydration therapy

Reduced osmolarity ORS	*Grams/liter*	*Reduced osmolarity ORS*	*mmol/liter*
Sodium chloride	2.6	Sodium	75
Glucose anhydrous	13.5	Chloride	65
Potassium chloride	1.5	Glucose, anhydrous	75
Trisodium citrate, dehydrate	2.9	Potassium	20
		Citrate	10
		Total osmolarity	245

Adjuncts to Therapy

Antibiotics used in the treatment of cholera (Table 4.32)

Table 4.32: Antibiotics used in the treatment of cholera

Antibiotics (a)	*Children*	*Adults*
Doxycycline once	—	300 mg (b)
Tetracycline 4 times a day for 3 days	12.5 mg/kg	500 mg
Trimethroprim (TMP) sulfamethoxazole (SMX) twice a day for 3 days	TMP 5 mg/kg and SMX 25 mg/kg (c)	TMP 160 mg SMX 800 mg
Furazolidone 4 times a day for 3 days	1.25 mg/kg	100 mg (d)

a. Erythromycin and chloramphenicol may also be used when none of the other recommended antibiotics are available, or when Vibrio Cholerae 01 is resistant to the latter.
b. Doxycycline is the antibiotic of choice for adults (excepting pregnant women since a single dose suffices.
c. TMP-SMX is the antibiotic of choice for children. Tetracycline is equally effective, but is not available everywhere in pediatric form.
d. Furazolidone is the antibiotic of choice for pregnant women.

Disinfection

Both concurrent and terminal disinfections are important in respect of cholera. This can be done by the following measures:

a. Mix with cholera stools and vomit an equal quantity of 5 percent lysotol of 5 percent cresol or 30 percent bleaching powder. Allow to stand for 2 hours and bury the mixture.
b. If stools and vomit fall on the floor, the area around the patient should be covered with a thin layer of lime or bleaching powder.
c. A practical and cheap method is to immerse the pans and receptacles containing vomit and stools in boiling water.
d. Immerse the soiled clothes in boiling water or in 2 percent lysotol for some time.
e. Whitewash the walls and floors with lime or throw boiling water on them. Mud floors may be burnt with cowdung cakes.
f. Boil the utensils and burn cheap fomites.
g. Cots and linen may be disinfected by 10 percent formalin, 5 percent lysotol spray or exposure to sun. Steam disinfection may also be done.
h. Wash hands with soap and water. Dipping hands in 1 percent lysotol is also useful.
i. Well or tank water should be disinfected with bleaching powder so as to get 1.5 to 2.0 ppm of chlorine. This should be the first step when a report is received about occurrence of cholera. Potassium permanganate should not be relied upon.

Diarrheal Diseases Control Program

The National Cholera Control Program is now termed has diarrheal diseases control program

Investigation of an Epidemic

The occurrence of an epidemic always signals some significant shift in the existing balance between the agent, host and environment. It calls for a prompt and thorough investigation to prevent further spread. Emergencies caused by epidemics remain one of the most important role to play in the investigation of epidemics. The objectives of an epidemic investigation are:

a. To define the magnitude of the epidemic outbreak or involvement in terms of time, place and person.
b. To determine the particular conditions and factors responsible for occurrence of the epidemic
c. To identify the cause, source(s) of infection, and modes of transmission to determine measures necessary to control the epidemic
d. To make recommendations to prevent recurrence.

An epidemic investigation calls for inference as well as description. Frequently, epidemic investigations are called for after the peak of the epidemic has occurred. In such case, the investigation is mainly retrospective. No step by step approach applicable in all situations can be described like a " cook - book" . However, in investigating an epidemic, it is desired to have an orderly procedure or practical guidelines as outlined below which are applicable for almost any epidemic study.

Verification of Diagnosis

A clinical examination of a sample of cases may well suffice. Laboratory investigations wherever applicable, are most useful to confirm the diagnosis but the epidemiological investigations should not be delayed until the laboratory results are available.

Confirmation of the Existence of an Epidemic

This is done by comparing the disease frequencies during the same period of previous years. An epidemic is said to exist when the number of cases (observed frequency) in excess of the expected frequency for the population, based on past experience. An arbitrary limit of two standard errors from the endemic occurrence is used to define the epidemic threshold for common diseases such as influenza, often the existence of an epidemic is obvious needing no such comparison, as in the case of common—source epidemics of cholera, food poisoning and hepatitis A.

Defining the Population at Risk

Obtaining a map of the area: Before beginning the investigation, it is necessary to have a detailed and current map of the area. It should contain information concerning natural landmarks, roads and the location of all dwelling units along each road or in isolated areas. Within each section, the dwelling units (houses) may be designed by numbers.

Counting the population: The denominator may be related to the entire population or sub groups of a population. It may also be related to total events. Without an appropriate denominator of "population at risk" attack rates cannot be calculated.

Rapid Search for all Cases and their Characteristics

Medical survey: Concurrently a medial survey should be carried out in a defined area to identify all cases including those who have not sought medical care, and those possibly exposed to risk.

Epidemiological case sheet: The epidemiologist should be armed with an "epidemiological case sheet" for collecting data from cases and from persons apparently exposed but unaffected. The epidemiological case sheet or "case interview form" should be carefully designed (based on the findings of a rapid preliminary inquiry) to collect relevant information. This includes: name, age, sex, occupation social class, travel, history of previous exposure, time of onset of disease, signs and symptoms of illness, personal contacts at home, work, school and other places, special events such as parties attended, foods eaten and exposure to common vehicles such as water, food and milk; visits out of the community, history of receiving injections or blood products, attendance at large gathering, etc. The information collected should be relevant to the disease under study. For example, if the disease is food-borne, detailed food histories are necessary. A case review form will ensure completeness and consistency of data collection. If the outbreak is large, it may not be possible to interview all the cases (e.g. influenza). In such cases, a random sample should be examined and data collected.

Searching for more cases: The patient may be asked if he knew of other cases in the home, family, neighborhood, school, work place having an onset within the incubation of the index case. Cases admitted to the local hospitals should also be taken into consideration. This may reveal not only additional cases but also person-to-person spread. The search for new cases (secondary cases) should be carried out everyday, till the area is declared free of epidemic. This period is usually taken as twice the incubation period of the disease since the occurrence of last case.

Evaluation of Ecological Factors

An investigation of the circumstances involved should be carried out to undertake appropriate measures to prevent further transmission of the disease. Ecological factors which have made the epidemic possible should be investigated such as sanitary status of eating establishments, water and milk supply; breakdown in the water supply system; movements of the human population, atmospheric changes such as temperature humidity and air pollution, population dynamics of insects and animal reservoirs. The outbreak can be studied in a case control fashion. One of the primary concerns of the epidemiologist is to relate the disease to environmental factors to know the source(s) of infection, reservoirs and modes of transmission.

Further Investigation of Population at Risk

A study of the population at risk or a sample of it may be needed to obtain additional information. This may involve medical examination, screening tests, examination of suspected food, faces, blood samples, biochemical studies, assessment of immunity status, etc. The approach may be retrospective or prospective. For example, serological study may reveal clinically inapparent cases and throw light on the pathogenesis of the condition. Healthy individuals (those who are not ill) from the same universe may be studied in a case control fashion. This will permit classification of all members as to:

a. Exposure to specific potential vehicles
b. Whether ill or not.

Data Analysis

The data collected should be analyzed on ongoing basis, using the classical epidemiological parameters time, place and person. If the disease agent is known, the characteristics of time, place and person may be rearranged into the Agent-Host-Environment model.

Time: Prepare a chronological distribution of dates of onset and construct an "epidemic curve", Look for time clustering of cases. An epidemic curve may suggest: (a) a time relationship with exposure to a suspected source, (b) whether it is common-source or propagated epidemic, and (c) whether it is a seasonal or cyclic pattern suggestive of a particular infection.

Place: Prepare a "spot map" (geographic distribution) of cases, and if possible their relation to possible, sources of infection, e.g. water supply, air pollution, foods eaten, occupation, etc. Clustering of cases may indicate a common source of infection. Analysis of geographic distribution may provide evidence of the source of disease and its mode of spread.

Person: Analyze the data by age, sex, occupation and other possible risk factors. Determine the attack rates/case fatality rates, for those exposed and those not exposed and according to host factors. For example, in most food borne outbreaks, food-specific attack rates must be calculated for each food eaten to determine the source of infection.

The purpose of data analysis is to identify common event or experience, and to delineate the group involved in the common experience.

Formulation of Hypotheses

On the basis of time, place and person distribution or the Agent-Host-Environment model, formulate hypotheses to explain the epidemic in terms of:

a. Possible source
b. Causative agent
c. Possible modes of spread, and
d. The environmental factors which enabled it to occur.

These hypotheses should be placed in order of relative likelihood. Formulation of a tentative hypotheses should guide further investigation.

Testing of Hypotheses

All reasonable hypotheses need to be considered and weighed by comparing the attack rates in various groups for those exposed and those not exposed to each suspected factors. This will enable the epidemiologist to ascertain which hypotheses is consistent with all the known facts. When divergent theories are presented, it is not easy to distinguish immediately between those which are sound and those which are merly plausible. Therefore, it is instructive to turn back to arguments which have been tested by the subsequent course of events.

Writing the Report

The report should be complete and convincing with all the information of the epidemic in prescribed format.

SCABIES

It is a contagious disease more common in low socioeconomic group, who have poor personal hygiene, more so in children.

Epidemiology

Agent

Sarcoptes scabiei

Source of infection: Infected patients and their clothes and linen.

Mode of Transmission

1. Direct contact with patients
2. Fomites.

Period of communicability: Till such time as the infection persists in untreated cases, usually four to six weeks. Patient becomes noninfective within three days of effective treatment.

Incubation period: Usually seven days.

Secondary attack rate: Around 80 percent in children and around 30 percent in adult contacts.

Host

1. *Age:* Maximum incidence in school going children and occurs at all ages.
2. *Sex:* Equal in both sexes.
3. Poor personal hygiene.

Environmental and Social Factors

1. Maximum incidence in winter season
2. Over crowding
3. Low socioeconomic living style
4. Limited availability of water for washing.

Clinical Features

1. Severe itching, which is worse at night.
2. Common with other family members.
3. Burrow is the greyish, serpentine, dotted line on the skin which represents the tunnel made by the female mite.
4. Sites of Burrows are:
   a. Interdigital folds
   b. Flexor aspects of wrists
   c. Anterior axillary folds
   d. Umibilicus
   e. Lower abdomen
   f. Genitalia
   g. Buttocks and thighs.

Complications

1. Secondary infections
2. Urticaria and eczema
3. Glomerulonephritis.

Variants

1. Scabies in clean and healthy person.
2. Scabies incognito: It occurs in a patient taking steroids.
3. Norwegian scabies: It occurs in immunocompromised persons.
4. Facial scabies in infants.
   a. Secondary infections should be treated.
   b. All the drugs used locally should be applied below the neck on three consecutive days.

Control of Scabies

1. Benzyl Benzoate
   a. First application with 25% BB Lotion
   b. Second application 12 hours after 1st application
   c. Bath given 12 hours after 2nd application.
2. HCH 0.5 to 1.0 percent (Lindane)—should be rubbed on affected skin at an interval of two to three days.
3. Tetmosal 5 percent—3 daily applications.
4. Sulphur ointment—2.5 to 10 percent—daily for four days.

SEXUALLY TRANSMITTED DISEASES

The sexually transmitted diseases are a group of communicable diseases that are transmitted predominantly by sexual contact and caused by wide range of bacterial, viral, protozoal and fungal agents and ectoparasites.

What are Sexually Transmitted Diseases?

- Sexually transmitted diseases, commonly called STDs, are diseases that are predominantly spread by sexual contact.
- One can get sexually transmitted disease from sexual activity that involves the mouth, anus, vagina, or penis.
- There are at least 25 different types of common STDs. Most of these are curable.
- Some of the viral STDs, which cannot be cured, are preventable. for example hepatitis B can be prevented by vaccination.

Why is STD Control an Important Component of HIV/AIDS Prevention?

- STDs increase the risk of acquiring HIV or transmitting HIV
- Treatment of STD reduces the risk of transmission of HIV
- Prevention of STD will prevent the sexual transmission of HIV, which is the main route of HIV transmission
- STDs present earlier than HIV/AIDS. Hence, it offers an opportunity to counsel the patient for behavior change and condom use

- In a person with HIV/AIDS, repeated STD increases the HIV viral load and therefore shortens the life span of HIV
- STDs do not become AIDS.

What are the Symptoms of STDs?
At Least Half of STDs in Women do not produce any Symptoms

Some of the common symptoms of STD are:

- *Ulcers,* sores or, warts near the penis or vagina. In a person who practices oral or anal sex, these ulcers or blisters may be present around the mouth or anus.
- *Discharge* from the urethra (males) or vagina or more specifically cervical discharge in women. This group of individuals may also complain of pain or burning sensation while passing urine.
- *Swellings* in the groin , swelling of the scrotum in males.
- *Chronic lower abdominal pain* in women, may be a symptom of STD.

How can One Protect Oneself from STDs?

Here are some basic steps that one can take to protect oneself from STDs:

- Abstinence or not having sex or sexual relations: This is the only sure way to prevent STDs. However, this is not practical for a lifetime. Abstinence could be recommended pre-maritally. Delaying sexual debut can reduce the risk of STD/HIV transmission.
- Practice monogamy: This means have sex with only one person who is also mutually faithful.
- Use a latex condom every time one has sex (If one uses a lubricant, make sure it is water-based).
- Limit the number of sexual partners. The more partners one has, the more likely such a person is to get an STD.
- Choose sex partners with care. Don't have sex with persons who have multiple sexual partners or have an STD.
- Get checked for STDs.
- Don't use alcohol or drugs, before having sex. One may be less likely to use a condom if one is drunk or high.
- Know the signs and symptoms of STDs. Look for them in both the sex partners.

How can Reinfection of STDs be prevented?

Reinfection is very common, especially among women. Men and women can prevent reinfection by:

- Getting prompt, correct and complete treatment if they do have an STD. Any genital symptoms such as discharge or burning during urination or an unusual sore or swelling should be a signal to stop having sex and to consult a doctor immediately. Even if there are no symptoms

but one thinks that he/she is infected, it is recommended to avoid sexual contact and to consult a health care provider.
- Getting the sexual partner also treated concurrently. If one is told that he/she has STD and receives treatment, such person should notify all of his/her recent sex partners, so that they can see a doctor and be treated.
- Avoiding sex during treatment for a STD or use condoms during this time.
- Using condoms *correctly, continuously (from the beginning of sex to the end) and consistently (every time)* one has sex. The use of latex or ployurethane condoms during vaginal intercourse can prevent the transmission of STDs. However, condoms do not provide complete protection from all STDs. Sores and lesions of STDs on infected men and women may be present in areas not covered by the condom, resulting in transmission of infection to another person.
- Reducing the number of sex partners, reducing the frequency of change of partner, practicing sexual abstinence, or limiting sexual contact to one uninfected partner, are other options.

What are the Approaches to STD Management?

Etiological Diagnosis

An attempt is made to identify the specific cause based on laboratory investigations . Note that VDRL test is a test that can only tell whether a person has been infected with syphilis or not. It is not a test that detects all VDs or STDs.

Clinical Diagnosis

Diagnosis is made on the basis of clinical symptoms. It is possible to diagnose many STD and on the basis of clinical presentation. But misdiagnosis can lead to failure of treatments and continued transmission. Hence, syndromic approach is the most useful and effective approach.

What is the Syndrome Approach?

It is a scientific method of treating STDs in health fecilities that lack laboratory equipments or skills to make an etiological diagnosis.

A syndrome is a combination of the symptoms complained by patients and signs found on examination. Even though different organisms cause STDs these organisms give rise to only a limited number of syndromes.

Syndromic management is based on the identification of a consistent group of symptoms and easily recognizable signs.

The provision of treatment will deal with the majority of organisms responsible for producing the syndrome.

The Steps Involved in Adopting a Syndromic Approach

- Classify the main causative agents by clinical syndromic they produce.
- Choose the appropriate treatment flow-chart for each syndrome.
- Choose the appropriate treatment flow-chart if laboratory investigations are available.
- Treat the patients for all the important causes of the syndrome as per directions on the respective flow-chart, after examination of the patient.
- Ensure that the partners are treated, patients are educated, and that the use of condoms promoted.

Syndromic Case Management necessitates Clinical Examination of the Patient

It is not symptomatic treatment! identifying the syndromes in STD (Table 4.33).

Table 4.33: The syndromes in STD are grouped

	Common clinical signs	*Most common causes*	*Etiology*
Genital ulcer in males or females	Genital ulcer on penis or scrotum in men, on labia, vagina or cervix in women	Syphilis Chanchroid Genital Herpes Lymphogranuloma venereum, Donovanosis	*Treponema pallidum* *Hemophilus ducreyi* *Herpes simplex* virus, *Chlamydia trachomatis* (L1-L3) *Calynomato-bacterium, granulomatis*
Urethral discharge, dysuria in males	Urethral discharge on milking urethra	Gonorrhoea Non-gonococcal urethritis	*N. gonorrhoea* *C. trachomatis* or ureplasma urealyticum
Vaginal discharge	Abnormal vaginal and/or cervical discharge Vaginal inflammation cervical friability cervical motion tenderness	Cervicitis: Gonorrhoea Chlamydial infection Vaginitis: Trichomoniasis Bacterial-vaginosis Candidiasis	*N. gonorrhoea* *C. trachomatis* *Trichomonas vaginalis* *Gardenella vaginalis,* anaerobes *Candida albicans*
Lower abdominal pain in women, dyspare-unia, irregular bleeding	Adnexal + cervical motion tenderness Vaginal or cervical discharge (sometimes) fever	Gonorrhoea Chlamydial infection Anaerobes	*N. gonorrhoea* *C. trachomatis* Anaerobes
Inguinal swelling or bubo in males or females	Inguinal lymphadenopathy with or without ulceration	Lymphogranuloma-venereum	*C. trachomatis* (L1-L3)
Scrotal swelling or pain in males	Red + edematous scrotum Urethral signs	Gonorrhoea Non-gonococcal Urethritis	*N. gonorrhoea* *C. trachomatis* or Ureplasma Urealyticum

Syndromic Case Management

The aim of syndromic case management is to identify one of these six syndromes and manage it accordingly. It includes only those syndromes that are caused by organisms, which both respond to treatment and lead to severe consequences if left untreated. Some STD syndromes such as genital warts are not included in this program, as the presence of these lesions contributing to the transmission of HIV has not been adequately documented.

Roles and Responsibilities of the Doctors while giving Quality Care for Patients with STD

Compliance: Ensure that the patient takes full course of treatment as prescribed. This means that you need to spend some time communicating with him/her the importance of completing the treatment.

Contact treatment: Treat the sexual partner (s) for the same STD condition and initiate the treatment of the partner at the same time as the patient. Partner treatment is necessary even if the partner does not have symptoms.

Condom promotion: Advice, prescribe, distribute or demonstrate how condoms must be used correctly. Insist on use of condoms every time there is sexual contact.

Counseling counsel: The patient or refer him/her for counseling. Counseling includes risk reduction counseling and pre-test counseling for HIV/AIDS.

Continued support: Follow-up the patient to ensure that there is total cure of the condition, not only disappearance of syndromes. During follow-up once more emphasize on safer behaviors. Refer the patient to a STD specialist if there is no improvement after treatment or developing of complications such as super- added infection or sequel of the condition.

Collection of essential data: Maintenance of basic records for STD patients will not only help to document follow-up but will also be useful to track social, demographic and behavioral characteristics of patients with STD.

Advantages of the Syndromic Case Management

- The treatment for each syndrome is immediate and is given at the first line health facility.
- There is wider access to treatment catering to a large needy population.
- There are ample opportunities for preventive measures and promotion of condom use.

Syndromic Case Management

- Scientific
- Simple
- Free from errors in clinical judgment

- Effective against mixed infections
- Cost-effective in the long run as it does not require laboratory tests.

Treatment for the Most Common STD Associated Syndromes

Treatment of Urethral Discharge

Ciprofloxacin 500 mg as a single oral dose

- Alternatively, the patient may be treated with:
- **Norfloxacin** 800 mg single oral dose, or
- **Cefixime** 400 mg single oral dose, or
- **Ceftriaxone** 250 mg single IM dose, or
- **Spectinomycin** 2 g single IM dose.

Plus

Give **doxycycline** 100 mg orally twice daily for 7 to 14 days for (chlamydial urethritis). Alternatively, the following drugs may be used:

- **Tetracycline** 500 mg orally 4 times a day for 7 days, or
- **Erythromycin** 500 mg orally 4 times a day for 7 days.

Genital Ulcers

Treatment for syphilis

- Give **Benzathine pencillin** 2.4 million units intramuscularly
- Alternatively, if the person is allergic to penicillin, use;
- **Tetracycline** 500 mg orally 4 times a day for 15 days , or
- **Doxycycline** 100 mg orally twice daily for 15 days, or
- **Erythromycin** 500 mg orally 4 times a day for 15 days.

Plus

Treatment for chancroid

- Give **Erythromycin** 500 mg orally 4 times, daily for 7 days
- Alternatively, the following may be used:
- **Ciprofloxacin** 500 mg single oral dose, or
- **Ceftriaxone** 250 mg single IM dose, or
- **Spectinomycin** 2 g single IM dose, or
- **Trimethoprim** 160 mg/**Sulfamethoxazole** 800 mg (2 tablets) orally twice daily for 7 days.

Treatment for herpes
Acyclovir 200 mg orally 5 times daily for 7 days.

Treatment of Vaginal Discharge

- **Metronidazole** 2 g as a single oral dose, or
- **Metronidazole** 400 mg given orally twice daily for 7 days.
  Note: Do not use Metronidazole in the first trimester of pregnancy.

Plus

- **Nystatin** (100,000 units one pessary), inserted intravaginally daily at night for 14 days (for vaginal candidiasis), or
- **Miconazole** or **Clotrimazole** 200 mg may be inserted into the vagina daily for 3 days, or
- **Clotrimazole** 500 mg is inserted into the vagina once only.
- **Ciprofloxacin** 500 mg in a sinlge oral dose for gonococcal infection, or
- **Norfloxacin** 800 mg single oral dose, or
- **Cefixime** 400 mg single oral dose, or
- **Ceftriaxone** 250 mg single IM dose, or
- **Spectinomycin** 2 g single IM dose.
- **Doxycycline** 100 mg orally twice daily for 7 to 14 days for chlamydial infection, or
- **Tetracycline** 500 mg orally four times a day for 7 days, or
- **Erythromycin** 500 mg orally four times a day for 7 days.
  Note: **Ciprofloxacin, Doxycycline** and **Tetracycline** should not be used in pregnancy.

Treatment of Lower Abdominal Pain in the Female

Treatment for gonorrhea

- **Ciprofloxacin** 500 mg single oral dose, or
- **Norfloxacin** 800 mg single oral dose, or
- **Cefixime** 400 mg single oral dose, or
- **Ceftriaxone** 250 mg single IM dose, or
- **Spectinomycin** 2 g single IM dose.

Plus

Treatment for chlamydial infection:

- **Doxycycline** 100 mg oral twice daily for 14 days, or
- **Tetracycline** 500 mg orally four times daily for 14 days ,or
- **Erythromycin** 500 mg orally four times daily for 10 days.

Treatment for anaerobic bacterial infection:

- **Metronidazole** 400 mg given orally twice daily for 14 days.
  Note: **Ciprofloxacin, Doxycycline** and *Tetracycline*, should not be used during pregnancy and lactation, **Metronidazole** should not be used in the first trimester of pregnancy.

National STD Control Program

It was started in India as a pilot project in 1949. It has following main components:

a. Teaching and training
b. Research
c. Community education
d. Epidemiology

The control of STD now forms part of the National AIDS Control Program.

BIBLIOGRAPHY

1. A Guide to Leprosy Control WHO, 1980.
2. Annual Report: Ministry of Health and Family Welfare, Govt of India, 1998-99.
3. Das BC, Malini Shobha, Text of Community Medicine with Recent Advances, 1st edn, 2003.
4. Govt of India, Leprosy—National Leprosy Eradication Programme in India 1989. Guidelines for Multidrug Treatment in Endemic Districts, Leprosy, Division, DGHS, New Delhi, 1989.
5. Govt of India. TB India: RNTCP Status Report. Central TB Division, DGHS, Ministry of Health and Family Welfare, New Delhi, 2001.
6. Govt of India—SIDA, WHO. Review Committee Report, 1992.
7. Govt. of India. Annual Report 2001-2002. Ministry of Health and Family Welfare. Govt of India.
8. Gupta MC and Mahajan BK Textbook of Preventive and Social Medicine, 3rd edn, 2003.
9. Job CK, et al Leprosy: Diagnosis and Management, Hind Kusht Nivaran Sangh, New Delhi, 1975.
10. Kishore J , National Health Programmes of India, 4th edn, 2002.
11. WHO. Revising challenges towards the elimination of leprosy (Leprosy Elimination Project. Ind Join Lepr 2000; 72(1 :2000).
12. WHO: Techn Rep Ser 675, 1982.
13. WHO: Techn Rep Ser 542, 1974.
14. WHO: Techn Rep Ser 702, 1984.
15. WHO: Techn Rep Ser 768, 1988.
16. Worndorff van Diepen. Clafazimine resistant leprosy. A case report. Int Join. Lepre 1982; 50:139-42.

Chapter 5 Noncommunicable Diseases

CHAPTER OUTLINE

- CORONARY HEART DISEASE
- OBESITY
- MENTAL HEALTH
- CANCER
- NATIONAL CANCER CONTROL PROGRAM (NCCP)
- HYPERTENSION
- RHEUMATIC HEART DISEASE
- DIABETES MELLITUS
- CAUSES OF CANCER

Chronic noncommunicable diseases are assuming increasing importance among the adult population in both developed and developing countries. The impact of chronic disease on the lives of people is serious when measured in terms of loss of life, disablement, family hardship and poverty and economic loss to the country. Some cases of non-communicable diseases are kept for case presentation. They are discussed briefly in the following pages.

CORONARY HEART DISEASE

Coronary heart disease (CHD) is becoming a major health problem in India. The WHO has drawn attention to the fact that CHD is our modern "epidemic". However, there is no national program on prevention in the offing. As per current estimates at least 50 million people are suffering from CHD.

Prevalence rate (Age group 35-64 years).

10.9% in urban male
5.5% in rural male
10.2% in urban female
6.4% in rural female.

Definition

Coronary heart disease has been defined as "impairment of heart function due to inadequate blood flow to heart compared to its needs, caused by obstructive changes in the coronary circulation to the heart".

Manifestations

a. Angina pectoris of effort
b. Myocardial infarction

c. Irregularities of heart
d. Cardiac failure
e. Sudden death.

Measurement the Burden of Disease

It can be done by:

a. Proportional mortality ratio—in men 30 percent of deaths and women in 25 percent of deaths in western countries
b. Loss of life expectancy
c. CHD incidence rate
d. Age specific death rate
e. Prevalence rate
f. Case fatality rate
g. Measurement of risk factor levels
h. Medical care.

Epidemiology

No single agent can be pinpointed as the causative agent for coronary heart disease. The disease is caused by interaction of a variety of factors web of causation of myocardial infarction.

Risk Factors for CHD

Nonmodifiable Risk Factors

- Age—40 plus
- Sex—predominantly male
- Post—menopausal female
- Personalities—type A
- Family history of CHD
- Genetic factors are probably the most important determinants of a given individuals TC and LDL levels.

Modifiable Risk Factors

- Cigarette smoking—it is responsible for 25 percent of CHD death under 65 years in men.
- Hypertension—accelerates the atherosclerotic process
- Serum cholesterol—>220 mg/dl is risk for CHD
- Diabetes—the risk of CHD is two-three times higher in diabetes.
- Obesity and sedentary habits—physical exercise increases the HDL levels
- Stress.

Complications of Myocardial Infarction

Early

a. Arrhythmias
b. Cardiac failure
c. Embolization
d. Cardiac rupture
   i. Ventricular septal defect
   ii. Rupture through free wall causing cardiac tamponade.
e. Papillary muscle dysfunction
f. Cardiogenic shock.

Late

a. Ventricular aneurysm.
b. Dressler's syndrome
c. Shoulder hand syndrome.

Medical Treatment

For Angina

a. Control of risk factors like hypertension, diabetes, etc.
b. Bedrest and sedatives
c. Nitrates—isosorbide dinitrate-nitroglycerine ointment two percent
d. β-blockers
e. Calcium channel blockers.

For Unstable Angina and Myocardial Infarction

Relief of pain

i. Complete bedrest
ii. Nitrates sublingually and intravenously
iii. Analgesics
iv. Heparin
v. Thromobolytic therapy.

Supportive treatment

i. Prevention of deep vein thrombosis
ii. Proper laxatives
iii. Liquid diet initially during attack
iv. Sedative to allay the anxiety
v. Treatment of complications like cardiac failure, arrhythmia, etc.

Percutaneous Transluminal Coronary Angioplasty (PTCA)

Surgical treatment
Coronary arterial bypass grafting (CABG).

Prevention and Control

WHO expert committee recommended the following strategies:

a. Population strategy
   i. Prevention in whole populations
   ii. Primordial prevention in whole populations.
b. High-risk strategy
c. Secondary prevention.

Population Strategy

Population strategy is based on mass approach focussing mainly on the control of underlying causes (risk factors) in whole populations not merely in individuals, small changes in risk factor levels in total population can achieve the biggest reduction in mortality.

Specific Intervention

1. Dietary changes
   a. Reduction of fat intake by 20 to 30 percent of total energy intake
   b. Consumption of saturated fats must be limited to less than 10 percent of total energy intake
   c. A reduction of dietary cholesterol to below 100 mg per 1000 Kcal per day
   d. An increase in complex carbohydrate consumption.
2. Regular exercises and yoga practices
3. Hypertension and diabetes kept under control
4. Avoid undue stress
5. Avoid smoking and alcohol consumption.

Legislation

1. Banning the sale of cigarettes and alcohol
2. Making compulsory the printing of the statutory warning that smoking and drinking alcohol is injurious to health
3. Banning the advertisement of cigarettes and alcohol.

Secondary Prevention

1. Early diagnosis
   a. High-risk screening
   b. Routine periodic investigation
2. Prompt and effective treatment.

Tertiary Prevention

1. Disability limitation
   a. Balloon angioplasty and cardiac bypass surgery
   b. Laser and ultrasonic destruction of clots
2. Rehabilitation
   a. Physical rehabilitation
   b. Occupational rehabilitation
   c. Psychological rehabilitation.

HYPERTENSION

Hypertension is an iceberg disease, it has worldwide prevalence. Rules of halves or 50 percent of the patients were aware of their state.

- Fifty percent of those aware were taking treatment
- Fifty percent of those being treated, were treated properly.

Prevalence

59.9 per 1000 — In urban male population
69.9 per 1000 — In urban female population
35.5 per 1000 — In rural male population
35.9 per 1000 — In rural female population

The sixth report of the Joint National Committee (JNC) on detection, evaluation and treatment of high blood pressure, provides new guidelines for hypertension control (Table 5.1).

Table 5.1: Classification of blood pressure for adults aged 18 years and older *

Category	Blood pressure, mm Hg		
	Systolic		diastolic
Optimal +	< 120	and	< 80
Normal	< 130	and	< 85
High-normal	130-139	or	85-89
Hypertension 2+			
Stage 1	140-159	or	90-99
Stage 2	160-179	or	100-109
Stage 3	≥ 180	or	≥ 110

* When systolic and diastolic blood pressures fall into different category, should be selected to classify the individual's blood pressure status.

\+ Unusually low readings should be evaluated for clinical significance.

2+ Based on the average of two or more readings taken at each of two or more visits after an initial screening

Risk Stratification

The risk of cardiovascular disease in patients with hypertension is determined not by the level of blood pressure but also by the presence of target organ damage (TOD), clinical cardiovascular disease (CCD) or other risk factors such as smoking, dyslipidemia and diabetes. These factors independently modify the risk of subsequent cardiovascular disease. Based on the BP reading, the patient's risk factors and presence or absence of TOD/CCD, hypertensive patients have been stratified into risk groups. The treatment to be initiated depends on the risk group of the patient (Table 5.2).

Pharmacologic Treatment Initiation

The decision to initiate pharmacologic treatment requires consideration of several factors: the degree of BP elevation, the presence of target organ damage (TOD) and the presence of clinical cardiovascular disease (CCD) or other risk factors (Flow chart 5.1 and Table 5.3).

Table 5.2: Risk stratification and treatment *

Blood pressure stages (mm Hg)	*Risk group A (No risk factors; no TOD/CCD)* [2+]	*Risk group B (At least 1 risk factor, not including diabetes, no TOD/CCD)*	*Risk group C (TOD/CCD and/or diabetes with or without other risk factors)*
High – normal (130-139/85-89)	Lifestyle modification	Lifestyle modification	Drug therapy ξ
Stage 1 (140-159/90-99)	Lifestyle modification (up to 12 months)	Lifestyle modification (up to 12 months)	Drug therapy
Stage 2 and 3 (≥ 160/ ≥100)	Drug therapy	Drug therapy	Drug therapy

* Major risk factors include smoking, dyslipidemia, diabetes mellitus, age > 60 years, sex (men and postmenopausal women), family history of cardiovascular disease; and includes heart diseases (left ventricular hypertrophy, angina or prior myocardial infarction, prior coronary revascularization, heart failure), stroke or transient ischemic attack, nephropathy, peripheral arterial disease, retinopathy.

2+ For patients with multiple risk factors, clinicians should consider initial drug therapy plus lifestyle modifications.

ξ For those with heart failure, renal insufficiency or diabetes.

Table 5.3: Concomitant condition and antihypertensive drug of choice

Concomitant condition	*Antihypertensive drug of choice*
Angina	β-blockers, long-acting calcium antagonists
Postmyocardial infarction	β-blockers, with intrinsic sympathomimetic activity, ACE inhibitors, verapamil/diltiazem ACE inhibitors in conjunction with digoxin/diuretics, hydralazine plus isosorbide dinitrate, carvedilol, losartan
Renal disease	ACE inhibitors ACE inhibitor plus diuretic, loop diuretic, loop diuretics plus long acting thiazide diuretic
Dyslipidemia	α-blockers
Diabetes mellitus	ACE inhibitors, α-blockers, calcium channel blockers, diuretics (in low doses)
Elderly	Thiazide diuretics β-blockers plus thiazide diuretics, long-acting calcium channel blockers

Flow chart 5.1: Algorithm for the treatment of hypertension

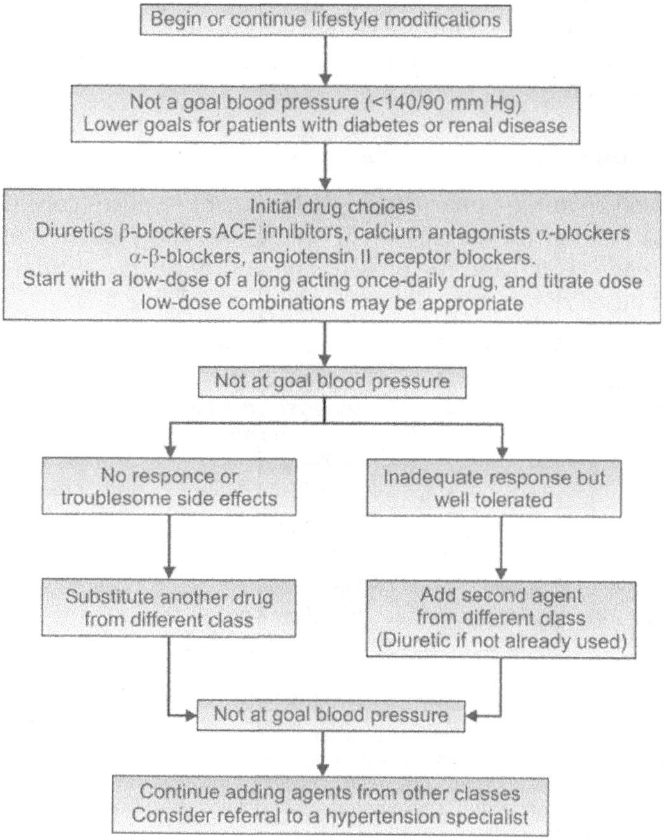

OBESITY

It is defined in terms of a body mass index (BMI) of 30 or more in male and 28.6 or more in female indicate obesity.

Types

- Hypertrophic obesity—increase in number of fat cell
- Hyperplastic obesity—increase in size of fat cell.

Prevalence

In adult—twenty to forty percent.
In children—ten to twenty percent.

Epidemiological Factors

Age

It can occur at any age and generally increase with age. Infants with excessive weight gain have an increased incidence of obesity in later life.

Sex
Men were found to gain more weight between the age of 29 and 35 years. Women gain most between 45 and 49 years of age.

Socio-economic factors
Directly proportional to the per capita income.

Family tendency
1. Due to rich diet pattern
2. Overeating associated with pregnancy and lactation in well to do families.

Individual eating habits
1. Preference for energy rich diets in marked excess to the daily requirement
2. Frequent eating
3. Alcohol consumption
4. Psychological overeating as a result of anxiety neurosis, depression, etc.
5. Junk food.

Physical exercise (enquire about)
1. Nature of job
2. Time devoted to sports or other physical activity
3. Recent illness particularly those which lead to long-term restriction of physical activity, e.g. fractures.

Endocrine Disorders

1. Cushing's syndrome
2. Cretinism and hypothyroidism
3. Pituitary disorders
4. Maturity onset diabetes mellitus
5. Insulinoma
6. Hypothalamic disorders.

Drug Intake

1. Corticosteroids
2. Estrogens.

Assessment of Obesity

Some indicators that are commonly used to measure obesity.

Broca's Index

The individual height in cms minus 100 = maximum permissible weight of the individual in kg.

For example: For a person with a height of 182 cm. 182-100 = 82 kg is the max permissible weight. Anything in excess of 82 kg will make the person to be considered as obese.

Body Mass Index

$$BMI = \frac{\text{Weight (in kg)}}{[\text{Height (in meters)}]^2}$$

Males

1. Twenty to twenty-five desirable range
2. Twenty-two desirable ideal
3. Greater than 30 obese

Females

1. Nineteen to twenty four desirable range
2. Twenty one desirable ideal
3. Greater then 28.6 obese

Corpulence Index

$$CI = \frac{\text{Actual weight (in kg)}}{\text{Desirable weight (in kg)}}$$

In obesity this should exceed 1.2.

Ponderal Index

$$PI = \frac{\text{Ht (in cms)}}{\sqrt[3]{\text{Wt (in kg)}}}$$

Lorentz's Formula

$$\text{LF (Males)} = [\text{Ht (in cms)} - 100] - \frac{[\text{Ht in(cms)} - 150]}{4}$$

$$\text{LF (Females)} = [\text{Ht (in cms)} - 100] - \frac{[\text{Ht in(cms)} - 150]}{2}$$

Fat Fold Thickness (Skin Fold Thickness)

The fat fold thickness is measured using skin callipers at the following sites, mid triceps, biceps, subscapular and suprailiac region.

The sum total of the above measurements from all four sites should not be more than 40 mm for adult males and 50 mm for adult females.

Normograms showing the ideal for males and females at various ages are available.

Total Body Mass

The total body mass is also calculated by weight/volume studies using water displacement technique.

Clinical Features of Obesity

1. Weight gain
2. Buffalo hump
3. Moon face
4. Prone to develop
   a. Diabetes
   b. Hyperlipidemia
   c. Gallstones

Complications

1. Respiratory
   a. Pickwickian syndrome
2. Cardiovascular
   a. Hypertension
   b. Cor pulmonale
   c. Varicose veins
3. Gastrointestinal
   a. Hiatus hernia
   b. Fatty liver
   c. Gallstones
4. Musculoskeletal
   a. Osteoarthritis
   b. Sciatica
   c. Flat foot
5. Miscellaneous
   a. Hernia

Treatment

1. Treatment of the secondary causes, like hypothyroidism, Cushing's syndrome, etc.
2. Diet:
   a. Restrict the calorie intake.
   b. Excessive eating should be avoided particularly at night.
   c. Small and frequent meals should be preferred.
   d. High roughage diet (which will have less calories) is preferred.
3. Exercise: It selectively decreases the body fat, while preserving the lean body mass.
4. Behavior modification: It is advisable to treat abnormal patterns of eating behavior.
5. Drugs:
   a. Fenfluramine: 20 mg/day
   b. Diethylpropion: 25 mg thrice a day

   c. Biguanides
   d. Thyroid extract
   e. Amphetamine
6. Other methods:
   a. Body massage
   b. Steam-bath (sauna)
7. Surgery:
   a. Gastric pouch by gastroplasty.
   b. Jejunoileal shunt.
   c. Gastric balloon: Balloon is introduced through gastroscope and kept inflated, so that the patient gets a sense of satiety (feeling of fullness) after a small feed.
   d. Lipectomy: Removal of omental fat by laparotomy or liposuction.

Prevention and Control

Primordial Prevention

Avoidance of lifestyles leading to obesity and inculcation of habits for a healthy lifestyle:
1. Dietary control
2. Physical exercises.

Secondary Prevention

Identification of risk individuals:
1. Obese children
2. Those with familial tendencies and starting them on obesity management regimes at an early age.
3. Treatment as outlined above.

Tertiary Prevention

1. Physical rehabilitation, e.g. physiotherapy.
2. Occupational rehabilitation.

RHEUMATIC HEART DISEASE

Rheumatic fever and rheumatic heart disease cannot be separated from epidemiological point of view. The antecedent streptococcal pharyngitis causes rheumatic fever that may lead to rheumatic heart disease. Once heart disease is established, patient has to be treated surgically or by other interventions and the financial burden increases.

Prevalence

Two per thousand population.

Epidemiological Factors

Agent—group A *streptococcus*

Special emphasis is M type 5 which is frequently associated with rheumatic fever.

Recently coxsackie B-4 has been suggested as a causative factor and streptococcus acting as a conditioning agent.

Host and Environmental Factors

- Age— in 5 to 15 years
- Sex—both sexes equally
- Socioeconomic status—common in low socioeconomic status
- Environmental factors:
  - Overcrowding
  - Poor housing conditions
  - Poor health care facilities (Particularly school health facilities).

Clinical Features

1. Fever
2. Polyarthritis—in 90 percent cases in large joints
3. Carditis—in 60 to 70 percent cases
4. Nodules—small painless non-tender
5. Brain—abnormal jerky purposeless movement
6. Skin—various types of skin rashes.

Diagnosis

A WHO expert committee in 1988 has recommended use of revised Jones criteria (Table 5.4) for diagnosis of acute rheumatic fever.

The presence of two major or one major and two minor manifestation plus evidence of preceding streptococcal infection indicate high probability of rheumatic.

Table 5.4: Jones criteria (revised) for diagnosis of acute rheumatic fever

Major manifestations	*Minor manifestations*
Carditis	**Clinical**
Polyarthritis	Fever
Chorea	Arthralgia
Erythema marginatum	Previous history of RF or RHD
Subcutaneous nodules	**Laboratory**
	Abnormal ESR
	C-reactive protein
	Leukocytosis
	Prolonged P-R intervals

Prevention and Control

Primary Prevention

a. *Health promotion:* Health education regarding RF, RHD, to school children, teachers and parents.

b. *Specific protection (throat swab):* If culture facility is not available, it is justified to treat all sore throat with penicillin. For this purpose one injection of penicillin containing 300,000 units of crystalline penicillin, 300,000 units procaine penicillin and 600,000 units benzathine penicillin (available as one injection).

Secondary Prevention

1. *Early diagnosis*
   a. Surveillance of school children for RF and RHD
   b. Throat swab for detection of group A Streptococci.
2. *Prompt and effective treatment*
   a. Injection penidure 1.2 mega unit deep IM once in three weeks
   b. Salt and water restriction and diuretics
   c. Bed rest.

Tertiary Prevention

1. *Disability limitation:* Cardiac surgery
2. Rehabilitation, physical rehabilitation, occupational rehabilitation, psychological rehabilitation.

MENTAL HEALTH

Mental health disorder is defined as a clinically significant behavior or psychological syndrome or pattern that occurs in a person and that is associated with a significantly increased risk of suffering death, pain, disability or an important loss of freedom.

Prevalence

In India 18 to 20 per 1000.

Classification

1. Depressive disorders
2. Schizophrenia
3. Substance abuse disorders
4. Disorders of childhood and adolescence
5. Suicidal tendencies.

Etiology

1. Idiopathic
2. Organic condition
3. Sociopathological cause
4. Heredity.

Organic Conditions

Prenatal Causes

a. Chromosomal anomalies
   i. Down syndrome
   ii. Turner's syndrome
b. Inborn errors of metabolism
   i. Phenyl ketonuria
   ii. Galactosemia
   iii. Mucopolysaccharidoses
c. Cranial malformations
   i. Microcephaly
   ii. Hydrocephaly.

Perinatal Causes

a. Infections, e.g. TORCH
b. Physical causes
   i. Birth trauma
   ii. Radiation
c. Prematurity
d. Intoxications like bilirubin.

Postnatal Causes

a. Infections
   i. Meningitis
   ii. Encephalitis
b. Head injury
c. Malnutrition.

Social Pathological Causes

1. Worries
2. Anxieties
3. Stress
4. Broken home
5. Industrialization and urbanization.

Environmental Factors

1. Toxic substances
2. Psychotropic drugs
3. Radiation
4. Trauma.

Warning Signals of Poor Mental Health

1. Are you always worrying?
2. Are you unable to concentrate because of unrecognized reasons?
3. Are you continually unhappy without justified cause?
4. Do you lose your temper easily and often?
5. Are you troubled by regular insomnia?
6. Do you have wide fluctuations in your moods from depression to elevation, back to depression, which incapacitate you?
7. Do you continually dislike to be with people?
8. Are you upset if the routine of your life is disturbed?
9. Do your children consistently get on your nerves?
10. Are you "browned off" and constantly bitter?
11. Are you afraid without real cause?
12. Are you always right and the other person always wrong?
13. Do you have numerous aches and pains for which no doctor can find a physical cause?

Prevention and Control

Primary Prevention

Health promotion

a. Health education regarding causes and how to avoid some of them
b. Prospective genetic counseling
c. Marriage counseling
d. Specific prevention
e. Good quality of MCH care.

Secondary Prevention

Early detection

Screening programs in schools, universities, and industry.

Prompt treatment

By using antipsychotic drugs.

Tertiary Prevention

Disability limitation

Rehabilitation

a. Specialized institution to impart care and training for the mentally handicapped

b. Occupational therapy
c. Half-way homes and family service programs
d. Public education.

National Mental Health Program

The Government of India has launched the National Mental Health program in 1982, keeping in view the heavy burden of mental illness in the community, and the absolute inadequacy of mental health care infrastructure in the country to deal with it (a total of about 20764 beds available or 1 bed for 15400 population). Around 10 to 60 percent of the OPD patients have mental illness which is usually mild in nature. In the community the prevalence of mental illness range from 10 to 20 percent, whereas severe type of mental illness is around 1 to 2 percent of the population. The program envisages a primary health care approach in the rural areas supported by professional psychiatric supervision from the district level and referral services by the mental hospitals and mental health units of the general hospitals.

Aims

1. Prevention and treatment of mental and neurological disorders and their associated disabilities.
2. Use of mental health technology to improve general health services.
3. Application of mental health principles in total national development to improve quality of life.

Objectives

1. To ensure availability and accessibility of minimum mental health care for all in the foreseeable future, particularly to the most vulnerable and under-privileged sections of population.
2. To encourage application of mental participation in the mental health knowledge in general health care and in social development.
3. To promote community participation in the mental health services development and to stimulate efforts towards self-help in the community.

Strategies

1. *Diffusion of mental health skills to the periphery of the health services system:* Through the primary health centers which is the most extensive health care system reach up to the most remote rural and tribal areas the mental health can be provided. It requires the training of all level of primary health care workers.
2. *Appropriate appointment of tasks in the mental health care:* The tasks to be specified at all level of the health care delivery from village to District health center.

DIABETES MELLITUS

Diabetes is an "iceberg" disease. The prevalence of diabetes mellitus in adult is around 4 percent worldwide (1995), which will be 5.4 percent in 2025.

In India, 2.4 percent in rural, 4.0 to 11.6 percent in urban dwellers.

It is a one **Potential Diabetic** who has a risk of developing DM due to genetic reasons (e.g. having a first degree relative with DM).

Latent Diabetic

It is a one who has risk of developing DM due to stressful conditions like pregnancy, surgery, trauma, infections, etc. they may return to normal if stress is removed.

Black Zone

It is a state of affairs in a Type 2 DM patients in whom blood glucose levels are high but do not have symptoms, although the process of complications is going on.

The factors that allow the patients to slip into the black zone are:

- Lack of health services provided to diabetics
- Lack of knowledge in the patient
  (Or Defects in the health education program provided to diabetics)
- Negligence by the patient (i.e. not accepting the presence of disease and practicing a self-damage) behavior such as alcoholism.

Clinical Classification of Diabetes Mellitus as Adopted by WHO

1. Diabetes mellitus
   a. Insulin-dependent diabetes mellitus
      i. Juvenile diabetes mellitus
      ii. Adult diabetes mellitus
   b. Noninsulin dependent diabetes mellitus
   c. Malnutrition-related diabetes mellitus
2. Impaired glucose tolerance
3. Gestational diabetes mellitus.

Epidemiology

Agent

1. Pancreatic disorders—inflammatory, neoplastic, cystic fibrosis.
2. Defects in formation of insulin.
3. Decreased insulin sensitivity.
4. Autoimmunity.

Host

a. Age—any age
 NIDDM usually at middle age group
b. Sex—male-female ratio is about equal
c. Genetic factor
d. Genetic marker—HLA B8 and B15
e. Immune mechanisms
f. Obesity.

Environmental Factors

1. Sedentary lifestyle
2. Diet and alcoholism
3. Malnutrition
4. Viral infections (rubella, mumps, etc.)
5. Chemical agents
6. Stress.

Social Factors

a. Occupation
b. Marital status
c. Urbanization
d. Changes in lifestyle.

Clinical Features

1. Polyuria
2. Polydipsia
3. Polyphagia
4. Weight loss
5. Repeated infections—like skin infections, urinary infections and others
6. Fatigue.

Complications

1. Diabetic ketoacidosis
2. Hyperosmolar hyperglycemic nonketotic coma
3. Latic acidosis
4. Diabetic retinopathy
5. Diabetic neuropathy
6. Nephropathy
7. Dermopathy
8. Fungal infections.

Investigations

1. Urine sugar and ketone bodies.
2. Fasting and postprandial blood sugar.
3. Glucose tolerance test (GTT) (Table 5.5).
4. Glycosylated hemoglobin.

Prevention and Care

High-risk Screening

Screening of the whole population is not a rewarding exercise. However, screening of "High-risk" groups is appropriate.
These groups are:

- Individuals above 30 years of age
- Those with a strong family history of DM
- Obese individuals
- Sedentary workers with lack of exercise.

Other than high-risk group, the following group of persons should also be screened for diabetes as a routine.

- A patient with premature atherosclerosis
- A person complaining polyurea, polyphagia, polydipsia sudden loss of weight, repeated infections, nonhealing ulcer (purities vulvae in a lady).
- Patients undergoing surgery, including tooth extraction
- All expectant mothers attending antenatal clinic
- A pregnant mother gaining more than 3 kg body weight in any month
- A woman who has given birth to a baby weighing more than 3.5 kg at birth.

Primary Prevention

1. Population strategy
2. High-risk strategy—avoid alcohol, smoking, oral contraceptives.

Table 5.5: Diagnostic values for the oral glucose tolerance test (mg/dl)

	Whole blood		*Plasma*	
	Venous	Capillary	Venous	Capillary
Diabetes mellitus				
a. Fasting value	≥ 120	≥ 120	≥ 140	≥ 140
b. 2 hours after glucose load	≥ 180	≥ 200	≥ 200	≥ 200
Impaired glucose tolerance				
a. Fasting value	< 120	< 120	< 140	< 140
b. 2 hours after glucose load	120-180	140-200	140-200	160-200

Secondary Prevention

1. Maintain blood glucose level
2. Maintain ideal body weight.

Treatment

It is based on:
1. Diet alone—small balanced meals more frequently
2. Diet and oral antidiabetic drugs
3. Diet and insulin
4. Self-care—adherence to diet and drug regimens, examination of his own urine and blood glucose monitoring self-administration of insulin: maintenance of optimum weight, estimation of glycosylated hemoglobin at half yearly interval.

Tertiary Prevention

To prevent complication like:
1. Blindness
2. Kidney failure
3. Coronary thrombosis
4. Gangrene of the lower extremities.

National Diabetes Control Program

Government of India started National Diabetes Control Program on pilot basis during 7th five year plan in 1987 in some districts of Tamil Nadu, Jammu and Kashmir and Karnataka, but due to paucity of founds in subsequent years this program could not be expanded further in remaining years. However, a sum of 12 lakh during 1995-1996 was allocated for the program. In 1997 to 1998, an allocation of 1 crore was made.

Objectives

1. Prevention of diabetes through identification of high-risk subjects and early intervention in the form of health education.
2. Early diagnosis of diseases and appropriate treatment to reduce morbidity and mortality with reference to high-risk group.
3. Prevention of acute and chronic metabolic, cardiovascular, renal and ocular complications of the disease.
4. Provision of equal opportunity for physical attainment and scholastic achievement for the diabetic patient.
5. Rehabilitation of those partially or totally handicapped diabetic people.

CANCER

Cancer is a major cause of death in India.

Prevalence

Cancer in all forms are causing about 12 percent of deaths throughout the world.

In India, it is estimated there are approximately 2 to 2.5 million cases of cancer in India at any given point of time with around 7,00,000 new cases being detected each year nearly half of these dies each year (Fig. 5.1).

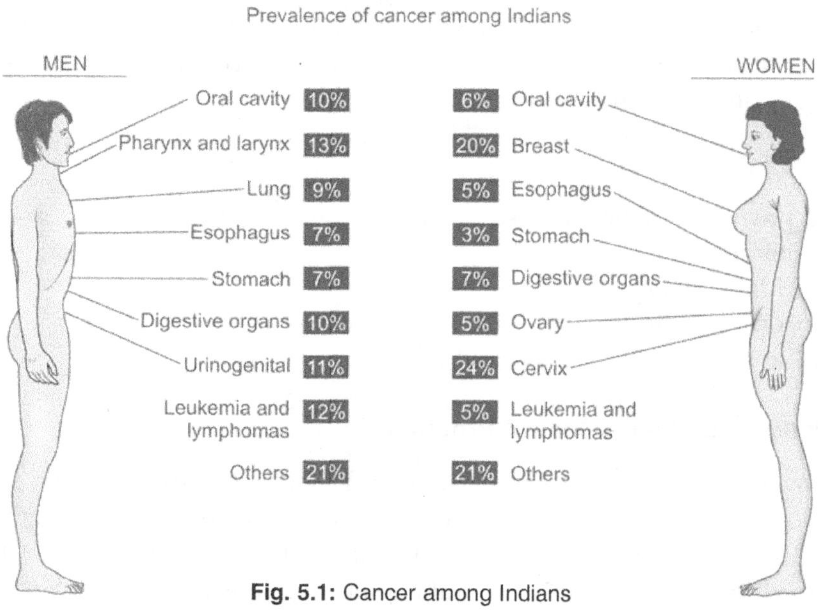

Fig. 5.1: Cancer among Indians

Cancer registration: It provides a base for assessing the magnitude of the problem and for planning the necessary services. There are two types of registers (Flow charts 5.2 and 5.3).

Sex Differences

Ranking order by site of eight selected cancer.

Flow Chart. 5.2: Cancer registration

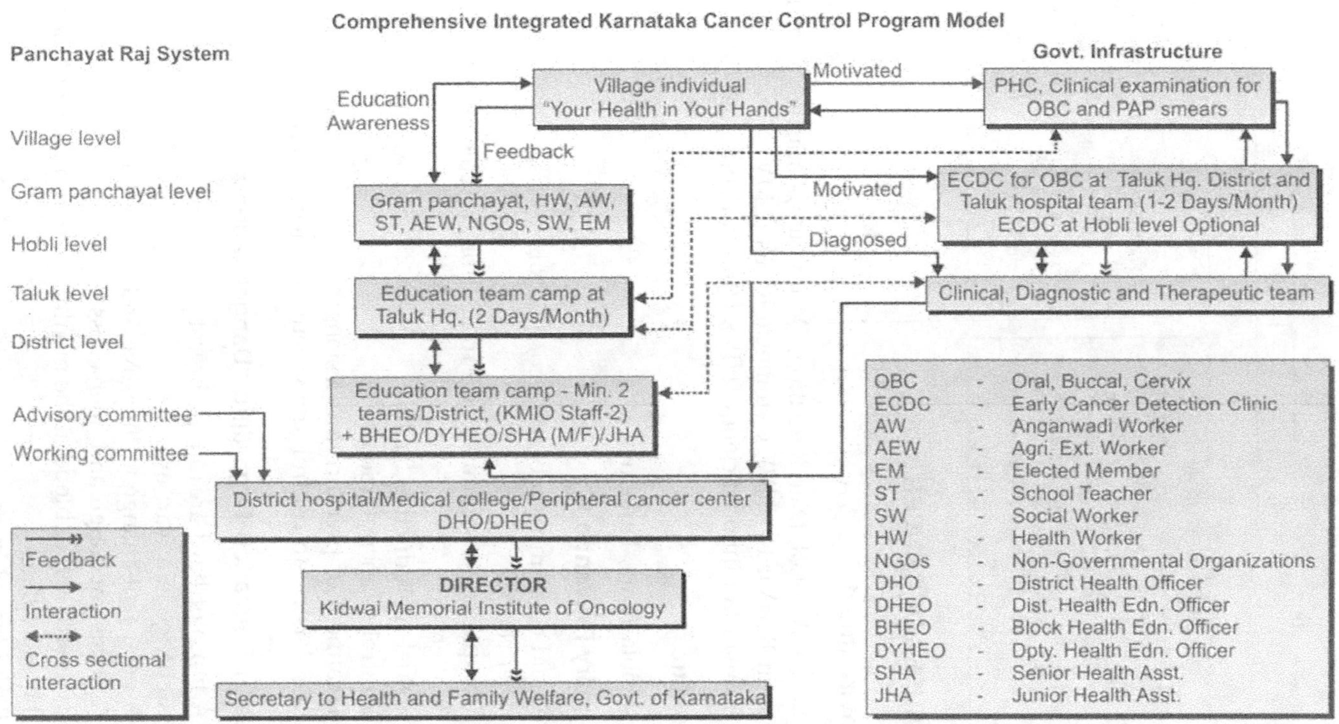

Flow chart 5.3: Cancer registration

Cancer registration

Hospital-based registers

1. It includes all in-patient and out-patients treated in particular hospital
2. Its use in epidemiological investigation purpose in limited
3. If there is long-team follow-up of patient, hospital based registries can be used for evaluation of diagnostic and treatment programs

Population-based registers

1. It includes all cancer patients in given geographic area
2. It is one of the best source for epidemiological investigation
3. Population based cancer registries have been established at Bangalore, Bombay and Madras under the National registry project of the ICMR

CAUSES OF CANCER

Environment

Tobacco, Alcohol, Diet, Radiation, Occupation, Parasites, Viral infection Ebstein Bar Virus (EBV), Cytomegalovirus (CMV).

Human Immunodeficiency (HIV), Human Papilloma Virus (HPV).

Genetic

Retinoblastoma, leukemia.

Primary Prevention

1. Avoid consumption of tobacco, alcohol
2. Diet control
3. Occupation, environmental (Protect from carcinogen)
4. Sunlight
5. Sexual reproductive factor
6. Control of air pollution
7. Treatment of precancerous lesions
8. Legislation—to control known environmental carcinogens.

Health Education Regarding "Danger Signals"

1. A lump or hard area in the breast
2. A change in a wart or mole
3. A persistent change in digestive and bowel habits
4. A persistent cough and hoarseness
5. Excessive loss of blood at the monthly period or loss of blood outside the exact date
6. Blood loss from any natural orifice

7. A swelling or sore that does not get better
8. Unexplained loss of weight.

Secondary Prevention

Early detection of cases.

Treatment for Cancer

1. Chemical therapy
2. Radiotherapy
3. Surgical therapy
4. Palliative care.

NATIONAL CANCER CONTROL PROGRAM (NCCP)

Basic Steps

1. Assess magnitude of National cancer problem
2. Setting measurable cancer control objectives
3. Evaluating possible strategies
4. Choosing priority of action.

Goals of NCCP

1. To prevent future cancers
2. To diagnose cancer early
3. To provide curative therapy
4. To ensure freedom from suffering
5. To reach all in population.

District Cancer Control Program

1. Cancer education
2. Cancer screening camps
3. Ca cervix—pap test

Carcinoma of Breast

1. Self-examination
2. Clinical
3. Thermography
4. Mammography.

Carcinoma of Lung

1. MMR
2. Sputum cytology.

Conceptual Framework of Safe Motherhood

Four important aspects are to be considered equity, accessibility, affordability, and accountability for quality care (Fig. 6.1).

Improvement of women's pre-pregnancy health is also important (Table 6.1)

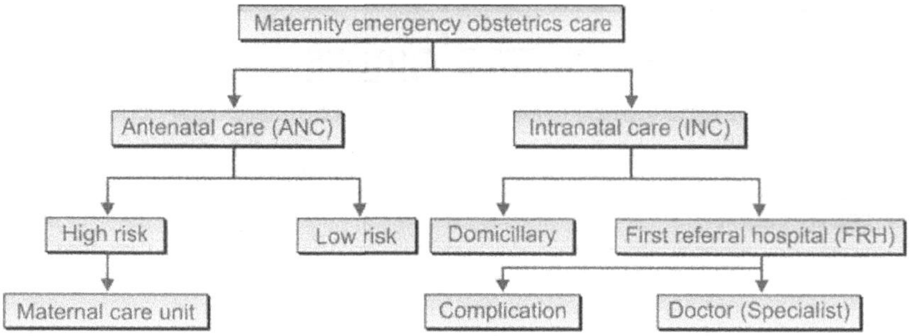

Fig. 6.1: Maternity emergency care

Risk Approach

The central purpose of antenatal care is to identify "High-risk" cases from a large group of antenatal mothers.

1. Elderly primi (30 years and over)
2. Short statured primi (140 cm and below)
3. History of previous cesarean or instrumental delivery
4. Antepartam hemorrhage threatened abortion
5. Twins—hydramnios
6. Pre-eclampsia and eclampsia
7. Previous stillbirth, intrauterine death, manual removal of placenta
8. Elderly grand multiparas
9. Prolonged pregnancy (14 days after expected date of delivery)
10. Anemia
11. Malpresentations, viz. breechs, transverse lie, etc.
12. Pregnancy-related general disease, viz. cardiovascular disease, kidney disease, diabetes, tuberculosis, liver disease, etc.

Table 6.1: Milestones of Family Welfare Program

1880	– Establishment of training for *dais* in Amritsar
1902	– Ist Midwifery Act to promote safe delivery
1930	– Setting up of Advisory Committee on Maternal Mortality
1951-56 1st Plan	Family Planning Program adopted by Government of India, first of its kind in the world
1961-66 3rd Plan	– Extension education approach – Department of Family Planning created in Ministry of Health – Created Target Oriented Approach – Lippe's loop introduced

Contd...

Contd...

1969-74 4th Plan	Family planning services under Primary Health Center – All India Hospital Postpartum Program – Medical Termination of Pregnancy (MTP) Act, 1971
1974-79 5th Plan	Renaming Family Planning to Family Welfare – Community Involvement – Child Marriage Restraint Act 1978
1983	National Health Policy
1980-85 6th Plan	Strengthening of Maternal and Child Health – Strengthening Family Welfare
1985-90 7th Plan	Further inclusion of various programs under MCH
1992-97 8th Plan	Child Survival and Safe Motherhood Program (CSSM)
1993-94	National Development Committee Report – International Conference on Population and Development (ICPD), Cairo 1994
1996	Target Free Approach Review of Safe Motherhood Component of CSSM
1997-02 9th Plan	Reproductive and Child Health (RCH) (CSSM plus STD and RTI components) RTI = Reproductive Tract Infections)

REPRODUCTIVE AND CHILD HEALTH PROGRAM

The Reproductive and Child Health (RCH) Program for the Ninth Plan is a very ambitious program which aims to effectively bring all the reproductive and child health services within easy reach of the community.

Reproductive and Child Health Program marks a significant paradigm shift in the India context—a change from a population control approach through a top-down, target-driven program, to one that provides high quality services that are gender-sensitive and responsive to the needs of clients, especially women who are the major users but have a serious problem of access, both physical and social to health services.

Definition of RCH

"People have the ability to reproduce and regulate their fertility, women are able to go through pregnancy and child birth safely, the outcome of pregnancies is successful in terms of maternal and infant survival and well being and couples are able to have sexual relations free of fear of pregnancy and of contracting diseases."

Components of RCH (Fig. 6.2)

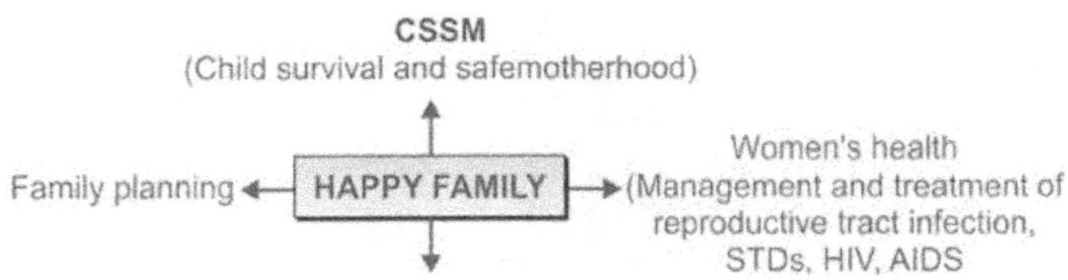
CSSM
(Child survival and safemotherhood)
Family planning
HAPPY FAMILY
Women's health
(Management and treatment of
reproductive tract infection,
STDs, HIV, AIDS

Fig. 6.2: Components of RCH

MAJOR ELEMENTS OF RCH PROGRAM

Reproductive Health Elements

1. Responsible and healthy sexual behavior
2. Intervention to promote safe motherhood
3. Prevention of unwanted pregnancies—increase access to contraceptives
4. Safe abortion
5. Pregnancy and delivery services
6. Management of RTI/STD
7. Referral facilities by government/private sector for pregnant woman at risk
8. Reproductive health services for adolescents
9. Screening and treatment of infertility, cancers and other gynecological disorders.

Child Survival Elements

1. Essential newborn care
2. Prevention and management of vaccine preventable disease
3. Urban measles campaign
4. Neonatal tetanus elimination
5. Surveillance of vaccine preventable diseases
6. Cold chain system
7. Polio eradication: Pulse polio program
8. Acute respiratory infections (ARI) control program
9. Diarrhea control program and ORS program
10. Prevention and control of vitamin A deficiency among children
11. Baby Friendly Hospital Initiatives (BFHI).

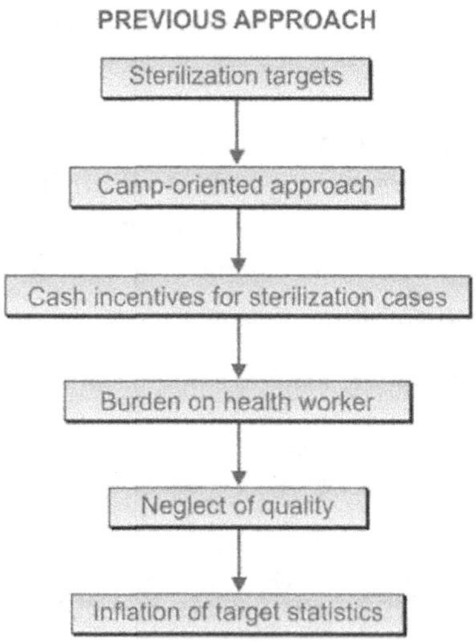

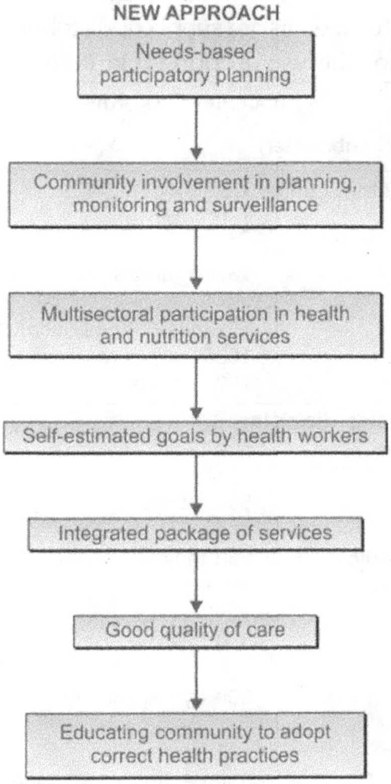

State Committee on Voluntary Action

For RCH implementation and flow of funds, the states who have established their ability for expenditure, utilization of funds and based on their performance will be provided funds through State Finance Department as at present. Otherwise, funds will be routed through a State Committee on Voluntary Action (SCOVA), a registered society with the State Chief Secretary as chairman and State Health Secretary (FW) as vice-chairman. This will provide flexibility in fund utilization on various activities like selection of contractual staff and experts.

Contents of Kits Supplied to Subcenter and First Referral Unit (FRU)

Under the CSSM program supplies of drugs are being made to the subcenters. These kits are supplied twice a year. There are two types of drug kits.

Drug kit A is supplied to all health workers while drug kit B is supplied to health workers in selected areas of the country only.

These kits will reach once in six months. The PHC/district medical officer, will have to ensure that the kits are supplied/distributed in turn to all health workers and monitor the use of individual items in the kits.

Subcenter Drug Kits

(Twice a year to each subcenter)

Drug Kit A (For all districts under CSSM)	
1. **IFA** (large) (100 mg)	15000 tablets
2. **IFA** (small) (20 mg)	13000 tablets
3. **Vitamin A**	6 bottles (100 ml each) (1 ml=1 lakh IU)
4. **Cotrimoxazole**	1000 tablets (pediatric)
5. **ORS packets**	150 packets
Drug Kit B (For selected districts)	
1. **Methylergometrine** (0.125 mgm)	500 tablets
2. **Paracetamol** (500 mg)	500 tablets
3. **Tablet antispasmodic**	250 tablets
4. **Methylergometrine** (0.2 mg/ml)	10 ampoule
5. **Mebendazole** (100 mg)	300 tablets
6. **Chloramphenicol** (1%)	500 eye applicants
7. **Cetrimide powder**	125 gms
8. **Providone ointment**	5 tubes (Iodine 5% tube of 25 gm each)
9. **Cotton bandage**	120 rolls (4 cm x 4 meter)
10. **Cotton absorbent**	One roll (500 gm)

Under RCH Program

Health facilities that can function as FRUs get kit E to kit P. The different types of kits are given below:

Kit E	Laparotomy set
Kit F	Mini-laparotomy set
Kit G	IUD insertion set
Kit H	Vasectomy set
Kit I	Normal delivery set
Kit J	Vaccum extraction set
Kit K	Embryotomy set
Kit L	Uterine evacuation set
Kit M	Equipment for anesthesia
Kit N	Neonatal resuscitation set
Kit O	Equipment and reagents for blood test
Kit P	Donor blood transfusion set

Methods to Estimate Requirements for MCH Services

- Probable number of pregnancies = Population of area × Birth rate of the area.
- Antenatal registration = Probable number of pregnancies + 10 percent (for pregnancy wastage)
- Fifteen percent of the antenatal women registered are high-risk
- Fifty percent of the registered antenatal mothers are anemic
- Ten percent of the live birth babies are sick or high-risk and need referral services
- Infants alive at one year in the area = number of live birth–infant mortality rate of the area
- Three percent of the total population is children below three years of age
- Thirteen percent of the total population is children below five years of age.

ANTENATAL CARE

Objectives of Antenatal Visit

1. Preventive services for mothers
2. Prenatal services
3. Prenatal advice
4. Specific protection
5. Mental health
6. Family planning
7. Pediatric care.

Prenatal Services

1. First visit—history, physical examination, investigation
2. Subsequent visit—physical examination, investigation
3. Distribution of iron and folic acid tablets
4. Immunization
5. Health education
6. Home visit
7. Referral services
8. High-risk approach
9. Maintenance of records.

Prenatal Advice

Prenatal advice regarding:

1. Diet
2. Personal hygiene—personal cleanliness, diet, rest, exercise, abstinence from smoking and alcohol, dental care, sexual intercourse.
3. Drugs

4. Radiation
5. Warning signals:
   a. Swelling of the feet
   b. Convulsions
   c. Headache
   d. Blurring of vision
   e. Bleeding and discharge per vagina
   f. Any other unusual symptom
6. Child care.

Specific Protection

1. Anemia
2. Nutritional deficiency disorder
3. Toxemia of pregnancy
4. Tetanus
5. Syphilis
6. German measles
7. Rh-Status
8. HIV infection
9. Prenatal genetic screening.

MATERNAL AND CHILD HEALTH

RCH-II and Family Planning

The RCH-II is the flagship program of the Government of India on reproductive, child and maternal health under National Rural Health Mission. The program has been reoriented and revitalized to give it a pro-outcome and pro-poor focus.

Under RCH-II it is envisaged that 50 percent of PHCs and all CHCs would be made operational as 24 hours delivery centers; in phased manner; by the year 2010. These centers would be responsible for providing basic emergency obstetric care and essential new born care and basic newborn resuscitation services round the clock. Beside these all the FRUs will also made operational for providing emergency obstetric care by the end of RCH-II.

New areas-components and elements in RCH-II at various levels:

1. *Village level:* One "Link worker" or ASHA in each village.
2. *Subcenter:* Location; analysis of subcenter and necessary relocation as per the need.
3. *PHC:* Location; analysis of PHC and necessary relocation as per the need.
4. *CHC:* Ensure full staff; five specialists (OBG, pediatrics, anesthetiology, general surgeon and physician) seven staff nurses, one pharmacist and two laboratory technicians and one radiographer. Gradually 50 percent of CHCs should become first referral units (FRUs) for emergency obstetric care.

5. *District:* The chief medical officer/civil surgeon will be provided adequate training and knowledge of public health functions.
6. *State:* To build capacity in management (planning and decentralization and management information and evaluation system).

Program Implementation Plan (PIP)

Differential approach for implementation of RCH-II program in empowered action group (EAG) states based on the level of infant mortality rate, institutional deliveries and strengthening of the health system.

i. Integrated management of neonatal and childhood illness (IMNCI) introduction in phased manner.
ii. Adolescent health initiative in selected districts (75 districts) for adolescent friendly health services and counseling and once a week clinic at PHC/CHC.
iii. Strengthening of social marketing of contraceptives in rural areas, through rural health practitioners and community mobilization through satisfied acceptor couples.
iv. Urban health: Provision of quality integrated primary health care services to urban poor by establishing urban health center for 1:50,000 population with one medical officer, 3-4 ANMs, one laboratory assistant, one public health nurse/lady health visitor, one clerk and one chowkidar and a peon.

    Second tier referral center it could be district hospital/maternity home/private and NGO nursing home (by public private partnership).
v. Tribal health will be given primacy.
vi. Establishing newborn care corner in phased manner in the existing FRUs/CHCs/PHCs/subcenters and priority will be given to EAG states.
vii. Hospital generated waste management/infection control.
viii. Incorporation of new areas (adolescent health, urban primary health care infrastructure, tribal health, adverse sex ratio in different states, PNDT Act) in the matrix of priorities for behavior change communication strategy (BCC).
ix. Revamping of training in RCH at various levels especially training under newer areas incorporated under RCH-II.

Janani Suraksha Yojana

Promoting hospital delivery among poor families. It is 100 percent centrally sponsored scheme to help all pregnant women (19 years and above) from 'below poverty line' families.

Janani Suraksha Yojana (JSY) has the main objectives of reducing maternal and infant mortality by focusing on promoting institutional delivery care during pregnancy, delivery and post-delivery by linking delivery care to antenatal check-up and neonatal care along with appropriate referral and transport assistance, in the BPL groups.

An Accredited Social Health Activist (ASHA) will be an effective link between the field level Government machinery and the poor pregnant women and they will make available the delivery services to the intended beneficiaries, encouraging antenatal care, institutional delivery, adopting small family norms. In addition, ASHA will escort the poor pregnant women and also stay with the women during delivery.

Important Features of JSY

a. The scheme is 100 percent centrally sponsored and intended all women from BPL families, of age 19 years or above. Benefit available up to two live birth. In 10 low performing states (LPS) (namely; Bihar, Chhattisgarh, Jharkhand, Orissa, UP, Uttarakhand, Rajasthan, Madhya Pradesh, Assam and Jammu and Kashmir) the benefit will be available for the woman on her own accord, chooses to undergo sterilization, after the delivery.

b. Scale of Assistance
NB 1: LPS: Low performing States (10 states)
HPS: High Performing States (Remaining states/ UTs)
NB 2: Cash benefit of Rs. 500/- per live birth is to be given to all pregnant women (BPL) after registration and at the time of delivery, irrespective of the place of delivery.
NB 3: Such eligible beneficiaries under the scheme who deliver in health institutions would get an additional cash benefit of Rs. 200/- if they belong to rural areas and Rs. 100/- if they belong to urban areas of ten low performing states (namely; Bihar, Chhattisgarh, Jharkhand, Orissa, UP, Uttarakhand, Rajasthan, Madhya Pradesh, Assam and Jammu and Kashmir).

c. The package for ASHA or an equivalent worker where ASHA has not been recruited includes:
   - The referral transport assistance to go to the nearest health center,
   - The compensation for ASHA or an equivalent worker if she stays with the pregnant woman in the health center for delivery.

d. *Placement of imprest money with the ANMs*: To quicken the process of disbursement, all ANMs will be having an imprest of Rs. 5000/to make all payment of cash assistance.

   Note: Where Panchayati Raj Institutions (PRIs) exist and an elected body is in place, the State Governments/District society will be at liberty to keep the money with Panchayati Raj Institutions and empower Auxiliary jointly with the Gram Panchayat through a simple procedures to recoup the imprest periodically. All disbursements should be made immediately after delivery, if possible, in the hospital itself.

e. *Disbursement of cash assistance:* As the scheme is targeting the poor women who would generally be short of cash, it is essential that the cash assistance provided under the scheme is made available to her in the shortest possible time. With a view to quicken the process of disbursement, ANM should keep a contingency amount of atleast Rs. 1500/- with the ASHA or AWW (if ASHA has not been recruited) and replenishment thereafter as already stated in the JSY guidelines.

f. *Linking antenatal check-up, institutional delivery and neonatal care:* Beneficiaries should register themselves with the Health Workers at the subcenter/primary health centers for availing of at least three antenatal check-ups, postnatal care and neonatal care.

g. *Encouraging pregnant women to undergo tubectomy/laparoscopy:* If hospitalization for delivery is followed immediately by tubectomy/ laparoscopy, the beneficiary will also get compensation money available under the existing family welfare scheme.

h. *Provision of cesarean section:* Where government specialists are not available, assistance up to Rs. 1500/- per case will be provided for hiring services of private experts to carry out the surgery either in a government medical facility or in private hospital, nursing home, etc.

i. *Partnership with private sector:* Benefits proposed under JSY would also be available to such beneficiaries delivering in an accredited private health institutions. Provision of five percent (4% for the district authorities and 1% for the state) of the fund released towards administrative expenses for monitoring, IEC and office expenses for implementation.

Mamta Scheme—An Example of Public Private Partnership in Health Care

India suffers from high maternal and neonatal mortality. One of the reasons of this high mortality is home delivery conducted by untrained personnel. In Delhi, approximately 3.2 lac deliveries take place every year and 63 percent (as per NFHS 3 survey report, 2005) of these are institutional deliveries and in some areas there are much lower rates of institutional deliveries. Government of NCT of Delhi is committed to provide equitable, quality health care for its citizens especially, the maternal and child segment of its population. An important component of health care aimed at reducing the maternal and infant mortality is provision of "Institutional Delivery" for pregnant women. The Government is trying to universalize institutional deliveries. However, there are constraints like lack of adequate Government health facilities equipped and functional to provide the comprehensive obstetric services for the mother and the newborn and overburdened Government hospitals. Therefore, PPP model was chosen wherein Private Hospitals were approached to express their intention to join the Mamta scheme. For comprehensive care, which includes antenatal Rs. 4000/- by the district societies, however, these are part packages also, wherein for institutional deliveries alone Rs. 3000/- is given. If only antenatal care is provided Rs. 2000/-is given (Kishore and Charu, 2008).

Health Care Services for the Beneficiaries under the Scheme

1. At least three antenatal check-ups with all necessary investigations including ultrasound of pregnant woman registered under the scheme.
2. Provision of injection TT and iron folic acid tablets to all pregnant women as per RCH schedule, provision of institutional delivery facilities, including emergency obstetric care to all care to the newborn including administration of birth doses of vaccines to newborns.
3. One postnatal check-up within first week of delivery but not later than 14 days.

Eligibility Criteria for Beneficiaries under the Scheme

a. The pregnant woman must belong to the BPL/SC/ST category and should be a resident of Delhi.
b. The pregnant woman should not be less than 19 years of age.
c. The pregnant woman should not have more than one living child.

Registration of Beneficiaries under the Scheme

The pregnant woman shall be enrolled under Mamta only after production of the following documents:

a. *Proof of age:* Ration card/school certificate/birth certificate/affidavit/any other relevant document/clinical assessment of the attending doctor in absence of any other proof. Proof that she is a resident of Delhi (Ration card/election I-card/any other document indication specific address).
b. Affidavits regarding number of living children.
c. Registration of pregnant women will be preferably done in the first trimester (12 weeks).
d. BPL card/certification of BPL status from the SDM/certificate of SC/ST issued by competent authority.

Prevention of Patient to Child Transmission (PPTCT)

Prevention of Parent to Child Transmission of HIV Infection

When a child or infant is infected with HIV from an infected mother it is known as vertical transmission and this can occur during pregnancy, child birth and through breastfeeding. In general, the level of transmission can vary in accordance with several variables, however, it is estimated that 35 percent of the children of seropositive women can acquire HIV, 10 percent in pregnancy, 10 percent during the child birth and 15 percent by breastfeeding.

In resource poor setting such as India the reported rate of mother-to-child transmission ranges from 13-60 percent. According to Kumar et al the vertical transmission rate in India is 48 percent. Another study conducted by ARCON in Mumbai, Dongaonkar et al reported a mother to child transmission rate of 36 percent.

1. All pregnant women attending the antenatal clinic are group counseled and offered HIV testing. Those who opt to be tested undergo pre-test counseling for HIV.
2. Testing is done as per NACO guidelines with 3 ELISA/Rapid test.
3. If the mother is found to be HIV positive, she is counseled after the test. The post-test counseling focuses on disclosing the results of the test, options to the mother with regard to breastfeeding of the child and about HIV. Confidentiality is maintained.
4. The spouse of the HIV positive women is offered HIV counseling and testing.
5. Nevirapine prophylaxis at the time of delivery is administered to both the mother at the time of delivery and to the child immediately after delivery, to reduce HIV transmission to the child.

Various Types of Antiretroviral Regimens

a. Short–Short course wherein the mother receives the ARV from 35 weeks of gestation and the infant for up to 3 days;
b. Long–Long course wherein the ARV from 28 weeks of gestation and the infant for up to 6 weeks;
c. Short–Long course wherein the ARV from 35 weeks of gestation and the infant for up to 6 weeks;
d. Long–Short course wherein the ARV from 28 weeks of gestation and the infant for up to 3 days.

Role of maternal and child health services in the prevention of HIV infection in infants and young children program.

Maternal and child health services:

- PPTCT programs need to be integrated as an essential part of MCH care. MCH care encompasses a broad range of educational and clinical services that help mothers, their children and their families lead healthy lives. Although, all four prongs of a comprehensive PPTCT programs are important, antenatal care is the most common entry point for women into those programs. MCH programs facilitate PPTCT by providing:
  - Essential antenatal
  - Family planning services
  - ARV prophylaxis
  - Safe delivery practices
  - Counseling and support for the woman's chosen infant feeding method.

Integration of PPTCT within Postnatal MCH Services

Effective integration of PPTCT within postnatal MCH services is likely to increase community acceptance of PPTCT programs and strengthen maternal care, infant care and family care.

- *Maternal care:* MCH postpartum care services help protect the mother's health by providing medical and psychosocial care.
- *Infant care:* MCH postnatal care services offer assessment of infant growth and development, nutritional support services may include ARV treatment.
- *Family care:* MCH services provide social support, testing and counseling for family members; referrals to community-based support programs; and assistance in dealing with stigma.

Key Points

- A comprehensive approach is needed to prevent HIV infection in infants and young children
- The four prongs of comprehensive care in PPTCT are:
  - Primary prevention of HIV-infection.
  - Prevention of unintended pregnancies in HIV-infected women
  - Prevention of HIV transmission from HIV-infected women to their infants
  - Provision of treatment, care and support to HIV-infected women, their infants and their families.
- Without intervention the risk of MTCT is 25 to 49 percent
- Combination interventions can reduce the MTCT rate by upto 40 percent in breastfeeding populations.
- Because ARV prophylaxis alone does not provide long-term benefit to the mother's infection, ongoing care and support are needed.
- MCH services can act as an entry point to the range of services that can provide care and support to HIV-positive women and affected family members.
- Linkages to community services provide enhanced care support PPTCT Services for the HIV-2 infected women. The HIV-2-infected women should have access to the entire range of neonatal, labor and childbirth, and postnatal services a linkages designed for HIV-1-infected women. Offering the HIV-2-infected other short-course ARV prophylaxis to prevent MCT should follow national and local policy, if such a policy statement exits. The following information, adapted from the US Centers Disease Control and Prevention (October 1998) provides pertinent background on HIV for consideration:
- HIV-2 infections are predominantly found in West Africa.
- HIV-2 infections:
  - Have the same modes of transmission as HIV-1
  - Are associated with the similar opportunistic infections

  - Develop more slowly and appear less virulent than HIV-1
  - Appear to be less transmissible from mother to child than HIV-1.
- Testing for both HIV-1 and HIV-2 should be considered in the following situations:
  - When demographic or behavioral risk factors are present
  - When illnesses (such as opportunistic infections) appear in someone whose HIV-1 test is negative
  - When an HIV-1 Western blot indicates certain indeterminate test band patterns.
- The best approach to clinical treatment of HIV-2 is unclear:
  - Not all drugs used to treat HIV-1 are as effective against HIV-2.
  - Treatment response is more difficult to monitor than in HIV-1; CD4 + T-cell counts and physical sings of immune *deterioration* are currently being used.
- Non-nucleoside reverse transcriptase inhibitors, such as nevirapine, are not effective against HIV-2; therefore, zidovudine therapy should be considered for HIV-2-infected expectant mothers and their newborn infants to reduce MTCT risk, especially for women who become infected during pregnancy.
- Woman's wishes: The healthcare provider should have a frank discussion with the HIV-2-infected woman to explain the prevailing policy and practice and support her incoming to a decision with which she is comfortable.
- Continued surveillance to monitor the further spread of HIV-2 is necessary.

Infant Feeding Formula (Table 6.2)

For infants from birth to six months old, modify animal milk to create infant formula following these directions:

Table 6.2: Infant feeding formula

60 ml (One feeding for a 1-month-old infant)			
Type of milk	Milk	Water	Sugar
Cow, goat, or camel	40 ml	20 ml	4 g (1 teaspoon)
Sheep and buffalo	30 ml	30 ml	3 g (3/4 teaspoon)
90 ml (One feeding for a 2-month-old infant)			
Cow, goat, or camel	60 ml	30 ml	6 g (1 ¼ teaspoon)
Sheep and buffalo	45 ml	45 ml	5 g (1 teaspoon)
120 ml (One feeding for a 3 to 4 -month-old infant)			
Cow, goat, or camel	80 ml	40 ml	8 g (2 teaspoon)
Sheep and buffalo			6 g (1 ¼ teaspoon)
150 ml (One feeding for a 5 to 6 -month-old infant)			
Cow, goat, or camel	100 ml	50 ml	10 g (2 teaspoon)
Sheep and buffalo	75 ml	75 ml	8 g (2 teaspoon)

INTRANATAL CARE

1. Thorough asepsis
2. Delivery with minimum injury to mother and child
3. Readiness to deal with complications such as prolonged labor, antepartum hemorrhage, convulsion, mal-presentation, prolapse of cord, etc.
4. Care of the baby at delivery.

Care at Birth

Five Cleans

Clean hands, clean surface, clean cord tie, clean razor blade and clean cord stump (no applicant).

POSTNATAL CARE

Care of the mother and baby after delivery.

Objectives of Postnatal Care

1. *To prevent complications of postnatal period*

Immediate	**Late**
a. Puerperal sepsis	Subinvolution
b. Thrombophlebitis	Retroverted uterus
c. Secondary hemorrhage	Prolapse uterus
d. Others	Cervicitis

2. *Restoration of mother to optimum health*
   a. Physical: Postnatal examination
      i. Twice daily for three days
         Once daily—till umbilical cord falls
         Once in month up to six months
         Once in two to three months up to 1 year
      ii. Anemia correction
      iii. Nutritional deficiency treatment
      iv. Postnatal exercises to strengthen perineal muscles
   b. Psychological: Eliminate anxiety, fear insecurity, Rx postpartum psychosis if it occurs.
   c. Social:
3. Breastfeeding
4. Family planning
5. Basic health education regarding—personal hygiene, environment hygiene, nutrition of mother and child, importance of health check-up, spacing, birth registration.

Warm Chain

The warm chain is a set of ten interlinked procedures carried out at birth and later, which will minimize the likelihood of hypothermia in all newborns. The elements of warm chain are:

1. Warm delivery room (25^{0}C)
2. Warm resuscitation
3. Immediate drying
4. Skin-to-skin contact between baby and the mother
5. Breastfeeding
6. Postpone bathing
7. Appropriate clothing and bedding
8. Mother and baby nursed together
9. Warm transportation
10. Training and awareness raising of health care providers.

At risk infants: Identification of these neonates and giving special care is important.

High-Risk Infants

1. Birth weight (1800-2500 gm)
2. Multiple births
3. Cesarean section
4. Suspected sepsis
5. At risk for isoimmunization
6. Born to mothers with previous bad obstetric history
7. At risk for hypoglycemia.

MALNUTRITION

Definition

Malnutrition has been defined as "a state resulting from a relative or absolute deficiency or excess of one or more essential nutrients".

Classification

1. Undernutrition
2. Overnutrition
3. Imbalance
4. Specific deficiency.

Children under 15 years of age are main victims.

Nutritional Problems (Table 6.3)

Table 6.3: Nutritional problems

Nutritional problem	*Prevalence*
a. PEM	By clinical examination 3% in (0-6 years children) By anthropometric 4% in (0-6 years children)
b. Vitamin A deficiency	Conjuctival xerosis 5-10% Corneal involvement 0.12% (in 0-6 years children)
c. Anemia	By Hb estimation 90% in pregnant women and 60% in 0-6 years children
d. Endemic Goiter	Thyroid enlargement in 33% of the community at risk.

Epidemiology

Conditioning Influences

1. Diarrhea
2. Intestinal parasites
3. Malaria
4. Measles
5. Whooping cough.

Cultural and Social Factors

Harmful cultural patterns and habits related to:

a. Breastfeeding
b. Weaning
c. Food taboos
d. Feeding of pregnant and lactating women
e. Repeated pregnancy.

Infections

a. Gastrointestinal infections
b. Worm infestation
c. Respiratory infection
d. Measles.

Health and Other Services

1. Nutritional surveillance
2. Nutritional rehabilitation
3. Nutritional supplementation
4. Health education.

PROTEIN-ENERGY MALNUTRITION

Definition

A range of pathological condition arising from deficiency of protein and energy, normally associated with infection.

Protein-energy malnutrition (PEM) is major health problem and a leading cause directly or indirectly of death during an emergency.

It is not only an important cause of childhood mortality and morbidity, but also leads to permanent impairment of physical and possibly of mental growth of those who survive.

Most commonly affecting children are between the age of six months and five years.

The condition may result from lack of food or from infections that causes loss of appetite while increasing the body's nutrient requirements.

Children between 12 and 36 months old are especially at risk since they are the most vulnerable to infections such as GIT infection and measles.

Incidence of PEM in preschool age children is one to two percent.

Types of PEM

1. Marasmus
2. Kwashiorkor
3. Dwarfism (Subnormal physical development)
4. Marasmus-Kwashiorkor.

Marasmus

If deficiency arises early in the infancy marasmus is likely to supervene. Marasmus is due to deficiency of protein and energy, characterized by severe wasting of fat and muscle, which the body breaks down for energy leaving skin and bones. This is most common form of PEM in nutritional emergencies.

Nutritional marasmus is due to prolonged starvation.

Secondary marasmus is due to the result from chronic or recurrent infection with marginal food intake.

Clinical Features

1. Low body weight for age
2. Loss of subcutaneous fat
3. One of the cardinal sign is muscle wasting [Signs—(a) old man face, (b) Baggy pants] (the loose skin of the buttocks hanging down).
4. No edema
5. Mental retardation
6. Infection.

In Kwashiorkor (Moonface)

In kwashiorkor, energy is adequate but lack of protein is the cause. Kwashiorkor is mainly due to lack of protein (hypoalbuminemia).

Clinical Features

1. Low body weight
2. Muscle wasting
3. Dermatitis
4. Enlargement of liver
5. Changes in hair
6. Mental retardation
7. Infection
8. Edema.

Signs

Tick Sign

In kwashiorkor, if you start treatment edema start disappearing which leads to weight loss, afterwards baby starts gaining weight, this sign is known as tick sign.

Flag Sign

The hair is thin, dry, brittle, easily pluckable, sparse and devoid of their normal shine. It becomes straight and hypopigmented.

The length of hair that grows during the period of nutritional deprivation appears reddish brown, during phases of better nutrition, the growing part of the hair gets appropriately pigmented. This gives appearance of alternate bands of hypopigmented and normally pigmented hair.

Classification of PEM

Gomez's Classification (Weight for Age)

Normal	90-110
Grade I	75-89 percent
Grade II	60-74 percent
Grade III	Less than 60 percent

Dr Udani's Classification (Calorie Deficiency Classification)

Grade I	Twenty percent less than expected
Grade II	Subcutaneous fat reduced in buttock
Grade III	Subcutaneous fat reduced all over the body except cheeks
Grade IV	Subcutaneous fat reduced all over the body including cheeks.

Waterlow's Classification defined Two Groups for PEM (Table 6.4)

- Malnutrition with retarted growth, in which a drop in the height/age ratio points to a chronic condition—shortness or stunted.
- Malnutrition with a low weight for a normal height in which the weight for height ratio is indicative of an acute condition of rapid weight loss or wasting.

wt/ht = wt of the child/wt of the normal child at same height × 100
ht/age = ht of the child/ht of normal child at same age × 100

Table 6.4: Waterlow's classification

Nutritional status	*Stunting (% of ht/age)*	*Wasting (% of wt/ht)*
Normal	> 95	> 90
Mild impaired	87.5-95	80-90
Moderate impaired	80-87.5	70-80
Severly impaired	< 80	< 70

Harward's Classification

Fifty percent Harward standard.

Arrange children of same birth date in ascending or descending order, take 50th child as Indian standard.

Jellyfish Classification

Grade I 81-90% of the 50th Harward
Grade II 71-80% of the 50th Harward
Grade III 61-70% of the 50th Harward
Grade IV Less than 60% of the 50th Harward

NSIAP (National Subcommittee of Indian Academy of Pediatric)

Grade I 71-80% of 50th Harward
Grade II 61-70% of 50th Harward
Grade III 51-60% of 50th Harward
Grade IV Less than 50% of 50th Harward

Waterlow's Classification

When child age is known, measurement of weight enables almost instant monitoring of growth (Table 6.5).

Table 6.5: Measures of height assess the effect of nutritional status on long-term growth

W/H *H/A*	*> m-2D*	*< m-2D*
> m –2D	Normal	Stuntend
< m – 2D	Wasted	Wasted and stunted

Epidemiology of Malnutrition

Poverty Cycle

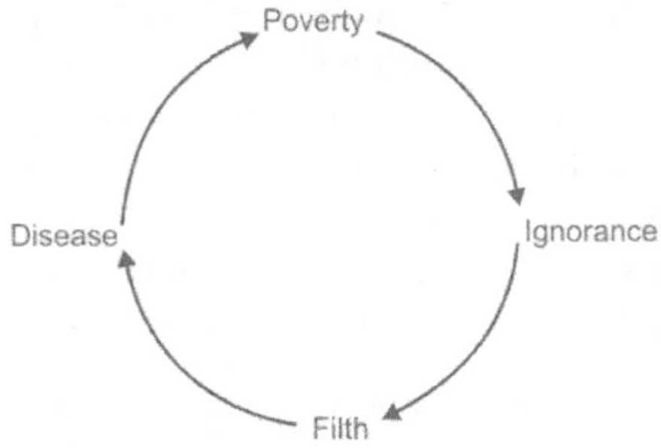

Vicious Cycle

1.

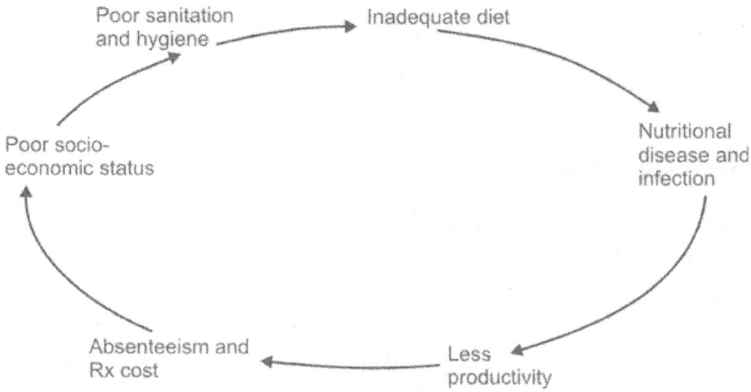

2.

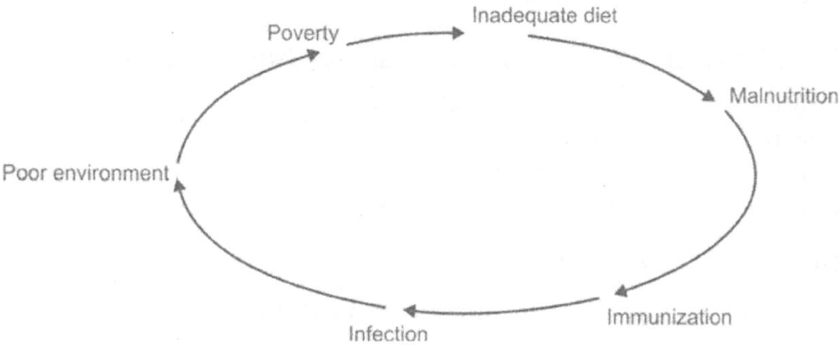

Agent Factor

1. Ignorance—of nutritional awareness in the country.
2. Inadequate diet—in terms of quality and quantity.
3. Infection—most common is diarrhea, ARI, measles, worm infestation
4. Weaning—gradual withdrawal of the child from the breast of the mother and introduction of supplimentary (semisolid) food.

Breast milk is—birth right of child

After four months breast milk alone is insufficient for development of child.

Next choice is cow's milk.

- Belief—customs and habits
- Misuse of antibiotics and self-medication.

Host Factors

1. Age—five years
   Six months to two years most vulnerable group
2. Sex—female children > vulnerable.
3. Birth order—chance of PEM increases with increasing birth order 1st child > PEM
4. Family size—larger the family size > PEM
5. Literacy state—PEM is more in baby of illiterate mother
6. Socioeconomic state—PEM > in low socioeconomic state
7. Knowledge Attitude Practice (KAP)—regarding PEM
   a. Cow dung application for umbilical cord
   b. Brand marking if child weeps, suspecting for abdominal pain and sometime purgatives are given
   c. Postnatal mother kept in for one month with child in dark room.
   d. Child is not put to breast during first three days of birth because of belief that colostrum might be harmful. Instead child is put on sugar solution and water.

Social Problems

A crucial role in the causation of PEM

1. Addiction in relation to alcohol
2. Reasons for smoking
3. Divorce and broken homes
4. Food habits and food fads
5. Cooking practices—open cooking pan lose all nutrients
6. Food storage
7. Food habits of mother.

Environmental Factors

1. Poor housing
2. Inadequate water supply
3. Food production and availability
4. Infection and malnutrition—against six killer diseases, i.e. DPT and MTP (Measles, TB and Polio)
5. Economical status—political will to improve economic status
6. Control of population explosion.

Examination of the Case

Hair : Luster, gray color, straight, easily pluckable
Face : Moon face in Kwashiorkor, pigmentation (due to specific vitamin deficiency) old man face in marasmus
Eye : Anemia
Bitot spots
Conjunctival—xerosis
Corneal—xerosis
Keratomalacia
Night blindness
Lips : Pigmentation, angular stomatitis
Tongue : Raw tongue, dry tongue pigmentation fissure
Teeth : Caries, mottled
Gum : Bleeding
Glands : Enlarged (inguinal glands)
Skin : Dermatitis
Flaky paint dermatitis
Nail : Koilonychia, brittle nail, bridged nail
Subcutaneous fat—edema
Musculoskeletal system—wasting
Frontal and parietal bossing
Hepatomegaly
Mental confusion
Sensory loss
Calf tenderness

Body Measurement Techniques

Responsible personnel should be trained to measure and record weight, height, and/or arm circumference as described in the following paragraphs.

Weight

Weight should be measured to the nearest 100 g (0.1 kg). Although, various types of scales are used for weighing infants in the field, the most commonly used is the hanging spring balance scale, which can weigh up to 25 kg.

Weighing Procedure (Fig. 6.3)

Note: If the parent or carer or other untrained person is acting as the assistant, the measurer should carry out the weighing and record the weight on the record form.

1. *Measurer or assistant*: Hang the scale from a tree branch, ceiling beam, tripod, or pole held by two people, using a rope if necessary, so that the scale is at eye level. Make sure that it is secure. Ask the parent or carer to undress the child.

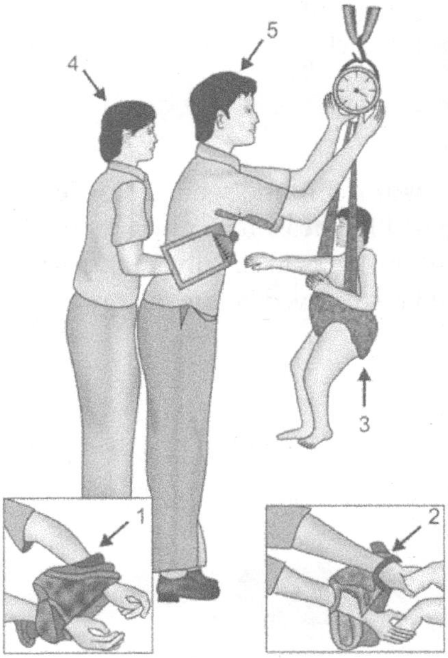

1. Put hands through leg holes
2. Grasp feet
3. Child hangs freely
4. Assistant with record form
5. Measurer reads scale at eye level

Fig. 6.3: Use of the hanging spring balance for weighing infants

2. *Measurer*: Attach a pair of weighing pants (or infant sling or basket) to the hook of the scale and adjust the scale to zero; then remove the pants.
3. *Measurer*: Put your arms through the leg holes of the weighing pants (if used) while the parent or carer holds the child, grasp the child's feet and pull his or her legs through the leg holes; make certain that the strap of the pants is in front of the child.
4. *Measurer*: Attach the strap of the pants to the hook of the scale. Do not carry the child by the strap alone. Gently lower the child and allow him or her to hang free.
5. *Assistant*: Stand behind and to one side of the measurer ready to record the weight (arrow 4). Have the record form and a pencil ready to hand.
6. *Measurer or assistant*: Check the child's position—make sure he or she is hanging free and not touching anything.
7. *Measurer*: Hold the scale and read the weight to the nearest completed 0.1 kg call out the measurement when the child is still and the scale needle has stopped moving; even the most active child will eventually become still long enough for a reading to be taken.
8. *Assistant*: Immediately record the weight and show your record to the measurer.
9. *Measurer*: Take hold of the child in one arm and gently lift him or her; release the state from the hook of the scale with your free hand. Do not lift the child by the strap of the weighing pants.

10. *Measurer*: Check the recorded weight on the form for accuracy and eligibility. If there are any errors instruct the assistant to erase and correct them.

Height or Length (Fig. 6.4)

Every effort should be made to measure children's height or length accurately, to the nearest 0.1 cm if possible. Measurement errors of 2 to 3 cm can easily occur and cause significant errors in classifying nutritional status. Shoes and other footwear should be removed before measurements are made.

Length

A child two years old or shorter than 80 cm (or 85 cm in a population that is not chronically undernourished) should be measured lying

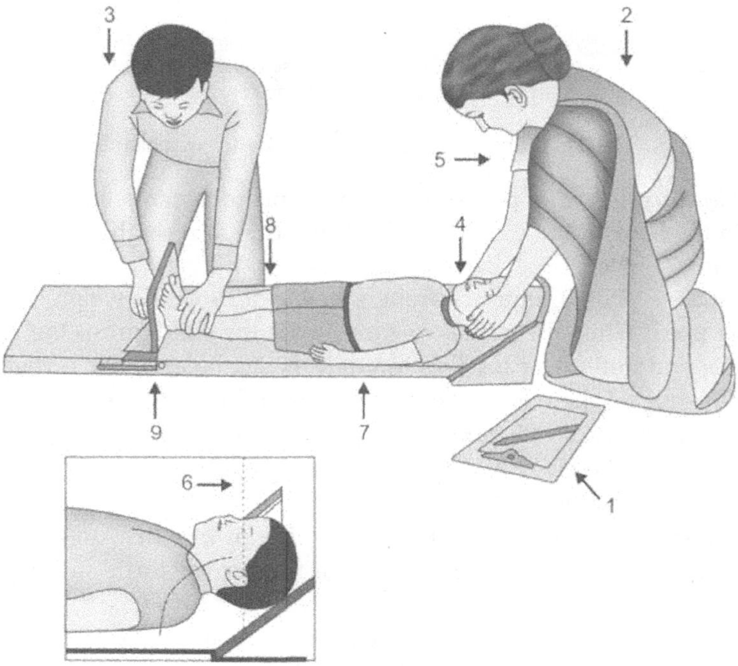

1. Record form and pen
2. Assistant on knees
3. Measurer on knees
4. Hands cupped over ears—head against base of board
5. Arms comfortably straight
6. Line of sight perpendicular to base of board
7. Child flat on board
8. Hands on knees or shins legs straight
9. Feet flat against foot piece.

Fig. 6.4: Measuring a child's length

on its back. The child should be quiet, relaxed, and lying straight, with the head resting against a fixed head-board; the child's should be looking vertically upwards. The help of the childs parent or carer is often valuable. Using one hand, the measurer should keep the legs straight by applying gentle pressure to both knees of the child and ensure that the movable slide is in contact with the surface of the soles and heels of the child's feet (not just the toes).

Height (Fig. 6.5)

A child over two-years old (or taller than 80 or 85 cm) should normally stand to be measured. The child's heels should be together, at the back of the fixed foot-board. The buttocks, the backs of the heels, the upper back, and the head should touch the measuring board, which should have a metal tape-measure attached. The child's knees should not be bent. The movable head-board, which must be horizontal, should be

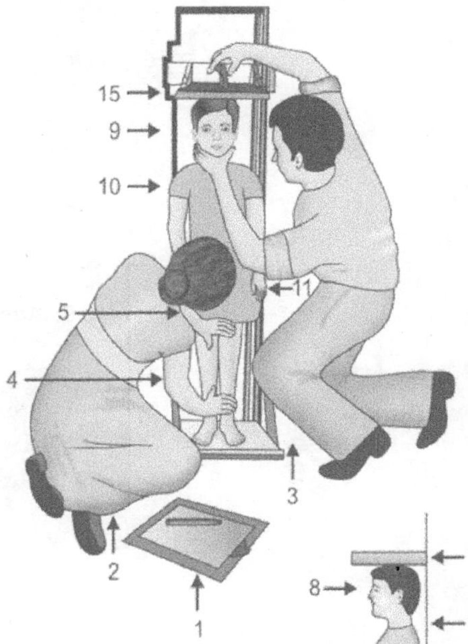

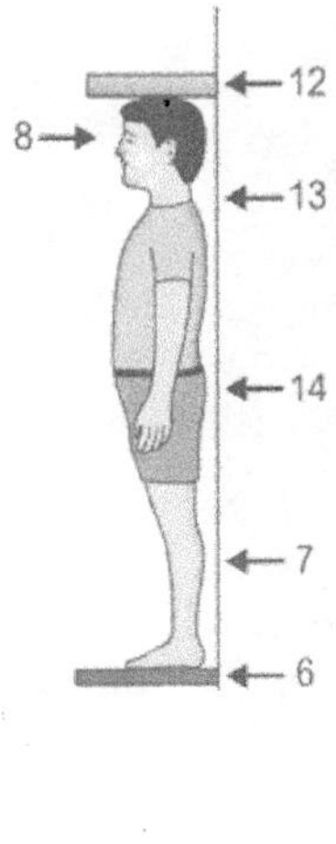

1. Record form and pencil
2. Assistant on knees
3. Measurer on knees
4. Right hand on shins heels against back and base of board
5. Left hand on knees. Knees together and leg straight
8. Line of sight
9. Hand on chin
10. Shoulder level
11. Hands at side

   6, 7, 12, 13, 14 Body flat against board
15. Head piece firmly on head.

Fig. 6.5: Measuring a child's height

slowly lowered until it rests firmly on the crown of the head (not just lightly on the hair). The vertical tape-measure is read opposite the highest point of the head when the child is looking straight ahead.

Midarm Circumference

Arm circumference is measured on the upper left arm. To locate the correct point for measurement, the child's elbow is flexed to 90 degree, with the palm facing upwards. A measuring tape is used to find the midpoint between the end of the shoulder (acromion) and the tip of the elbow (olecranon); this point should be marked. The arm is then allowed to hang freely, palm towards the thigh, and the measuring tape is placed snugly around the arm at the midpoint mark. The tape should not be pulled too tight (Figs 6.6 and 6.7).

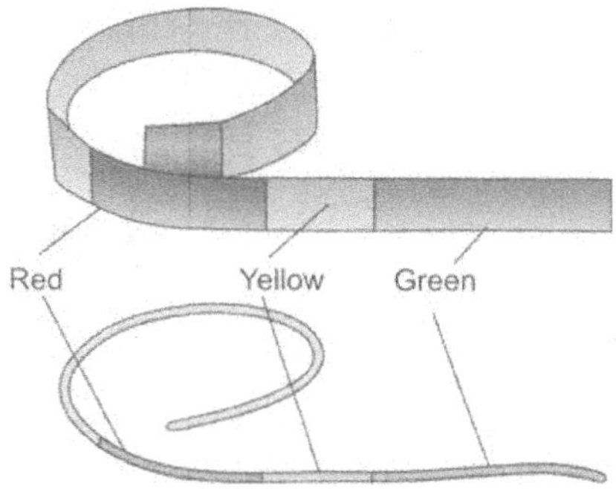

Fig. 6.6: Arm tapes

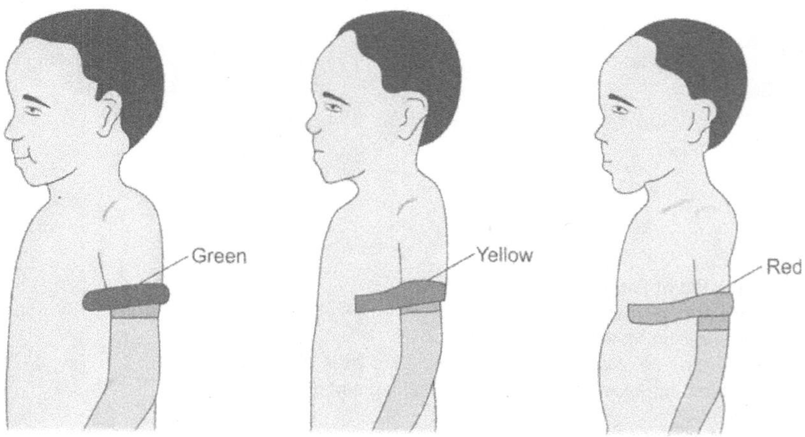

Fig. 6.7: These three children are being measured using an arm tape. Which child is weak and thin?

Head and Chest Circumference

At birth the head circumference is about 34 cm. It is about 2 cm more than the chest circumference. By six to nine months the two measurements become equal, after which the chest circumference overtaken the head circumference. In severely malnourished children, this overtaking may be delayed by three to four years due to poor development of thoracic cage. In a ICMR study, the crossing over of chest and head circumference did not take place unitl the age of two years and six months, this has been attributed to growth retardation in poor Indian children.

General Procedures for Treatment of Severe PEM

1. Initial treatment phase
2. Rehabilitation phase.

Initial Treatment Phase

Initial treatment phase begins with admission to the therapeutic feeding center and lasts until the child condition is stable and his or her appetite has returned (Usually after 2-7 days).

Growth chart is a visible display of the child's physical growth and development. The WHO prototype (home-based) chart is shown in Figure 6.8. It has two reference curve. The upper reference curve represents the median (50th percentile) for boys (slightly higher than that for girls), and the lower reference curve the 3rd percentile for girls (slightly lower than that for boys). Thus, the chart can be used for both sexes. The space between two growth curve in Figure 6.8 has been called the "road-to-health".

"Acute severe PEM" is as much a medical emergency, as say a heart attack even with utmost care, mortality rates are often 20 to 30 percent or higher. Deaths commonly occur during the first 24 to 48 hours after admission.

Complications

Commonly include:

1. Dehydration
2. Localized and generalized infection
3. Septic shock
4. Hypothermia
5. Hypoglycemia
6. Anemia
7. Vitamin A deficiency
8. Fluid and electrolyte imbalance.

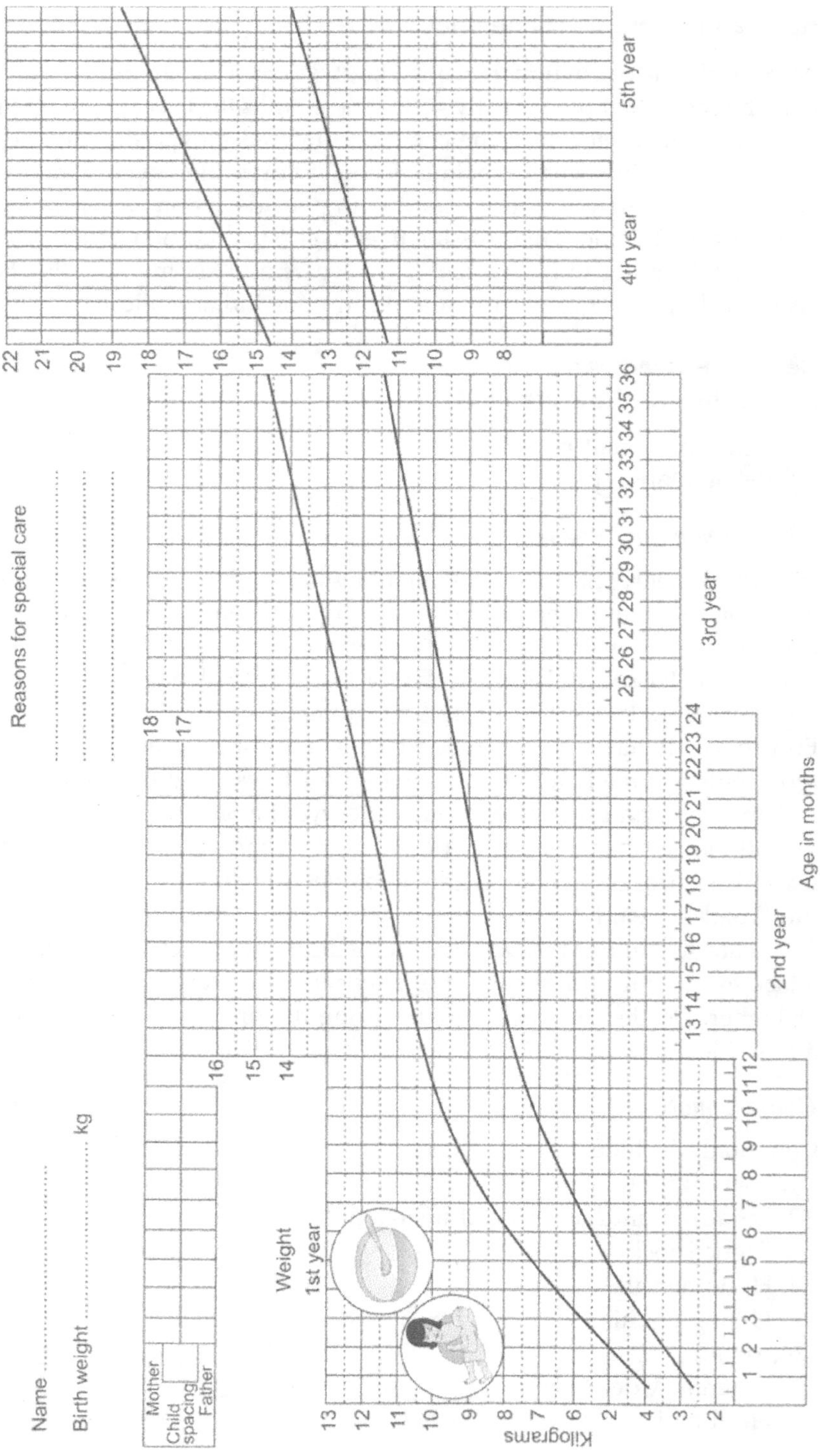

Fig. 6.8: The WHO prototype growth chart

Preventive Measures

There is no simple solution to the problem of PEM. Many types of action are necessary. The following is adopted from the 8th FAO/WHO expert committee on nutrition for the prevention of PEM in the community.

Health Promotion

1. Measures are directed to pregnant and lactating women (education, distribution of supplements like food, iron and folic acid tablets).
2. Promotion of breastfeeding
3. Development of low cost weaning foods, the child should be made to eat food at frequent intervals.
4. Measures to improve family diet
5. Nutrition education promotion of correct feeding practices
6. Home economics
7. Family planning and spacing of births
8. Family environment.

Specific Protection

1. Child's diet must contain protein and energy rich foods, milk, eggs. Fresh fruits should be given if possible
2. Immunization
3. Food fortification.

Early Diagnosis and Treatment

1. Periodic surveillance
2. Early diagnosis of any lag in growth
3. Early diagnosis and treatment of infection and diarrhea
4. Development of programs for early rehydration of children with diarrhea
5. Development of supplementary feeding programs during epidemics
6. Deworming of heavily infested children.

Rehabilitation

1. Nutritional rehabilitation services
2. Hospital treatment
3. Follow-up care.

Calculation of Expected Weight of the Child

For 3 to 12 months old child : $\dfrac{\text{Age (months)} + 9}{2}$

For 1 to 6 years of child : $(\text{Age in years} \times 2) + 8$

For 6 to 12 years of child : $\dfrac{(\text{Age in years} \times 7) - 5}{2}$

Calculation of Expected Height of the Child

At birth	: 50 cm
At one year of age	: 75 cm
For 2 to 12 years of age	: (age in years × 6) × 77

Surface Area According to Weight

Range	*Surface area (meter²)*
1-5 kg	: $(0.05 \times kg) + 0.05$
6-10 kg	: $(0.04 \times kg) + 0.1$
11-20 kg	: $(0.03 \times kg) + 0.2$
20-40 kg	: $(0.02 \times kg) + 0.4$

Calculation of Pediatrics Doses

Young's formula : $\dfrac{\text{Age}}{\text{Age} + 12} \times \text{Adult dose}$

Dilling's formula: $\dfrac{\text{Age}}{20} \times \text{Adult dose}$

BREASTFEEDING

A to Z Benefits for Baby

A—Antibodies
B—Brain development
C—Colostrum
D—Digestion
E—Easy
F—Fresh
G—Growth promoting
H—Healthy
I—Immunity factor
J—Joyful
K—Knotting with baby
L—Loving
M—Magnificent
N—Nutrition
O—Obesity prevention
P—Promotes development
Q—Quantity unlimited
R—Recommended
S—Satisfactory
T—Time tested
U—Unique
V—Valuable
W—White blood
X—Xenial
Y—Yummy
Z—Zephyr

Advantages to Mother

1. Feeling of motherhood
2. Reduces postpartum bleeding

3. Natural birth spacing method
4. Reduces risk of cancer
5. Economical
6. Reduces chances of osteoporosis
7. Helps to lose weight.

BIBLIOGRAPHY

1. Belavady B, Gopalan C. Indian J Med Res 1959;47:234.
2. Govt of India. RCH II and family planning—program implementation plan (PIP). New Delhi: Ministry of Health and Family Welfare, Govt of India: 2004.
3. Gopalan C, Kamala Jaya Rao. In: Prevention in childhood of health problem in adult life F, Falkner (Ed), Geneva, WHO, 1980.
4. Govt of India, Reproductive and Child Health Service in Urban Areas. Ministry of Health and Family Welfare, Nirman Bhawan, New Delhi.
5. Kohler KA, et al. Vaccine-associated paralytic poliomyelitis in India during 1999: decreased risk despite massive use of oral polio vaccine. Bull WHO 2002;80:210-6.
6. Lallemant M, Jourdain G, Le Couer S. A trial of shortend zidovudine regimens to prevent mother to child transmission of human immunodeficiency virus type 1. N Engl J Med 2000;343:982-91.
7. NFHS-3 IIPS, Mumbai, India, 2005-06.
8. Park's Textbook of Preventive and Social Medicine, 16th edn, Nov 2000.
9. Planning Commission. Tenth five year plan 2002-07. Vol II. New Delhi: Planning Commission GOI;2002.
10. The Management of Nutrition in Major Emergencies. Authorized reprint. WHO Geneva, 2002.
11. Venkatachalam PS, et al. Nutrition for Mother and Child, Spl Rep Ser, No 41, ICMR, New Delhi, 1971.
12. WHO. Risk Approach for MCH Care, WHO Offset Publication No. 39, 1978.
13. WHO. Techn Rep Ser, No. 600, 1976.
14. WHO. The Health Aspects of Food and Nutrition, A manual for developing countries in the Western Pacific Region, 1979,p49.
15. WHO. Techn Rep Ser, No. 477, 1971.
16. WHO. The World Health Report 1996, Report of the Director General.

Chapter 7 Reproductive and Child Health

CHAPTER OUTLINE

- SUBCUTANEOUS DMPA AND HOME INJECTION
- MANUAL VACUUM ASPIRATION (MVA)
- CALCULATION OF THE EFFECTIVE COUPLE PROTECTION RATE (ECPR)

INTRODUCTION

Birth control services involve guidance about the timing, spacing and number of children, education regarding contraceptive methods and provision of facilities for the same, unless we understand the exact technique of use, advantages and disadvantages. It is not possible to motivate eligible couples to use them. Every doctor is expected to know the use of contraceptives thoroughly.

Qualities of Good Contraceptives

The wide variety of contraceptives available today reflects the fact that an ideal contraceptive is yet to be developed. The desirable qualities in a good contraceptive are listed below.

1. Reliability — 100 percent effectiveness
2. Safety — Freed from associated side effect or complication
3. Reversibility — Complete return to fertility when the method is discontinued
4. Low cost
5. Convenience
6. Consumer control
7. Cultural acceptability.

Cafeteria Choice

That is to offer all methods from which an individual can choose according to his needs and wishes and to promote family planning as a way of life.

Conventional Contraceptive

Contraceptive is used to denote those methods that required action at the time of intercourse, i.e. condoms, spermicides, etc.

Contraceptive Failure Rate (CFR) (Table 7.1)

It is calculated as:

$$CFR = \frac{\text{No. of accidental pregnancies} \times 1200}{\text{No. of patients observed} \times \text{months of use}}$$

Example: If 100 couples have used a method for a period of one year and has resulted in 20 accidental pregnancies then the pregnancy rate (contraceptive failure rate) would be:

$$\frac{20 \times 1200}{100 \times 12} = \frac{20}{HWY},$$

where HWY is hundred women years.

Table 7.1: Failure rate of contraceptives

Contraceptive methods	*Failure rate (Pregnancies per 100 women years)*
None used	80
Natural methods	
Rhythm method	25
Withdrawal (coitus interruptus)	25
Barrier methods	
Condom	10-14
Spermicidal	30
Douching	40
Dutch cap	4-6
Today (nanoxynol-9)	9-30
IUCD	
Progestasert	0-3
Lippes loop	3
Copper-7	1.9
Cu-T-200	3.0
Cu-T-200c	0.9
Nova T	0.7
Multiload 250	0.5
Multiload 375	0.1
Oral pills	
Postcoital:	
– Ethinyl estradiol	1-1.5
– Stilbestrol 5 days	0-2.4
Combined (Mala N,D)	0.1
Minipills	2-3
Injected and implants	
Depot (Medroxyprogesterone acetate)	1.0
Depot (Norethisterone Oenanthate)	0.6
Norplant	1.1
Silastic vaginal rings (SVR)	3.5
Centchromen	1.83
Sterilization	
Mini-laparotomy (Pomeroy's method)	0.4
(Madlener method)	7.0
Laparoscopic sterilization	0.6
Hysteroscopic sterilization	1.5

Pregnancy Rate

It is calculated as:

CFR = Twenty per hundred women years (HWY) of exposure.

(Do not forget to write the rate in terms of HWY or you will lose valuable marks).

Methods of Family Planning (Flow chart 7.1)

Flow chart 7.1: Family planning methods

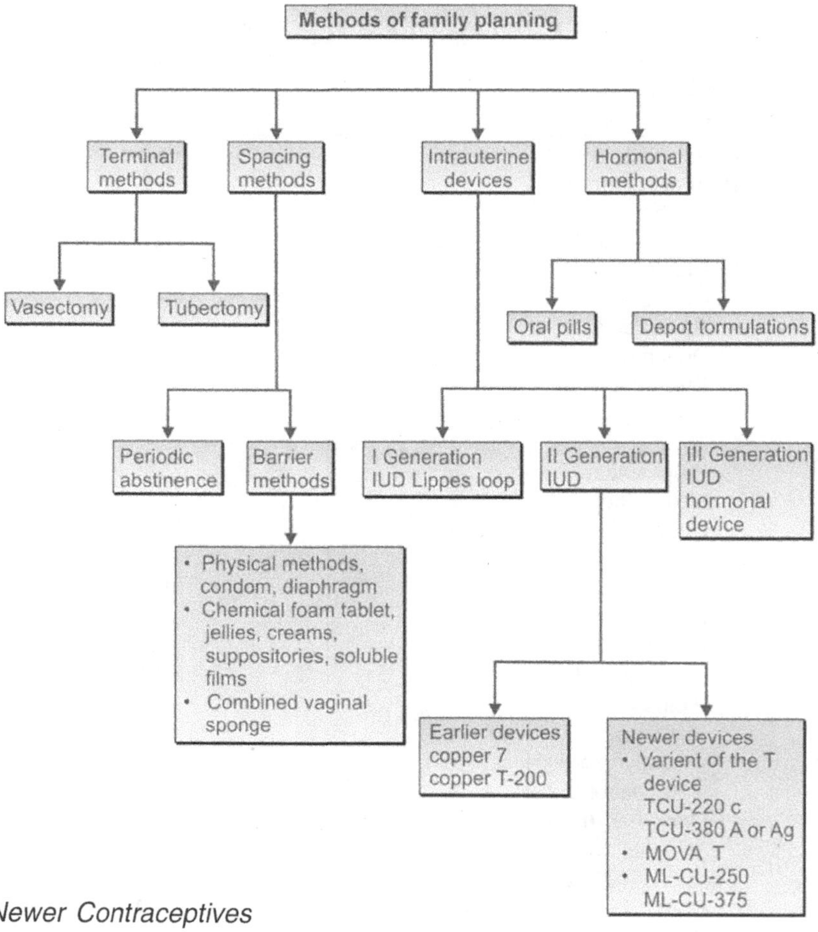

Newer Contraceptives

To expand choices for women, CuT 380A, a long-term intrauterine device has been added in the National Family Welfare Program. This will provide long-term (upto 10 years) protection for women and will be useful for women who have completed their family size but do not want to undergo for terminal methods (Table 7.2).

Table 7.2: A brief account of contraceptives

Method	*How it works*	*Advantages*	*Disadvantages*
Low-dose combined oral contraceptives (the pill)	When a woman swallows a pill each day, her ovaries stop releasing eggs. She cannot become pregnant without an egg. Effectiveness: Very effective if taken every day. Effective as usually used. • No STD protection. Also can be used for emergency contraception	No need to do anything at the time of sex. Monthly periods are regular, light short; milder, fewer cramps. Helps to prevent iron deficiency anemia, ectopic pregnancy ovarian and uterine cancer, and pelvic inflammatory disease (PID)	Some women have upset stomach (especially in first 3 months) and/or spotting or bleeding between menstrual periods, missed periods, mild headaches, breast tenderness and/or slight weight gain. Some women cannot remember pill a every day. In rare cases the pill causes stroke, heart attack, or clots deep in the especially in woman with high leg blood pressure and in woman who smoke and also are 35 or older.
Condom	A very thin, flexible sheath that covers the man's erect penis during sex. It keeps sperm out of the woman's vagina. Also prevents many STDs from passing between sex partners. Effectiveness: Effective if used correctly and every time. Only somewhat effective as usually used*. Best method for STD prevention.	Only method proved to prevent STDs, including HIV/AIDS, and also pregnancy when used correctly with every act of sexual intercourse. Helps prevent conditions caused by STDs, such as pelvic inflammatory disease (PID) in women and infertility in both women and men. No need to see a health care provider before using.	Must take the time to put condom on erect penis before sex. May decrease sensation. May cause itching for a few people allergic to latex rubber.

Contd...

Contd...

Method	*How it works*	*Advantages*	*Disadvantages*
Female sterilization	A specially trained health care provider makes a small surgical opening in the woman's abdomen and closes off both tubes that carry eggs from the ovaries to the womb. Then eggs cannot meet the man's sperm. The woman still has menstrual periods. Effectiveness: Very effective and permanent. * No STD protection.	A single procedure leads to effective, lifelong family planning. Nothing to remember and no repeated clinic visits needed. No known long-term side effects or health risks. A woman can still have sex as usual.	Usually painful for a few days after the procedure. Slight chance if infection or bleeding at incision, internal infection or bleeding, or injury to internal organs. Usually not reversible.
Vasectomy	A specially trained health care provider makes a small surgical opening in the man's scrotum (the sac of skin that holds the testes) and closes off both tubes that carry sperm from his testes. The man still produces semen, but it has no sperm in it to make a women pregnant. Effectiveness: Very effective and permanent. * No STD protection.	A single quick procedure leads to effective, lifelong family planning. A man can still ejaculate and have sex as usual. No known long-term side effects of health risks.	Not effective at once. Couple must use another method for at least the first 20 ejaculations or 3 months. Usually some discomfort for a few days after the procedure. Possibly also some pain, bruising in the scrotum. Usually not reversible.
Long-acting injectable contraceptives	Injectables Depo-Provera (DMPA) and Norethisteron enanate (NET EN) stop ovaries from releasing eggs. A woman cannot become pregnant without an egg. They also thicken cervical mucus so sperm cannot pass. Effectiveness: Very effective when	Private. No one else can tell that the woman is using contraception. Long-term yet reversible. Each injection lasts at least 3 months (DMPA) or 2 months (NET EN). The woman has to remember only to return for next injection.	Changes in menstrual bleeding are normal—such as light spotting at first and no periods after the first year of use. (Some women consider no periods an advantage). Some women gain some weight. (Some women consider this an

Contd...

Contd...

Method	*How it works*	*Advantages*	*Disadvantages*
	spaced 3 months apart (for DPMA) or 2 months apart (for NET EN)*.		advantage).
Norplant implants	Small plastic capsules placed under the skin of a woman's arm slowly release a hormone. The hormone thickness cervical mucus so sperm cannot pass. Sometimes also stops ovaries from releasing eggs. Effectiveness: Very effective. *No STD protection.	Lasts at least 5 years; fertility returns when capsules are taken out. Nothing to remember. No need to do anything at the time of sex. Helps prevent iron deficiency anemia and ectopic pregnancy.	Changes in menstrual bleeding are normal—especially spotting or bleeding between periods. Some women have no periods. (Some women consider no periods an advantage). Clinic procedure needed to start or stop use.
Intrauterine device (IUD)	A small, flexible plastic frame, often with copper wire or sleeves on it. A health care provider inserts the IUD into the woman's womb through her vagina. The IUD stops egg and sperm from meeting. Effectiveness: Very effective. *No STD protection.	Effective prevention of pregnancy for as long as 10 years; fertility returns when IUD is taken out. No need to do anything at the time of sex. Can be inserted just after childbirth.	Many women at first have longer, heavier menstrual periods, bleeding or spotting between periods, or more menstrual cramps or pain. Clinic procedure needed to start or stop use. Pelvic inflammatory disease is more likely to follow STD infection if a woman is using an IUD.
Fertility awareness based methods (Including periodic	A woman learns to recognize the fertile time of her menstrual cycle. To prevent pregnancy, a couple	No physical side effects. Very little or no cost. Most couples can use these	More effective methods take 2 or 3 months to learn. Calendar method takes 6 months of recording

Contd...

Contd...

Method	*How it works*	*Advantages*	*Disadvantages*
abstinence)	avoids vaginal sex during the fertile time or else uses a barrier method or withdrawal. Effectiveness: Effective if used correctly. Only somewhat effective as usually. *No STD protection	methods if committed to them. Acceptable to some religious groups that objects to other	cycle length before it can be used. Long abstinence may cause tension. Some methods may be less reliable or more difficult to use if woman is sick, has a vaginal infection, or is breast-feeding.
Vaginal methods (Spermicides, diaphragm, cervical cap)	A woman places a spermicide, or else a diaphragm or cap with spermicide, in her vagina before sex. Spermicides kill sperm or stop their movement. Diaphragms and caps keep sperm out of the womb. Effectiveness: Effective if used correctly and every time. Only somewhat effective as usually used. * Help prevent STDs.	Woman—controlled method for use when needed. May help prevent some STDs and conditions caused by STDs. Possibly some protection against HIV/AIDS, but this is not proved. No need to see a health care provider before using spermicides.	May cause irritation. Can make urinary tract infections more common. Woman must put method in vagina before every act of sexual intercourse.

What to do if you miss one or more pills (Flow chart 7.2)

Flow chart 7.2: Every time you miss one or more active pills (days 1-21:)

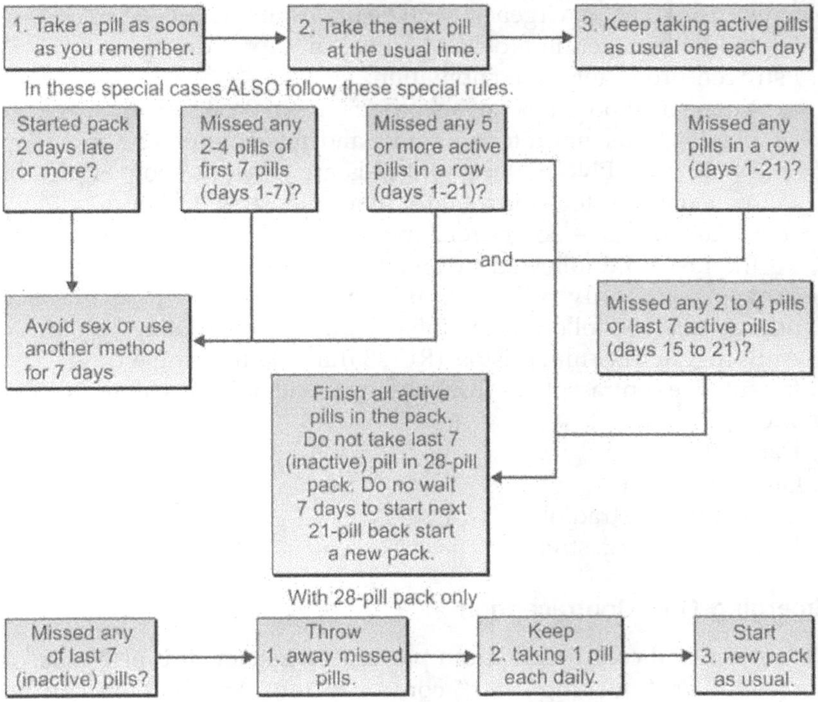

Anti-fertility Vaccines

Under development.

1. Anti-hCG Vaccines—β subunit of hCG linked chemically to a carrier protein.
2. Immunization of female using specific antigen-Zona pellucida, trophoblastic surface antigen, sperm-inhibine antigen.
3. Anti GnRH Vaccine—Hocks LHRH activity prevents spermatogenesis/ ovulation.

No Scalpel Vasectomy

It is an improvement on the conventional vasectomy as it is safe, convenient and more acceptable to male. In this operation the pair of scissors is used to pierce the skin and through small opening the vas is tied and cut. No stitch is required. This new method is being offered to men, who have completed their families on a voluntary basis.

Emergency Contraceptives

Experience gained from clinic-based trials is not adequate from the point of program operations. Without careful planning and preparation, the new methods may be poorly accepted and the dropout and pregnancy rates may be unacceptably high. It also damages the reputation of family planning program. Emergency contraceptives are as follows:

1. High-dose estrogen in a dose of 5 mg daily for 5 days
2. Estrogen-progesterone combination:
   a. Yuzpe method: EE 50 µg + LNG 250 µg of 2 pills given as soon as possible after unprotected coitus and repeat after 12 hours
   b. EE 30 µg + LNG 150 mg of 4 pills are taken as soon as possible after unprotected coitus and 4 more pills after 12 hours
   c. EE 200 µg + dl – norgestrel 2 mg or 1 mg/LNG 1 mg of one pill as the first dose followed by another pill after 12 hours.
3. Progesterone-only pill: LNG 0.75 mg as soon as possible after unprotected sex followed by another pill 12 hours later
4. Antiprogesterone-mifepriston (RU-486) in 600 mg single dose
5. Intrauterine contraceptives (IUD) insertion within 5 days of unprotected sex
6. Danazol
7. GnRH antagonist

   EE = ethinyl estradiol
   LNG = levonorgestrel

Emerging Oral Contraception

Emergency oral contraception can prevent pregnancy. It is also called as postcoital or "morning after" contraception. Any women can use emergency oral contraception if she is not already pregnant.

Emerging oral contraception should be started up to 72 hours after unprotected sex.

It mainly stops ovulation but perhaps also works in other ways. It does not disrupt existing pregnancy. It seems to prevent at least three-fourths of pregnancies that would otherwise have occurred. (Average chance of pregnancy due to one act of unprotected intercourse in the second or third week of the menstrual cycle is 8 percent; after emergency oral contraception—1-2%). The sooner emergency oral contraceptive are used, the better they prevent pregnancy.

Emergency oral contraception should not be used in place of family planning methods. It should be used only in an emergency for example:

- A woman has had sex against her will or has been forced to have sex (rape).
- A condom has broken.
- An IUD has come out of place.
- A woman has run out of oral contraceptives, has missed 2 or more progestin only oral contraceptives, or is more than a few weeks late for a DMPA injection and has had sex without using other family planning.

- Sex took place without contraception, and woman wants to avoid pregnancy.

Emergency oral contraception does not prevent sexually transmitted diseases.

Give Specific Instructions

1. Upto 72 hours after unprotected sex, the woman should take 4 low dose or 2 "standard dose" combined oral contraceptives, or else take 20 or 25 progestin contraceptives, and then take another equal dose 12 hours later.
   Important: If she takes pills from a 28 days packet of combined oral contraceptives, she must be sure to take hormone-containing pills. Show her which pills contain hormones.
2. If willing, she should start another method immediately, such as condoms and/or spermicide, or she should avoid sex until she can start her preferred methods.

Progestin-only pills better for emergency contraception.

A large WHO study has found that progestin-only pills are better than combined oral contraceptives (progestin + estrogen) for emergency contraception. Used for emergency contraception, progestin – only pills were more effective and caused less nausea and less vomiting.

Dosage: Either 20 or 25 progestin-only oral contraceptive tablets up to 72 hours after unprotected sex. Then 20 or 25 more tablets 12 hours later.

Note: Special-purpose pills, each containing 0.75 milligrams levonorgestrel may be available in some places.

Table 7.3 tells us how many pills to take according to their formulation:

Table 7.3: Pills and their formulation

Formulation (Examples of brands)	*Number of pills to swallow within 72 hours*	*Number of pills to swallow 12 hours later*
Progestin-only oral contraceptive containing 0.075 milligrams (75 micrograms) of norgestrel (Ovrette, Neogest, Norgeal)	20	20
Progestin-only contraceptives containing 0.03 milligrams (30 micrograms) of levonorgestrel (Follicle, Microval, Microlut, Microluton, Mikro–30 Wyeth, Mikro-30, Norgestin, Nortel).	25	25
Low dose COCs containing 0.15 or 0.25 milligrams of levonorgestrel or 0.5 milligrams of norgestrel plus 0.03 milligrams (30 micrograms) of ethinyl	4	4

Contd...

Contd...

Formulation (Examples of brands)	*Number of pills to swallow within 72 hours*	*Number of pills to swallow 12 hours later*
estradiol (Lo-feminal, Lo-ovral, Mala–D (India), Nordette, Microgynon-30)		
"Standard-dose" COCs containing 0.125 or 0.25 milligrams of **levonorgestrel** or 0.5 milligrams of norgestrel plus 0.05 milligrams (50 micrograms) of ethinyl estradiol (Eugynon 50, Nordiol, Ovral, Microgynon – 50, Nordette – 50)	2	2
Levonorgestrel 0.75 mg (Postinor – 2)	1	1

COC = Combined oral contraceptive

Important

Other combined oral contraceptive pills may work too but their effectiveness for emergency contraception has not been tested. (Note that equal weights of different hormones do not mean equal strength).

Give Advice on Common Problems

- *Nausea:* Suggest that she eat something soon after taking the pills to reduce any nausea. Prescription anti-nausea medicines such as Dramamine and Marezine can reduce the risk of nausea when taken half hour before taking emergency contraceptive pills and every four to six hours thereafter.
- *Vomiting:* If the woman vomits within two hours after taking the pills, she need to take another dose. Otherwise, she should not take any extra pills. Extra pills will not make the method more effective and they may increase nausea. If vomiting continues, she can repeat dose by vaginal replacement.
- Her next monthly period may start a few days earlier or later than expected. Reassure her that this is not a bad sign.

Explain Specific Reasons to Return to the Health Care Provider

1. Advise her to return or see another health care provider if her next period is quite different from unusual for her, especially if it is:
   - Unusual light (possible pregnancy).
   - Dose not starts within four weeks (possible pregnancy).
   - Unusually painful (possible ectopic pregnancy. But emergency oral contraception does not cause ectopic pregnancy).
2. Describe the symptoms of sexually transmitted diseases, for example, unusual vaginal discharge, pain or burning on urination. Advise her to see a health care provider if any of these symptoms occur.

Introduction to Injectable Contraceptives

- Depot-medroxyprogesterone acetate (DMPA) is given every three months. It contains a progestin, similar to the natural hormone that a woman's body makes. The hormone is released slowly into bloodstream also known as depot-medroxyprogesterone acetate, Depo-proverai, Depo and Mejestron.
- There are other injectable contraceptives. NET EN-also called Noristrat, norethindrone enanthate and norethisterone enanthate is given every two months.

Mechanism of Action

- Mainly stops ovulation (release of eggs from ovaries).
- Also thickens cervical mucus, making it difficulty for sperm to pass through.

DMPA does not work by disrupting existing pregnancy. Failure rate 0.3 pregnancies per women in first year of use (1 in every 333) when injections are regularly spaced three months apart. Pregnancy rates may be higher for women who are late for injection or who miss an injection if provider runs out of supplies.

Advantages and Disadvantages of Injectable Contraceptives

Advantages

- Very effective
- Private. No one else can tell that a women is using it.
- Long-term pregnancy prevention but reversible. One injection prevents pregnancy for at least three months.
- Does not interfere with sex.
- Increased sexual enjoyment because no need to worry about pregnancy.
- No daily pill taking.
- Allows some flexibility in return visits. Client can return as much as two week early or weeks late for next injection.
- Can be used at any age.
- Quantity and quality of breast milk do not seem to be harmed. Can be used by nursing mothers as soon as six weeks after childbirth.
- No estrogen side effect. Does not increase the risk of estrogen related complications such as heart attack.
- DMPA prevents ectopic pregnancies in user
- DMPA prevents endometrial cancer in user
- DMPA prevents uterine fibroids in user
- DMPA help prevents ovarian cancer in user.

- Special advantages for some women:
  - May help in preventing iron deficiency anemia.
  - May make seizures less frequent in women with epilepsy.
  - Makes sickle cell crisis less frequent and less painful.

Disadvantages

- Common side effects (not sign of sickness)
- Changes in menstrual bleeding are likely including:
- Light spotting or bleeding. Most common at first.
  - Heavy bleeding can occur at first but rare
  - Some women will have amenorrhea, especially after first year of use. It may cause weight gain (average of 1-2 kilo or 2-4 lbs each year). Some women see weight gain as advantage.
- Delayed return of fertility (until DMPA levels in the body drop). About four months longer wait before pregnancy than for women who had been using combined oral contraceptives, IUDs, condoms or a vaginal method.
- Requires another injection every three months.
- May cause headaches, breast tenderness, moodiness, nausea, hair loss, less sex drive and/or acne in some women.
- Does not protect against sexually transmitted diseases including HIV/ AIDS. Table formulations, injection schedules and availability of injectable contraceptives are given in Table 7.4.

Table 7.4: Injection schedules and availability of injectable contraceptives

Common trade names	*Formulation*	*Injection type and schedule*
	Progestin-only injectables	
Depo-provera, Mejestron, contracep, Depo-prodasone	Depot medroxyprogesterone acetate (DMPA) 150 mg	One intramuscular (IM) injection every three months
Depo-sub provera 140 (DMPA – SC)	DMPA 140 mg	One subcutaneous injection every three months
Noristrat, Norigest, Doryx	Norethisterone enanthate (NET- EN) 200 mg	One IM injection every two months
	Combined injectables (progestin + estrogen)	
Cyclofem, Ciclofeminina, Lunelle	Medroxyprogesterone scetate 25 mg + Estradiol cypionate 5 mg (MPA/E2V)	One IM injection every month
Deladroxate, Perlutal, Topasel, Patectro, Nomagest	Dihydroxyprogesterone (algestone) acetophenide 150 mg+ Estradiol enanthate 10 mg	One IM injection every month
Anafortan, Yectames	Dihydroxyprogesterone (algestone) acetophenide 75 mg + Estradiol enanthate 5 mg	One IM injection every month

SUBCUTANEOUS DMPA AND HOME INJECTION

A new lower dose formulation of DMPA, depo-subQ provera 104 (also called DMPA-SC) is injected under the skin rather than in the muscle. It contains 104 mg of DMPA rather than the 150 mg in the intramuscular formulation. Like the intramuscular formulation, DMPA-SC is given at three months intervals.

Approved first in the United States and the United Kingdom, subcutaneous injection of DMPA may be available in some developing countries by 2008. DMPA-SC is available only in prefilled, single use syringes. In developing countries it will be available only in prefilled Uniject devices designed as the formulation for subcutaneous injection.

DMPA-SC is just as effective as the formulation injected into the muscle and the patterns of bleeding changes and amount of weight gain are similar. One year continuation rates in clinical trails were high, 68 percent on average at sites in North and South America and 80 percent in Europe and Asia. Despite the lower dose, DMPA-SC is effective for over weight or obese women.

Injections of DMPA-SC are given in the upper thigh or abdomen. DMPA-SC should not be injected intramuscularly and intramuscular formulation should not be injected subcutaneously. The intramuscular formulation cannot be diluted to make the lower dose subcutaneous formulation.

Injectables work mainly by preventing the development and release of eggs from the ovaries (ovulation). They also thicken cervical mucus, which blocks sperm from meeting the egg. Both progestin-only and combined injectables are very effective when users return on time for their next injections.

Long-term studies of the health risks and benefits are under way, but few results are available yet. Still combined injectable contraceptives contain the same types of hormones as combined oral contraceptives (COCs). Therefore researchers assume that most of the findings about COCs also apply to combined injectables. A difference is that monthly injectables are not processed by liver before entering the bloodstreams, as are medication taken by mouth. As a result, monthly injectable have less effect.

Centchroman

This oral contraceptive does not contain any steroidal hormones, developed by the Central Drug Research Laboratory, Lucknow. It is marked under the brand names "Saheli" and "Centron". It is taken twice weekly for intial two months and thereafter once a week and has no known side effects, except that in about 8 percent of users there is delay in menses. It is advised to use barrier method for the initial two months of start. Fertility typically returns within six months of discontinuation of Centchroman. However 80 percent of the women do not know about them (Vatsayan A et al, 1996).

Family Planning Insurance Scheme

Government of India is introducing a Family Planning Insurance Scheme for acceptors of sterilization and indemnity cover for doctors performing sterilization procedures in both government and private/NGO/ corporate health facilities. The insurance scheme will be operated by the Oriental Insurance Company Ltd. (OCIL). The insurance scheme is as follows:

Section I:

1. Death due to sterilization in hospital Rs.1,00,000
2. Death due to sterilization within 30 days of discharge from hospital Rs. 30,000
3. Failure of sterilization (including first insurance of conception after sterilization) Rs. 20,000
4. Medical complication occurring within 60 days of sterilization operation Rs. 20,000

   *To be reimbursed on the basis of actual expenditure incurred, not exceeding Rs. 20,000.

Section II:

All the doctors/health facilities including doctors/health facilities of central, state, local-self governments, other public sectors and all accredited doctors/health facilities of non-governmental and private sectors rendering Family planning services, conducting such operations shall stand identified against the claims arising out of failure of sterilization, death or medical complication resulting there from up to a maximum amount of Rs. 2 lakhs per doctor/health facility in court, which would be borne by the insurance company within certain limits.

All persons undergoing sterilization operation in public health facility/ accredited health facility in private/NGO sector are covered under section I of the policy. The consent form filled by the person at the time of enrolling himself/herself for sterilization operation shall be proof of coverage under the scheme.

The scheme is uniformly applicable for all States/Union territories. Government of India has paid entire premium for Insurance policy. States do not have any expenditure under this scheme.

The claim settlements has been decentralized at state and District levels and nominated officers of third party administrators (TPAs) will co-ordinate with existing machinery of the States/UTs.

The present scheme will do away with the complicated process of payment of ex-gratia to the acceptors of sterilization for the treatment of postoperative complications, medical complications or deaths attributed to the procedure of sterilization or deaths resulting from sterilization but would also provide indemnity cover to the Doctor/ health facility affirming sterilization procedure.

Medical Methods of Abortion

Medical abortion methods are especially effective in the first trimester, most effective before 49 days of pregnancy. This is due to the fact that both Mifepristone and Methotrexate cause detachment of the trophoblast (outer layer of developing embryo which ultimately forms the placenta) from the uterine wall, which is easier to accomplish the less developed the pregnancy.

Mifepristone and Misoprostol

Mifepristone (aka RU486) is more effective, earlier in the pregnancy it is used: "women with pregnancy durations of seven weeks or less LMP experience a complete abortion about 95 percent of the time. Success rates decrease to about 80 percent in the ninth week LMP."Mifepristone acts primarily as an anti-progestational agent. The progesterone receptors in the endometrium are blocked, and the disruption of the embryo and trophoblast lead to a decrease in human chorionic gonadotropin (hCG) produced by the placental tissues and therefore a withdrawal of hormonal support for the corpus luteum. This provides the rationale for why this method is more effective the earlier the pregnancy, because the more dependent the pregnancy is on progesterone produced by the corpus luteum, the more likely the action of the progesterone antagonist, mifepristone, will result in abortion. The regimen involves three visits to an abortion provider. On the first visit, the woman takes 600 mg mifepristone orally. She returns two days later for administration of Misoprostol, a prostaglandin which serves to soften and open the cervix and cause contractions of the uterus, expelling the contents of the pregnancy. In five percent of pregnancy, mifepristone alone is enough to induce abortion, but in all other cases 400 to 800 ug of misoprostol is administered orally or vaginally. Following administration of misoprostol, "three-fourths experience expulsion within 24 hours and 80 to 95 percent abort within two weeks." The third visit is for follow-up.

Side Effects

Most of the side effects when using this early abortion option are caused by the second medication, misoprostol. Side-effects may include heavy bleeding, headache, nausea, vomiting, diarrhea, and heavy cramping.

Criteria

Abortion medication may be an option if you:

- Are less than eight weeks since your last menstrual period.
- Are willing and able to give informed consent.
- Have the support you need such as access to reliable transportation and ability to communicate with the clinic by telephone.
- Live no more than two hours away from emergency medical care (a hospital).
- Are able to come back to the clinic for one to three follow-up appointments.
- Agree to have a surgical abortion if the misoprostol does not induce termination.

Contraindications

- Blood clotting problem or women on anticoagulant medicine.
- Severe anemia.
- Adrenal failure.
- Long-term systemic corticosteroids.
- Ectopic pregnancy.
- Mass in the tubes or ovaries.
- Inherited porphyria.
- Allergy to mifepristone, misoprostol or other prostaglandin medicine.
- Severe diarrhea.

Future Fertility

According to studies of the Food and Drug Administration (FDA) and the National Abortion Federation, there are no known long-term risks associated with using mifepristone and misoprostol. Therefore, women may pursue another pregnancy whenever they feel the time is right after having a Medical Abortion.

MANUAL VACUUM ASPIRATION (MVA)

Methods of Uterine Evacuation

Surgical Methods of Evacuation

The primary surgical methods of uterine evacuation following incomplete abortion in the first trimester are dilation and curettage (D and C) and vacuum aspiration (VA).

The decision on which method should be used to empty the uterus should be based on:

- The duration of gestation
- Availability of equipment and supplies
- Training and skill level of staff and facility.

D and C also called sharp curettage uses mental surgical instruments to empty the uterus. The use of D and C may entail operating theater facilities and staff trained in surgical techniques and general anesthesia.

VA uses a vacuum of at least 55 mm Hg with a cannula made of flexible plastic, rigid plastic or metal to evacuate the uterus. This technique has low complication rates and involves very little trauma. It can often be performed in a clinic or outpatient setting that requires fewer resources and fewer staff.

Currently VA is preferred to D and C because of the lower complication rates and the reduced need for transporting the woman to a high level facility with an operating theater.

Types of Vacuum Aspiration

Two types of vacuum aspiration (VA) are available:

1. Electric vacuum aspiration uses an electric pump and rigid cannula for uterine evacuation in the first trimester.
2. Manual vacuum aspiration (MVA) uses a hand held vacuum syringe and flexible plastic cannula. Foot-operated pumps also available in some areas. MVA was developed in the early 1970s in the US. MVA is a safe, effective and low cost method of uterine evacuation. MVA is a very similar to the better known technique of menstrual regulation (MR).

Mechanism of MVA

The MVA cannula is inserted through the cervix and attached to a syringe that contains a vacuum. A valve or two valves are compressed which creates this vacuum. When the valve is released, the contents of the uterus are emptied by suction into the syringe. The syringe aspirates (provides suction), while the cannula reaches into the uterus.

Key Aspects of MVA Mechanism

- It does not require electricity
- It is portable
- The syringe has two functions: source of vacuum and a container
- The syringe (double and single valve) holds 60 cc of aspirated fluid and tissue.

The Government of India has approved the use of MVA for termination of pregnancy up to eight weeks of gestation. The MTP Act special provision for this and Ministry of Health and Family Welfare (MOHFW) has issued guidelines for use of MVA.

Uses of MVA Equipment

The single and double valve syringes may be used for performing abortion or for treatment of incomplete abortion up to 8 weeks from the last menstrual period (LMP) (confirmed by bimanual examination), and the double valve syringes may be used for MVA for abortion or treatment of incomplete abortion up to 12 weeks LMP.

The single valve syringes are also appropriate for use in obtaining an endometrial biopsy. MVA can be used in outpatients setting, thus increasing women's access to care.

Advantages of MVA

- Incidence of hemorrhage, pelvic infection, cervical injury and uterine perforation are lower than with D and C.
- Because no general anesthesia is used, the recovery time is quicker.
- Less cervical dilation is necessary.
- Heavy sedation is required.
- Costs for procedure, time of staff and resources are lower.

CALCULATION OF THE EFFECTIVE COUPLE PROTECTION RATE (ECPR)

Suppose a village is having a population of 2000, with 320 eligible couples. Sixty of the eligible couples were using condoms, ten were using oral contraceptives, ten got IUCD inserted, four have got vasectomy and sixteen tubectomy. Calculate the effective couple protection rate of this village?

Effective Protection

Effective protection of contraceptive accepted:

- Sterilization (Vasectomy/Tubectomy): 100%
- Oral contraceptive: 100%
- IUCD: 95%
- Conventional contraceptives: 50%

Based on these rates the effective protection is calculated:

- Sterilization $= \frac{20 \times 100}{100} = 20$
- Oral contraceptive $= \frac{10 \times 100}{100} = 10$
- IUCD $= \frac{10 \times 95}{100} = 9.5$
- Conventional contraceptives $= \frac{60 \times 50}{100} = 30$

- $ECPR = \frac{20 + 10 + 9.5 + 30}{320} \times 100 = 21.7\%$

Pearl Index

Pearl index give rise to the failure rate of the contraceptives. It is calculated by the formula:

$$= \frac{\text{No. of accidental pregnancies}}{\text{No. of women observed} \times \text{months of use}} \times 1200$$

Important Facts about Contraceptives (Tables 7.5 and 7.6)

Table 7.5: Important fact about contraceptives

Intrauterine contraceptive devices (IUCD)	
• Removal rate at the end of one year due to complication and side effects	15.16%
• Expulsion rate	5.15%
• Perforation rate	1-3 per 1000 insertion
• Ectopic pregnancy	1-30 pregnancies
• Copper T 200 effective for	3 years
• Copper T 380 effective for	6-8 years
• NOVAT	5 years
Vasectomy reversibility	
• After anastomoses	60-70%
Tubectomy reversibility by tuboplasty	
• For laparoscopic sterilization	70%

Table 7.6: Choice of contraceptives

Subject	*Contraceptive*
Newly married	Pill
Postabortal	Pill
Postpartum nonlactating	Pill
Women below 35 years of age	Minipill or injectable steroid
Above 35 years of age	Pill
Women who smoke and above 35 years of age	IUCD
Diabetic mothers/overt diabetic	IUCD
Pulmonary tuberculosis on chemotherapy	Barrier methods (condom)
Heart disease (incomplete family)	IUCD
Heart disease decompensated with complete family	Barrier methods (condom) Permanent sterilization of husband

BIBLIOGRAPHY

1. Clive Wood. Contraception Explained, Geneva, WHO, 1975.
2. Dalsimer I, et al. Barrier Methods, Population Report Series H:I, 1973.
3. Medical methods for first trimester abortion Cochrane review on methods available for first trimester abortions.
4. Medical methods for termination of pregnancy report of a WHO scientific group technical report series, No. 871.
5. National Population Policy Action Plan 2002-2003, Department of Family Welfare, Ministry of Health and Family Welfare, Government of India.
6. Park's Textbook of Community Medicine, 16th edn.
7. Sherris JD. Barrier Methods, Population Report Series H:6, 1982.
8. WHO. The Work of WHO 1976-77, Biennial Report, 1978.

Chapter 8 Immunization

CHAPTER OUTLINE

- NATIONAL IMMUNIZATION SCHEDULE

NATIONAL IMMUNIZATION SCHEDULE

The age at which the vaccines are best given and the number of doses of each vaccine is called the immunization schedule. The immunization schedule is framed keeping in view the epidemiological pattern of the diseases, the types of vaccines available and the administrative and economic feasibility of providing the services. In our country we give:

- Two doses of TT to pregnant women
- Three doses each of DPT and OPV and one dose each of BCG and measles vaccines to infants
  School children are given DT and TT vaccines.

Immunization of Pregnant Woman

The pregnant woman develops adequate antibody titers to protect herself and her child after birth from tetanus (NNT) only two to three weeks after the second dose. It is recommended that the first dose be given on first contact during pregnancy. The second dose should be given ensuring at least one month's interval after the first completing the schedule as early as possible.

Reactions after Vaccination

Reactions after vaccination are in general mild and of a short duration. These may be:

- Mild fever
- Local pain, swelling at the site of injection
- Mild rash one week after measles vaccination
- A lump or papule appears in the third or fourth week after BCG vaccination.
- It is generally not painful but is tender to touch. The papule increases in size to 6 to 10 mm in diameter by the sixth week. The nodule softens with the formation of pus. No treatment is necessary. At the end of 10 to 12 weeks only a small scar is visible .

In rare cases convulsions or collapse after DPT vaccination have been observed. In such cases further doses of DPT should be stopped. Instead, one dose of DT may be given (second dose). If two doses of DPT have already been administered, further doses are not required.

Complications

Abscess formation is usually due to the use of unsterilized or inadequately sterilized syringes and needles.

The injections are painful if blunt needles are used.

Determine Needs and Requirement

Estimation of Eligibles

Your aim is to provide universal immunization coverage in your area. In order to do this you must have an estimate of the total annual number of pregnant women and infants. The numbers can be calculated by using the formula given below:

Population × Birth rate = No. of pregnant women

Population × BR × (1-IMR) = No infants at one year of age.

For example,

If the population served by a health center is 50,000, the birth rate-30/1000.

And IMR 100/1000 live births, the expected number of pregnant woman and infants will be:

50,000 × 0.03 = 1500

50,000 × 0.03 × (1-0.01) = 1350

The estimates of the pregnant women and infants should be worked out at each level locally and compare with the list maintained by the health worker to ensure completeness of registration.

The health workers should have a list of the pregnant women and infants in the areas covered by them. The list should be kept up to date. The information can easily be obtained during, their visits to the villages and also through the village level workers such as *dais*,VHGs, *anganwadi* workers (AWWs) and others. The name of the child should be registered soon after birth, the vaccinations being given when the child reaches the right age.

At any given time, 100 percent of the total estimated annual number of infants and 60 percent of the pregnant women should be registered. If the numbers do not fall within 10 percent of your estimates, it is your responsibility to get the lists updated immediately. You may already have the required information in the Eligible Couples and Child Register (ECCR).

Estimation of Number of Contacts

The number of vaccination sessions to be scheduled depends upon the number of children to be vaccinated in the area served by the health center or vaccination site. If there are ten or more children to be vaccinated each day, schedule daily sessions. This will ensure that all children can be vaccinated at the earliest acceptable age and will therefore, give them the best protection against disease. If there are fewer than ten children to be vaccinated each day,the vaccines and the time of the health staff may be wasted by holding daily sessions, so it is better to plan fewer vaccination sessions.

To determine the number of children to receive vaccinations per month (monthly target population), divide the number of children to receive vaccinations for the year by 12 and multiply by the number of doses of the vaccine which need to be given.

Contaminated vaccines can lead to severe reactions including death. Use only sterile syringes and needles to mix vaccines and to draw them from the vials or ampoules (Measles and BCG vaccines). Use a single sterile syringe and needle for each injection. Do not use opened vials in subsequent sessions. Display these instructions at all sites where immunization sessions are conducted.

The parents should be informed of the expected side effects so that they do not worry. If there is any anxiety they should be encouraged to return to the health center for consultation.

Difference between EPI and UIP

Expanded Program of Immunization (EPI)

- Started in 1978
- High coverage of children under two years and pregnant women
- DPT, BCG and TT vaccines
- DT and TT vaccines for school children
- Oral polio vaccine added in 1979.

Universal Immunization Program (UIP)

- Started in 1985
- Universal coverage of infants and pregnant women
- Measles vaccine added to the program
- Strengthen cold chain
- Take up districts in phases.

National Immunization Schedule (Tables 8.1 and 8.2)

Table 8.1: Schedule of National Immunization

a. For Infants	
At birth (for institutional deliveries)[$]	• BCG and OPV-O dose Hepatitis B*
At 6 weeks	• BCG (if not given at birth) Hepatitis B
	• DPT-1 and OPV-1 Hepatitis B
At 10 weeks	• DPT-2 and OPV-2 Hepatitis B
At 14 weeks	• DPT-3 and OPV-3 Hepatitis B
At 9 months	• Measles

Contd...

Contd...

b. At 16-24 months	• DPT and OPV (Booster 1)
c. At 5-6 years	• DPT (Booster 2) OPV #
d. At 10 and at 16 years	• *Tetanus toxoid*—The second dose of TT vaccine should be given at an interval of one month if there is no clear history or documented evidence of previous immunization with DPT, DT or TT vaccines
e. For pregnant women Early in pregnancy One month after	• $TT_1 - TT_2$

Note: i. Interval between two doses should not be less than one month.
ii. Minor cough, colds and mild fever are not a contraindication to vaccination
iii. In some states Hepatitis B vaccine is given as routine immunization.

$ For institutional delivery OPV and Hepatitis B is considered as zero dose.
# Initially DT used to be given recently DPT is advocated

Table 8.2: Some more vaccines in the immunizations schedule

Vaccine	*Dose*	*Age*	*Cost per dose*
1. Hepatitis A	1st Dose	Before 1st year of birth	
	2nd dose	After 1 year of birth	Rs 900
2. Chickenpox	One dose	After 1st year within 2 years	Rs 1,300-1,500
3. Typhoid		After 3 years, repeated every 3 years	Rs 150
4. Meningitis	1st dose	1½ months	Rs 450
	2nd dose	2½ months	
	3rd dose	3½ months	

Note: i. Interval between doses should not be less than one month
ii. The dose of all vaccines is 0.5 ml except BCG which is 0.1 ml polio vaccine is given by mouth in 2 drops.
iii. Check the label of the vial before use.

The Indian Association of Pediatrics recommends four more vaccines in the immunization schedule which is not recognized by the WHO. Although these are optional, it is safe to get them done.

A PHC would roughly be required to keep 400 to 500 vials a month. Such quantities can be easily stored in an ordinary refrigerator.

Cold boxes, vaccine carriers and day carriers would be needed to carry vaccines to the lower formations and to the field. The total numbers will depend on the number of the centers, the staff in position and the strategies adopted for coverage.

Estimation of Requirements of Syringes and Needles

The total number of syringes and needles that you would require will depend on the number of pregnant women and infants you plan to immunize. It is expected that an ordinary glass syringe would be used at least 50 times and a needle 10 times before replacements are made. Reusable plastic syringes are also being supplied to the UIP districts. Such syringes can be steam sterilized up to 200 times.

The calculations of syringes and needles is quite simple:

Total number of pregnant women and infants to be covered

× number of doses of each vaccine (total number of injections)

– ÷ 50 (glass syringes)

– ÷ 200 (plastic syringes)

– ÷ 10 (number of needles)

This calculation gives annual requirement of syringes and needles. However, for any session syringes to be carried will depend on the expected number of injections to be given. At this rate about 500 syringes and needles are required for each PHC.

A sterile syringe and needle should be used for each injection. The total number of syringes and needles at each PHC session should not be less than the expected number of children and pregnant women during the session. The syringes and needles should be sterilized before the session.

You must ensure that adequate quantities of the syringes and needles have been distributed to the field workers and replacements are made to them periodically or autoclaved syringes and needles should be provided on the day of session.

Estimation of Requirements of Sterilization Equipment

Arrangements must be made for the sterilization of syringes and needles for the immunization sessions.

Each visit to the health center or vaccination site for vaccination is called as contact. Minimum four contacts are required for one child to receive the complete series of vaccinations, so the total number of contacts will be four times greater than the number of children in the target population. Two contacts with each pregnant woman are expected.

Estimation of Vaccine Needs

Estimation of vaccine requirements and ordering for the right quantities of vaccine is critical for the success of your program. The requirements depend on the population to be covered and the number of sessions to be held (periodicity of supply).

The vaccine requirements will depend on the number of pregnant woman and children and on the number of sessions held.

The calculations for vaccine requirements are simple:

Total number of infants/pregnant women to be covered

- No. of doses of the vaccine
- WMF (Wastage Multiplication Factor)*
- No. of sessions proposed to be held.

* WMF: 1.33 for DPT, DT, TT and OPV, 2 for BCG and Measles.

The vaccines are supplied in 10 or 20 doses vials or ampoules. The required number of doses are divided by 10 or 20 and rounded off to the next nearest number of vials or ampoules.

You must always check your previous balance stocks before placing order for fresh.

You must monitor the performance reports from the centers to which you supply vaccines to ensure that the expected number of pregnant women and infants are being immunized and the vaccines are not wasted. If the attendance is low, vaccine supplies must be suitably reduced till you can find out the reasons and take corrective measures to step up coverage.

Health centers should not keep more than one month's requirements and no vaccine should be stored at a subcenter.

Estimation of Cold Chain Requirements

All vaccines must be kept at +2°C to + 8°C otherwise they lose their effectiveness to protect against diseases. The cold chain requirements will depend on the quantities of vaccines to be stored and the period for which they will be stored.

It is estimated that cold storage facilities for roughly 30,000 to 40,000 vials of all vaccines will be necessary at the district level (>3 month's requirements of an average district of 2.5 million population).

Storage capacity of around 900 to 1200 liters is required to store the above quantities of vaccines.

Each task described in the task description must be included somewhere in a job description of an individual staff member. Otherwise it will not be clear who is to perform which tasks and some steps may not always be performed or may not even be performed at all.

Make a list of the activities and allocate job responsibilities to the staff. Ensure that the following tasks are covered:

a. Vaccination coverage of pregnant women and infants.
b. Stores including vaccines. The person concerned should indent the required quantities of vaccines and other supplies in time. He should be responsible for the distribution of the required quantities to the lower formations and also for monitoring that the supplies are used properly.
c. Monitoring and supervision of services.
d. Preparation and display of health education material, advance plan for health talks in the community prior to outreach operation and compaigns.
e. Recording and keeping reports in order, compilation and analysis of the reports. Forwarding the reports to the higher formations and providing feedback.
f. Surveillance of diseases.

Although, you may delegate some of the duties to others, the final responsibility for ensuring that the immunization sessions are organized efficiently and effectively is yours.

Determine Training Needs

You are expected to immunize all pregnant women and infants in your area. This means that you must contact all the eligibles. Since some of the vaccines require repeated dose, each child must be contacted at least five times.

It is clear that unless the quality of the services is high it will not be possible to achieve universal immunization coverage. The planning and implementation of the program must be meticulous. There is no scope for any default in the services. Even temporary dislocation can prove disastrous. Critical to the success of the program will be the high quality and easy accessibility of the services.

It is expected that the Medical Officers at the PHC level responsible for the immunization program will attend four day course at the district level. The course will cover the modules on surveillance, cold chain and organization of immunization sessions. In addition, the manual for the health workers should also be covered.

All the MPWs and their supervisors are expected to undergo a two day task oriented course and cover the manual for the health workers. The course should include practical demonstration of all the items covered in the manual. The manuals are available in the regional languages.

Each PHC has been provided with an autoclave. The syringes and needles required for the sessions held at the PHC can be autoclaved the previous evening.

Three or four subcenters may organize vaccination sessions on the same day. These subcenters must be supplied vaccines from the PHC on the day of the sessions. The feasibility of autoclaving the required number of syringes and needles at the PHC and supplying them to the subcenters along with the vaccines must be seriously considered. This will ensure proper sterilization of the syringes and needles, save the time of the ANMs at the subcenters and also avoid the logistics of supplying kerosene and sterilization equipment to the subcenters.

Where the above arrangements are not operationally feasible stoves and pressure sterilizers must be provided to the subcenters. It will also be your responsibility to ensure that adequate stocks of kerosene are available. This should be replenished regularly.

Boiling of syringes and needles at outreach sites should be done only as an emergency and not on a routine basis. Sufficient number of sterilised syringes and needles should be taken by the health staff to the outreach sessions. The numbers taken should be at least 10 percent more than the expected number of children and pregnant women to be vaccinated on that day.

Estimation of Requirements of Immunization Cards

Vaccination cards must be given to all the pregnant women and infants. The card used for the pregnant women can be later used for the infant after the birth of the child. The cards should be in the regional language. During the first year of the program you will, however, need more cards for the infants.

The number of cards you would need is as follows:
- First year—total number of pregnant women and infants +10 percent
- Later—total number of pregnant women + 10 percent.

Manpower Needs

You must clearly define:
Task description of all the steps to be performed in order to carry out each major step. Task descriptions describe what must be done.
Job responsibilities describe the tasks to be performed by the staff member. Job responsibilities describe who will do the work.

Enumerate Eligibles

The vaccine requirements depend on the eligibles and the number of sessions to be held. The simplest and best way to know the eligible is house to house enumeration of pregnant women and infants. The village wise enumeration at a particular period should get the information of infants according to month of birth. Though enumeration can be done at any time in the year, it is ideal to do in the first week of April every year. Thereafter, regular updating of the eligibles must be done during the routine visits. However, the number of eligibles in the future months can be assumed to be same as the corresponding period of the previous year. Pregnant women should be registered at the earliest period of pregnancy and expected date of delivery (EDD) should be worked out.

Obtain Vaccines

Estimation of the vaccine requirements and ordering for the right quantities of vaccines is critical for maintaining the cold chain. The requirements depend on the population to be covered and the number of sessions to be held (periodicity of supply). Estimation based on the following formula will enable the supervisors to assess the vaccine requirements and to verify the correctness of enumeration.

Estimation of Vaccine Requirements

Total number of pregnant women/infants in the area.
× Proposed coverage
× Number of doses of the vaccine to be given (including booster dose)

- Vaccine administration rate *(VAR).
- Periodicity of supply (depending on the number of sessions held per month).

For example, in an area with a population of 5,000 birth rate of 30/1000 and IMR of 100/1000 live births, the estimated number of pregnant women and infants is calculated as follows:

Eligibles:

Pregnant women	=	Population × BR
Infants	=	Population × BR × (1 – IMR)
Pregnant women	=	5,000 × 0.03 = 150
Infants	=	5,000 × 0.03 × (1 – 0.0) = 150 × 9 = 135

Vaccine requirements are calculated based on the following formula:

Number of vials required = Number of eligibles × expected coverage Number of doses ÷ VAR ÷ Number of doses per vial.

Instead of dividing by VAR you can multiply by wastage multiplication factor (WMF) as indicated by equivalents below:

VAR	WMF
50%	2
75%	1.33
90%	1.11

Thus, the formula using WMF will be:

No. of eligibles × expected coverage × No. of doses × WMF ÷ No. of doses per vial continuing with the example on previous page.

Requirement of TT = 150 × 100/100 × 2 × 1.33 = 400 doses.

This is annual requirement of TT for pregnant women.

Monthly requirement = 400 ÷ 12 = 34 doses ÷ 10 = 4 vials.

If sessions are held fortnightly, divide by 24 and if weekly, divide by 52.

Although minimum coverage required for DPT, OPV, BCG and measles is 85 percent, it is better to calculate vaccine requirements for 100 percent. Accordingly in the example cited, requirement of DPT/OPV will be:

135 × 100/100 × 4 × 1.33 = 720 doses (4 doses include 3 primary and one booster)

Accordingly, monthly and fortnightly requirements will be 60 and 30 doses.

BCG/Measles = 135 × 100 ÷ 100 × 1 × 2 = 270 doses.

Accordingly, monthly and fortnightly requirements will be 25 and 13 doses.

The vaccines are supplied in 10 or 20 dose vials or ampoules. The required number of doses are divided by 10 or 20 and rounded off to the next higher number of vials or ampoules.

Since, the subcenters are not supposed to keep vaccines there will be no balance stocks from previous supplies.

(*Note*:*Vaccine administration rate: It is the number of doses actually administered to beneficiaries out of one hundred doses of the vaccine).

You must monitor the performance reports from the subcenters to ensure that the expected number of pregnant women and infants are being immunized and the vaccines are not wasted. If the attendance is low, vaccine supplies must be suitably reduced till you can find out the reasons and take corrective measure to step up coverage.

Maintain Vaccines

When administrating vaccine to expectant mothers and infants at the vaccination site, you must take great care not to expose the vaccine to heat and sunlight. To do this:

- Select a vaccination site that is as cool as possible, preferably inside a room. If a room is not available, vaccinate in the shade. Do not vaccinate in the sunlight.
- Open the carrier only when necessary
- Remove vaccine and diluent from the vaccine container, only when you need it.
- Take only vial of one type of vaccine from the container at a time. Do not take the second vial from the carrier until it is needed.
- Secure the lid tightly after opening as soon as possible
- Wrap the BCG ampoules in a dark paper to protect them from heat and light.
- When you take vaccine out of the container, place vials inside a cup containing ice. If the ice melts and no mothers and children are waiting, put the vials back into the cold chain container until a mother arrives. Then place the vials inside the cup with ice.
- When the vaccination session is completed, return all vials to the health center store, if ice packs in the carrier still contain ice, mark unopened vials by putting rubber band, and return them to the refrigerator. Be sure to use these marked vials during the next vaccination session.

  Do not take the same vial of the vaccine out to the field more than three times. If a vial of vaccine has been taken to the field third time, return it to the PHC after marking 'Discard'. You must, however, be careful that vaccines are not wasted in this way too often.
  - Keep opened vials in plastic bag and return these to PHC at the end of the session for discarding by an identified person.
  - If the ice in the cold chain container is completely melted for less than one day:
    i. Discard polio vaccine, so that no one else can use.
    ii. Mark the remaining DPT, tetanus toxoid, measles and BCG vaccine, return it to the refrigerator, and use it during the next vaccination session.
  - If the ice in the cold chain container is completely melted for more than one day throw away all vaccines.
- Keep a record of the vaccine you administer.

- Keep record of the batch numbers and the expiry dates of the vaccines used.
- Keep a record of vaccines returned to PHC.

The administration rate of the vaccines will depend on the number of sessions held and the attendance at the sessions. The fewer the number of pregnant women and infants per session the lower will be the administration rate. This is because opened vials must be discarded at the end of the session. On an average, the administrative rates of all vaccines is estimated to be 75 percent except BCG and measle-vaccines for which the administration rate is around 50 percent.

Sometimes the services may have to be intensified to cover up the back logs. On the other hand, due to various reasons, such as heavy rains, priorities of other programs, vacant posts, etc. services may be considerably reduced during some months of the year. Thus, the monthly requirements will be more in some months and less in others. The supplies to the subcenters must be adjusted accordingly with less vaccines being supplied over some months and more during the others. This must be part of your planned activities.

Before the vaccines are despatched, make sure to check the ice packs of the vaccine carriers. These should be frozen solid. If using thermocol carrier, these should be packed at least 1/3rd with ice.

Check that the types and amounts of vaccine and diluent are the same as you estimated.

Check that the expiry date on each vial of vaccine has not passed.

Check that DPT, DT, TT vaccines have not been frozen. The solution of such vaccines, on shaking is not uniform. Small granules or floccules will be seen. Such vaccine also forms sediment faster than the normal vaccine (shake test).

If you are sending vaccines to more than one subcenter see that the subcenters fall on the same route and if one person can deliver the vaccines taking the shortest route. The vaccines should reach the subcenters in time for the vaccination sessions.

Any unused vaccine left at the end of the day should be returned to the PHC on the same day. No vaccine should be stored at the subcenter. These vials should be kept in a separate box in the refrigerator marked "returned". Put a rubber band around the vial to indicate that it was taken out once, two rubber bands if taken out twice. Any vial which has been taken out three times and not used, must be discarded. You must, however, be careful that this does not happen too often.

Maintain Equipment

Vaccine and diluent taken from cold storage can be kept for several hours if packed properly in well insulated cold chain containers. To do this, three types of cold chain containers are available for your use:

- A cold box

- Vaccine carrier
- A day carrier.

Vaccine

BCG

History: Developed in the year 1927 by Calmette and Guérin from bovine bacilli after 230 subcultures (Table 8.3).

Table 8.3: Milestones in vaccination

1796 -	First vaccination. Jenner tests for smallpox resistance
1883 -	Vaccination for children against rabies
1892 -	Cholera vaccine
1913 -	Toxoid, antitoxin immunization against diphtheria
1921 -	BCG vaccine
1923 -	Diphtheria toxoid
1923 -	Pertussis vaccine
1927 -	Tetanus toxoid
1937 -	Influenza vaccine
1937 -	Yellow fever vaccine
1949 -	Mumps vaccine
1954 -	Salk's polio vaccine
1957 -	Sabin's oral polio vaccine
1960 -	Measles vaccine
1962 -	Rubella vaccine
1968 -	Type C *meningococcus* vaccine
1970 -	Researchers in Israel proved that injection of a peptide from a virus or disease can induce the production of antibodies that recognize the entire virus or disease
1971 -	Type A *meningococcus* vaccine
1980 -	First commercial vaccine for Hepatitis B
1982 -	First vaccine produced through genetic engineering (vaccines for diarrhea in pigs)
1982 -	First synthetic vaccine created at Institute Pasteur and at Weizmann Institute from diphtheria toxin.

Aim: To induce benign artificial primary infection which will stimulate an acquired resistance to possible subsequent infection with virulent TB bacilli and thus reduce mortality and morbidity from pulmonary TB among those most at risk.

Vaccine

- It is a live bacterial vaccine. It consists of living bacteria derived from an attenuated bovine strain of TB *bacilli*
- Vaccine is prepared from "Danish 1331" strain since Jan 1967 at BCG laboratory Guindy, Chennai.

Potency

- Vaccine is stable for up to one year if stored below 10°C
- At room temp—one month
- During summer—one weeks
- After reconstitution with normal saline—three hours.

Protection

Protect it from sunlight.

Types of vaccine: Liquid vaccine (fresh) and freeze dried vaccine

Storage: Wrapped in a double layer of red or black cloth.

Dosage:
- 0.1 ml for infant
- 0.05 ml for neonate (< 4 weeks)
- 0.1 ml in neonate penetrats into deeper tissue and gives rise to local abscess formation and lymphadenopathies (axillary).

Route of Administration

Intradermal using a tuberculin syringe—omega microstate syringe fitted with 1 cm steel 26 gauge intradermal needle.

Site: Just above the insertion of the deltoid muscle. A satisfactory injection should produce a wheal of 5 mm in diameter. The vaccine must not be contaminated with an antiseptic or detergent.

Age: Immediately after birth for institutional delivery or at six week of age simultaneously with DPT and polio, it should always be completed by one year. It can be given up to 20 years irrespective of tuberculine status.

Complication

Ulceration at site and suppurative lymphadinitis occur in—1 to 10 percent of vaccination.

Osteomyelites, disseminated infection occur in—<1 percent/million vaccination.

Abscess formation—Rx incision and drainage—Rx with PAS or INH powder.

Protective value: Range of protection 0-80 percent is from 15 to 20 years, it gives protection against childhood TB, tubercular meningitis.

Contraindications

1. Generalized eczema
2. Infective dermatitis

3. Hypogamma globulinemia
4. History of deficient immunity.

Oral Polio

Oral polio vaccine was described by Sabin in 1957.

- It contains live attenuated vaccine (Type 1, 2 and 3)
- Grown in monkey kidney HDCC (Human Deploid Cell Cultures). The vaccines contain:
  - i. 300000 TCID 50 g type 1 polio virus
  - ii. 100000 TCID 50 g type 2 polio virus
  - iii. Over 30000 TCID 50 g type 3 polio virus per dose.

National Immunization Schedule

BCG may be given at the same time as the oral polio vaccine. DPT vaccine may also be given at the same time as BCG but in different areas:

- Three doses of OPV at one month interval commencing first dose when the child is 6 weeks old.
- It is very important to complete vaccination for all infants before six months of age.

Because most of the polio cases occur at the ages of six months and three years one booster dose OPV is recommended 12 to 18 months later.

If vaccine is spoon fed spoon should be boiled in water and cooled in ice water before administering vaccine. Don't use disinfectant for sterilization of spoon.

Development of Immunity

Live vaccine strains infect intestinal epithelial cells after replication, the virus is transported to the payer's patches where secondary multiplication with subsequent viraemia occurs. The virus spreads to other areas of body, resulting in production of circulating antibodies and prevent paralytic polio.

Intestinal infection stimulates the production of IgA secretory antibodies which prevent subsequent infection of the alimentary tract with wild strains of polio virus and is effective in limiting virus transmission in the community.

Oral Polio Vaccine (OPV)

It includes both local immunity and systemic immunity. Virus is excreated in feces and secondary spread occurs to house hold contacts and susceptible contacts in the community. Nonimmunized persons may therefore be immunized. Thus, widespread "herd immunity" results, even if only 66 percent approximately of community is immunized.

Therefore, this property of OPV has been exploited in controlling epidemics of polio by administration of vaccine simultaneously in a short period to all susceptibles in a community. This procedure, virtually eliminates wild polio strains in the community. Wild polio is replaced by attenuated strains.

Failure of Three Dose Regimen

The proportion of children developing antibody after three doses of trivalent vaccine can be as low as 30 percent in tropical countries as against the more usual 90 percent in temperate climate countries.

Failure of OPV

Increased gradually from – 5 percent in 1960 to 30 percent currently.

To overcome this failure Indian academy of pediatric has recommended five dose of OPV in clinic based programs. Some have recommended yearly dose up to eight years.

At the vaccination clinic, the bottle containing the OPV should not be frozen and thawed repeatedly. It would be preferable to keep the vials of the vaccine in ice during its administration to children.

Breastfeeding does not impede the effectiveness of OPV. However, hot water, hot milk or hot fluids should be with held for about half an hour after the administration of the vaccine. The vaccine should be administered preferably in a cool room, rather than in a hot, humid and crowded room.

Complications

Risk of vaccine associated paralysis is 1 case/1 million vaccination. Risk of close contact of vaccine developing paralytic polio is about 1 case/5 million dose of vaccination.

Contraindications

For administration of OPV are fever, diarrhea, dysentery, leukemia's, malignancy, those receiving corticosteroids. These are only relative contraindications.

Storage

OPV(Heat stabilized) can be stored without losing potency for a year at 4°C and for a month at room temperature. Nonheat stabilized vaccine should be stored at –20°C in a deep freeze. If deep freeze is not available it might be stored temporarily in freezing chamber of refrigerator.

Salk Polio Vaccine

Inactivated by formaline. It contains 20, 2, and 4 D antigens unit—type 1, 2 and 3 respectively.

third dose—at an interval of one to two months

fourth dose—6-12 months after 3rd dose

Additional doses—recommended prior to school entry and then every five years until the age of 18 years. One or two dose of OPV are given safely as booster after an initial course of immunization.

- Induce—humeral antibodies (IgM and G, A) serum antibodies.

Advantages

Safe to administer in:

1. Person with immune deficiency disease.
2. To person undergoing corticosteroid and radiation therapy.
3. For those over 50 years who received vaccine for 1st time.
4. During pregnancy.

Strategies for Polio Eradication

1. Conduct Pulse Polio Immunization (PPI) days every year for three to four years or until polio myelitis is eradicated.
2. Sustain high level of immunization coverage.
3. Monitoring OPV coverage at district level and below.
4. Improve surveillance capable of detecting all cases of Acute Flaccid Paralysis (AFP) due to polio and non-polio etiology.
5. Ensure rapid case investigation, including the collection of stool samples for virus isolation.
6. Arrange follow-up of all cases of AFP at 60 days to check for residual paralysis.
7. Conduct outbreak control for cases confirmed or suspected to be polio myelitis to stop transmission.

Even a single case is treated as an out break and preventive measures are initiated, usually within 48 hours of notification of case. Reporting of all cases of acute flaccid paralysis in children under 15 years of age is mandatory and line lists of all reported cases of polio are maintained.

Current Four Basic Strategies to Eradicate Polio

Routine Immunization

Immunize every child aged < 1 year with at least four doses of oral polio vaccine.

National Immunization Days (NIDs)/Pulse Polio Immunization (PPI) Program

Conduct by giving additional doses of OPV, four to six weeks apart to every child aged < 5 years. Intensification of the Pulse Polio Immunization

Program can be done by adding additional rounds, house-to-house "search and vaccinate" component to the fixed post approach. Intensification of PPI needs a meticulous planning of the program along with intensive supervision and monitoring besides social mobilization effort.

National Immunization Days

In India, transmission of polio has dramatically reduced from 1934 laboratory confirmed cases in 1998 to 1126 in 1999 and just 263 in 2000. It is decided that there is a need to make extra-efforts to reach the unreached during Pulse Polio Immunization Days. For that reason **Intensified Pulse Polio Immunization** was proposed and just after the National Immunization Day a immunisation team would go to house to check whether the child has received pulse polio vaccine and if not given then child must be given a dose. An elaborative work plan has been proposed for each supervisor to ensure that no child is left without polio vaccine.

Surveillance of Acute Flaccid Paralysis (AFP)

To identify all reservoirs of wild poliovirus transmission.

Objective

To find places with circulation of wild poliovirus.

Components

Establishment and maintenance of reporting units (RUs): Reporting units form the backbone of surveillance network. These are hospitals, pediatricians, doctors, and medical/health establishments in government or private sectors who are likely to see a case of Acute Flaccid Paralysis (AFP). The reporting units are well distributed to cover all areas in the country. Apart from reporting AFP cases immediately, the RUs send a weekly AFP surveillance report to the District Immunization Officer (DIO) irrespective of whether or not they see a case of AFP during the work. Each RU has a nodal officer responsible for reporting and upkeep of records. At present, 8,453 RUs are participating in AFP surveillance throughout India. Apart from these, numerous small clinics, private practitioners, doctors of Indian systems of medicine, quacks (all together termed as **informers**) report AFP cases whenever they see them. Both the Surveillance Medical Officer (SMO) and DIO are involved in the creating of a sound reporting network and visiting regularly to the reporting units in their area and conducting active case searches in the RUs at regular intervals to look for any cases that might not have been reported.

AFP case notification: The RUs and informers notify AFP cases immediately to the DIO. Since very important activities like stool specimen collection, outbreak response immunization, active case search in the community, etc. should occur early, rapid notification is very essential.

AFP case investigation: An AFP case is immediately investigated, usually within 48 hours of notification, by DIO or SMO. After confirming the case as AFP, the DIO clinically examines the child, takes history and fills a standard Case Investigation Form (CIF).

Stool specimen collection and transportation: From every case of AFP, 2-stool specimens are collected. The aim is to get these specimens at the earliest, within 14 days of onset of paralysis (or maximum of eight weeks) and at least 24 hours apart. Each specimen is 8 grams or about adult thumb size collected in a clean, dry screw capped container. The container need not be sterile and no preservative/transport media is used. The specimens are collected, labeled and transported in cold chain to the designated national lab. A standard Lab Request Form (LRF) is filled that accompanies the stool specimen. Special stool specimen carriers have been provided to districts for this purpose. Stool specimens are collected from all AFP cases detected within eight weeks from the onset of paralysis.

Virological Classification Scheme (Flow chart 8.1)

Flow chart 8.1: Virological classification scheme

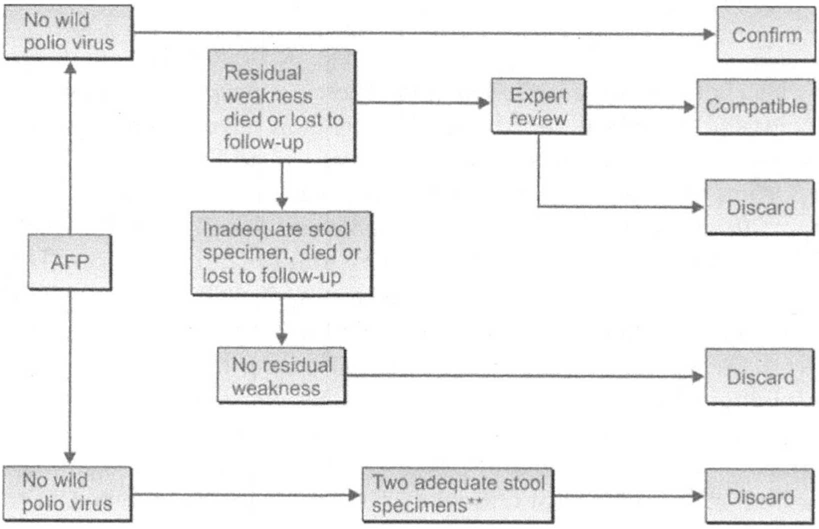

** 2 Specimen at least 24 hours apart and within 14 days of onset paralysis: each specimen must be of adequate volume (8-10 grams) and arrive at a WHO accredited laboratory in good condition (i.e. no desiccation, no leakage; adequate documentation and evidence that the cold chain was maintained)

Process of AFP Surveillance (Flow chart 8.2)

Outbreak response immunization (ORI): Following stool specimen collection, outbreak response immunization is organized in the community. All 0 to 59 months old children are given one dose of oral polio vaccine irrespective of their previous immunization status while going house to house. The recipients include all target children in the village/locality. At least 500 children are vaccinated. The ORI is performed as soon as possible. The travel history of the child may suggest additional places of stay where ORI should also be conducted. While conducting the house-to-house immunization during ORI active case search is conducted in the community.

Active case search in the community: In the community where an AFP case lives, a house-to-house active case search is organized to find more AFP cases if they have occurred. This activity is carried out immediately along with Outbreak Response Immunization (ORI). The case definition used during searches is: Flaccid/floppy paralysis in a child between 0-15 years of age with onset within last 60 days. All the cases that are found are investigated immediately and have two stool specimens taken before the child is given Oral Polio Vaccine (OPV). The purpose of the search is to fully uncover additional polio cases, if any, in the community.

Sixty days follow-up examination: The District Immunization Officer or Surveillance Medical Officer revisits every case of AFP 60 days after the onset of paralysis to confirm the presence or absence of residual weakness. Child is assessed for weakness, asymmetrical skin folds, and difference in left/right mid-arm/mid-thigh circumference. The child has residual weakness, if any of the above is present, even if minimal. This activity is completed before 70th day of onset of paralysis.

Cross notification and tracking of cases: The cases are investigated anywhere in India irrespective of where the child lives. A very advanced communication system (telephone/fax/e-mail) has been established that sends information to DIO of the resident district of AFP case immediately. The AFP case is constantly tracked by SMOs to complete all the activities related with surveillance. This also leads to realistic and complete epidemiological picture at district level.

Data management and analysis: At the end of each week, DIO reports to the State EPI Officer the line of all new AFP cases, reported during that week. He summarizes the activities and reports the current status of investigation and the follow-up of AFP cases. Reporting takes place even when no cases of AFP have been identified. The data is entered into computers at National Polio Surveillance Unit (NPSU) and is used for program monitoring, checking quality of data and assessing progress towards eradication. The data is analyzed for taking appropriate action.

Flow chart 8.2: Process of AFP surveillance

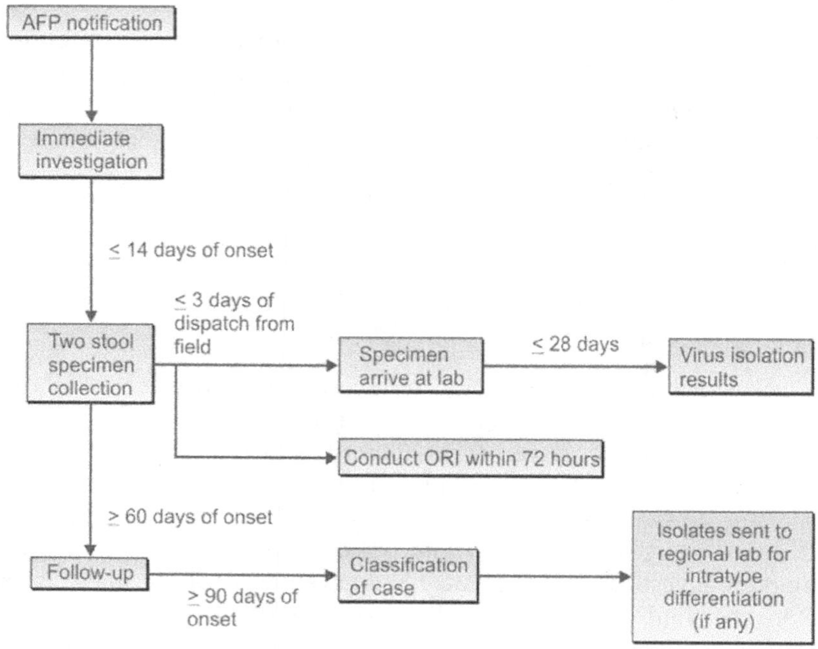

Case classification: When lab results and 60 days follow-up examination reports are available, the cases are classified at NPSU as polio or non-polio. Until 1999, the clinical system of classification was being used. According to this scheme, a case is classified as polio if wild poliovirus is isolated. If two adequate stool specimens have been collected (24 hr apart) from the case within 14 days of onset of paralysis and the stool results are negative then the case is non-polio. If the case had inadequate stool specimen and the AFP case had residual weakness, died or lost to follow-up then that case is classified as polio. From January 2000, India has shifted to the advanced virological system of classification. Cases with inadequate stool specimen and having residual weakness, died or lost to follow-up are subjected to special investigation and are presented for the review by the Expert Group at national level. The Expert Group classifies the case as compatible or discarded. This has been possible due to the achievement of a high level of surveillance of AFP.

Feedback: In order to give feedback, the reports and maps, which are generated by NPSU, are on the website. NPSU also sends line lists of the cases to the states twice a month.

Conduct Extensive House-to-House Immunization Mopping-up Campaigns

In the final stages in focal areas where wild poliovirus transmission persists.

Mopping-up: Conduct extensive house-to-house immunization mopping-up campaigns: Experience in previous years has shown that though the National Immunization Days (NIDs called as Pulse Polio Immunization or PPI in India) decrease polio transmission and delay the annual peak in high endemic states, the virus persists and bounces back in the later half of the year. But to achieve eradication quickly, it will be critical to target the remaining districts with extra rounds of house-to-house immunization early in 2001 before the onset of the hot summer and the subsequent high season of polio during the rains.

Mopping-up is not a Sub-National Immunization Day (SNID). SNIDs are done when there is widespread and dispersed transmission in a part of the country and is aimed at reducing the transmission to clearly delimited, focal areas. SNIDs are not an end-game strategy and can be repeated a few times if needed. On the other hand, mopping-up is aimed at stopping transmission in a defined area. This can't be repeated too many times. In mopping-up the virus from an area or population, there are no shortcuts to reaching all children. Going house-to-house or family-to-family are tools to achieve that elusive goal of reaching all eligible children.

Line Listing of Cases

Started in 1989.

Aim of line listing of cases

1. To check for duplication (Same case reported more than once).
2. Year of onset of illness to screen the children with residual paralysis.
3. Identification of high-risk pockets.
4. Documentation of high-risk age groups.

Intensive Pulse Polio Immunization (IPPI)

1. It will reduce number and size of high-risk areas.
2. Increase in the involvement of health official in the planning process. AFP surveillance information in planning of immunization activities by helping and monitoring of the technique.

Strategies Involved to Achieve Intensification of PPI

Conduct Nation wide four Pulse Polio Immunization (PPI) rounds based on June 1999 recommendation of "Global Technical" consultative group in polio myelitis eradication.

- Four rounds—with four weeks apart from 1999-2000
- First day—booth based 2nd and 3rd day—house-to-house search
- Aim—hundred percent immunization.

In addition—2 supplementary rounds in February 27th to 29th and March 26th to 28th in eight priority states Uttar Pradesh, Madhya Pradesh, West Bengal, Bihar, Rajasthan, Assam, Gujarat, and Orissa.

Vaccine Vial Monitoring

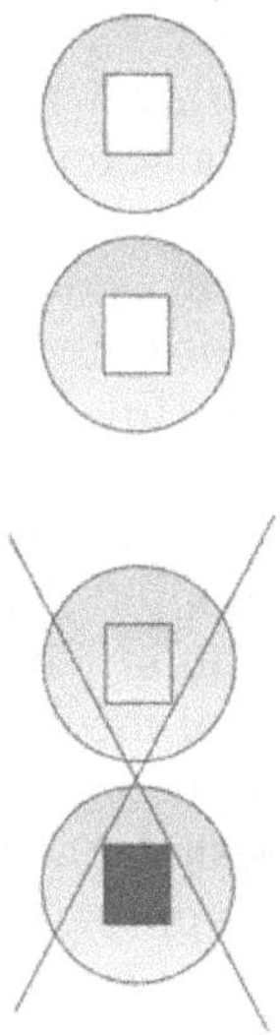

During the IPPI there is a need to reach every eligible child with potent oral polio vaccine. The Vaccine Vial Monitor (VVM) is a simple tool, which enable the vaccinator to know whether vaccine is potent at the time of administration.

On the vaccine vial there is a circle mark in which a small square is printed which is either white or lighter than the color of circle that indicate that the vaccine is potent and can be used. However, if the color of square is dark or of same color as circle mark then the vaccine should be discarded.

Measles Vaccine

Measles is best prevented by active immunization. Only live attenuated vaccines are recommended for use.

No egg culture vaccine are produced at all today.

- All are tissue culture vaccine—chick embryo, HDCC (Human diploid cell culture)
- It is a freeze dried product.

Age

1. The most effective compromise is immunization as close to the age of nine months as possible.
2. If there is measles outbreak in community, measles vaccine should be started at sixth month.
3. For infants immunized between six and nine months of age, a second dose should be administered as soon as possible after the child reaches the age of nine months provided that at least four weeks have elapsed since the last dose.
4. In countries where the incidence of measles has declined, the age of immunization is being raised to 15 months in order to avoid the blocking effect of persistent transplacentally acquired antibody.

Storage

Heat stable measles vaccines able to maintain their potency for more than 2 years at 2 to 8°C have been developed.

Administration

It is administered in a single subcutaneous dose of 0.5 ml.

Diluting fluid for reconstituting the vaccine must be kept cold at 4 to 8°C.

- The reconstituted vaccine should be kept on ice and used within one hour
- Measles vaccine has recently been adapted for aerosol administration.

Reactions

When injected into the body—attenuated virus multiplies and induces a mild "measles illness" (fever and rash) 5 to 10 days after immunization

- But reduced in frequency and severity. This may occur in 15 to 20 percent of vaccinees.
- Fever may last for—one to two days and the rash for one to three days.

  There is no spread of the virus from the vaccinees to contacts.

Immunity

Develops within 11 to 12 days after vaccination

- Appears to be of long duration probably for life.
- One dose of vaccine offers 95 percent protection.

Contacts

Susceptible contacts over the age of 9 to 12 months may be protected against measles if vaccine is given within three days of exposure. This is because incubation period of measles induced by vaccine is about seven days compared to 10 days for the naturally acquired infection.

Contraindications

1. Pregnancy is positive contraindication
2. Acute illness
3. Defective cell mediated immunity
4. Steroids and immunosuppressive drugs.

Adverse Effects of Vaccine

Toxic shock syndrome (TSS) occurs when measles vaccine is contaminated or same vial is used for more than one session on the same day or next day.

Vaccine should not be used after four hours of opening the vial. TSS is totally preventable. TSS symptoms are:

1. Fever (high degree)
2. Watery diarrhea

3. Vomiting within few hours of measles vaccination.
   Case fatality rates are high. May cause death within 48 hours.

Combined Vaccine

It can be combined with other live attenuated vaccines such as mumps and rubella vaccines (MMR vaccines) and such combinations are highly effective.

Immunoglobulin

Measles may be prevented by administration of immunoglobulin early in the incubation period, the dose recommended by WHO is 0.25 ml per kg of body weight. It should be given within 3 to 4 days of exposure. The person passively immunized should be given live measles vaccine 8 to 12 weeks later.

Eradication is possible because:
1. Highly potent vaccine is available
2. Need a single dose of vaccine
3. Vaccine can be stored for long time and gives long lasting immunity
4. Case detection and surveillance is possible
5. By primary health care approach-universal immunization program facilities are made available even in remote areas.

Urban Measles Campaign

Measles is a highly contagious viral disease occurring in overcrowded areas where poor people live and coverage of measles vaccination is poor. These areas are needed special vaccination drive initiated by UNICEF in 1998 covering 13 cities and in 1999-2000, 50 more cities are also covered. The main focus is on covering all unprotected children up to the three years.

Diphtheria Immunization

Current prophylactics. These may be grouped as below:

Combined or Mixed Vaccines

- DPT (Diphtheria, pertussis-tetanus vaccine)
- DT (Diphtheria and tetanus toxoid)
- dT (Diphtheria and tetanus, adult type).

Single Vaccines

- FT (Formal toxoid)
- APT (Alum-precipitated toxoid)

- PTAP (Purified toxoid aluminum phosphate)
- PTAH (Purified toxoid aluminum hydroxide)
- TAF (Toxoid-antitoxin floccules).

Antisera

Diphtheria antitoxin
- Combined vaccines DPT vaccine.

Advantages

1. The infant can be immunized simultaneously against—three diseases viz. diphtheria, pertussis and tetanus.
2. Pertussis component enhances the potency of the diphtheria toxoid.

   Two types of vaccines—plain and adsorbed. Adsorbtion is carried out on a mineral carrier like aluminum phosphate or hydroxide.

Composition of DPT Vaccines (Table 8.4)

Table 8.4: Composition of DPT vaccines

Contents	*Glaxo (Per/0.5ml)*	*Kasauli*
Diphtheria toxoid	25 Lf	30 Lf
Tetanus toxoid	5 Lf	10 Lf
B. pertussis (millions)	20,000	32,000
Aluminum phosphate	2.5 mg	3.0 mg
Thiomersal, BP	0.01%	0.01%

Storage

Vaccines should not be frozen. They should be stored in a refrigerator between 4 to 8°C.
- Optimum age is six weeks after birth
- No of doses: 2-3 doses
- Two dose of DT gives > 80 percent protection
- But two doses of pertussis gives—50 percent protection
- Three dose of DPT offers better protection than two doses of DPT.

Interval between Doses

An interval of four weeks between three doses with a booster injection at 1½-2 years followed by another booster dose (DT only) at age five to six years.

Mode of Administration

Deep IM upper outer quadrant of the gluteal region.

In 1984, Global Advisory Group recommended DPT vaccine for children under one year of age, DPT—should be administered in lateral aspect of thigh.

Reactions

Fever and mild local reactions are common two to six percent of vaccinees develop fever of 39°C or higher 5 to 10 percent experience swelling and induration or pain lasting more than 48 hours.

Neurological Complications

These are due to the pertussis component of the vaccine.
- Encephalitis
- Encephalopathy
- Prolonged convulsions
- Infantile spasms
- Reye's syndrome.

Contraindications

Minor illness such as cough, cold, mild fever are not considered contra-indications to vaccination.

DPT—should not be repeated if a severe reaction occurred after a previous dose.

Such reactions include collapse or shock like state, persistent screaming episodes, temp > 40°C, convulsions, anaphylactic reaction. In case of DPT subsequent immunization with a DT only is recommended without pertussis component.

Tetanus Toxoid

1. Active immunization
2. Passive immunization.

Aim

Protective level of antitoxin approximately—0.01 IU/ml serum throughout life.

All persons should be immunized regardless of age.

Two Preparations

1. Combined vaccine-DPT
2. Monovalent vaccines
   a. Plain or fluid (formal) toxoid
   b. Tetanus vaccine, adsorbed (PTAP, APT).

Monovalent

- 0.5 ml injected into arm—one to two months interval
- First booster dose—one year after the initial two dose
- Second booster dose—five year after 3rd dose

- It can be stored up to 5 hours at 4 to 10°C
- It must not be allowed to freeze at any time.

All wounds should receive surgical toilet (Flow chart 8.3)

Flow chart 8.3: All wound receive surgical toilet

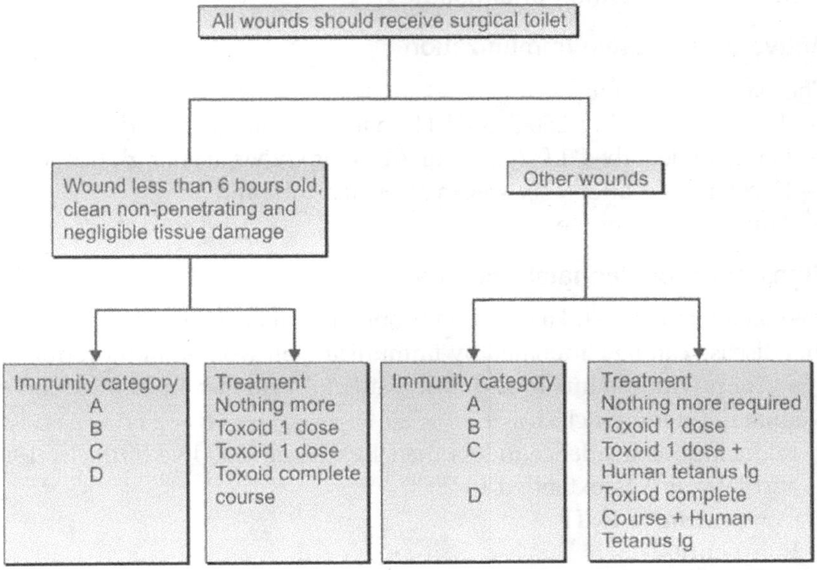

A = Has had a complete course of toxoid or a booster dose within the past five years.
B = Has had a complete course of toxoid or a booster dose more than five years ago and less than 10 years ago.
C = Has had a complete course of toxoid or a booster dose more than 10 years ago.
D = Has not had a complete course of toxoid or immunity status is unknown.

Passive Immunization

Temporary protection against tetanus can be provided by injection of Human tetanus hyperimmunoglobulin or ATS.

It is best prophylactic to use. The dose for all ages is 250-500 IU. It does not cause serum reactions. It gives longer passive protection up to 30 days or more compared to 7 to 10 days for Horse ATS. Human tetanus Ig is now available in India and it is produced by the Serum Institute of India, Pune.

ATS (Equine)

If human antitoxin is not available—equine antitoxin (ATS) is used. The dose is 1500 IU-SC after sensitivity testing.

- Gives passive protection for about 7 to 10 days.
- Being foreign protein ATS is rapidly excreted from the body and there may be very little antibody at the end of two weeks.

Therefore, it does not cover the tetanus incubation period (IP) in all cases. It causes sensitivity reaction in many cases. Person receiving first time may tolerate—subsequent injection with horse serum may lead to allergic reaction varying in severity from rash to anaphylactic reaction. It stimulates formation of antibodies.

Active and Passive Immunization

The patient is given:
- 1500 IU of ATS or 250-500 IU Human Ig in one arm, and
- 0.5 ml of adsorbed TT (PTAP or APT) into other arm or gluteal region
- Booster dose after—six weeks later (0.5 ml), and
- Third dose—one year later.

Elimination of Neonatal Tetanus

Neonatal tetanus is still a common problem in many districts. Fortunately this disease can be eliminated by immunising all women in reproductive age group with tetanus toxoid. The National Program of Elimination of Neonatal Tetanus includes:

- Reducing the incidence to less than 1 case per 1000 live births by 1995 and later it was extended to 2000
- Component of RCH
- Interventions:
  1. Coverage of all pregnant women with two doses of tetanus toxoid
  2. Extensive IEC efforts to promote clean deliveries: Five Cleans—Clean Hands, Clean Surface, Clean Blade, Clean Stump, and Clean Tie.
  3. Providing disposable delivery kits.
  4. Community based surveillance of neonatal deaths and investigation and control measures in case of neonatal deaths.

Anti-rabies Vaccine (Table 8.5)

Table 8.5: Dosage schedule

Class	*Adult*	*Children*	*Duration*	*Booster dose (Bd)*
Treatment recommended by Central Research Institute Kasauli				
Class I	2 ml	2 ml	7 days	No
Class II	5 ml	2 ml	10 days	1 Bd to be given 3 weeks or later after 10th inj.
Class III	5 ml	2 ml	10 days	1st Bd 7 days after 10th inj 2nd Bd 2 weeks or later after 1st Bd
Recommended by Pasteur Institute Coonoor				
Class I	2 ml	1 ml	7 days	No
Class II	3 ml	3 ml	10 days	
Class III	5 ml	3 ml	10 days	

Cell Culture Vaccine

Six doses 1 ml each on days—0, 3, 7, 14, and 28

- Bd on day 90. Injected IM on deltoid muscle.
- Multisite schedule
- Reduced multisite in regimen (2-1-1) (0.5/ml)
- (0.5/1 ml) deltoid
  - 2-1-1 regimen on days 0-7- 21
- Intradermal (Id): 2 Site regimen (2-2-2-0-1-1) on days 0, 3, 7, 28 and 90 dose: 1 Id dose = 1/5th of IM dose (1.0 or 0.5 ml) Id per site
- Intradermal regimen: 8 Site (8-0-4-0-1-1) on days 0,7,28,90 dose—1/5th of IM dose.

Pre-exposure Prophylaxis

Cell culture vaccine is given either as 1 ml IM of 0.1 ml Id on days, 0.7 and 28.

If serum titers of virus neutralizing antibodies are less than 0.5 IU/ml, booster doses of 1 ml IM or 0.1 ml intradermally should be administered until antibodies become demonstrable. Further booster injections should be administered at intervals of two years as long as exposed person remains at risk.

Re-exposure to Animals after Anti-rabies Vaccination

Re-exposure after six months of completion of course of anti-rabies vaccination (with nervous tissue vaccine). It should be considered as fresh case.

Re-exposure within six months:

Class I risk within 6 month—1 Bd 2 ml vaccine

Class I infected by class II and III wound

- Full course vaccine to be given.

If Patient has been treated earlier for class II and III wound next exposure is also same class—2 Bd of 5 ml—1st dose immediately and 2nd dose – after a week.

In tissue culture vaccine—Re-exposure after 5 years should be treated as fresh case.

Re-exposure within 5 years: 2 Bd—Spaced a week apart

No anti-rabies serum indicated up to 5 years following primary immunization.

Adverse Reactions

General: Headache, insomnia, giddiness, palpitation

Local: Pain, tenderness, redness swelling

Allergic: Urticaria, syncope, angioneurotic edema

Neuroparalysis: Post-vaccinal paralysis due to sensitization

Advice to Patients

1. They should abstain from alcohol during and one month after completion of anti-rabic Rx—it may facilitate paralytic accident.
2. Undue physical and mental strain should be avoided
3. Corticosteroid and other immunosuppressive agent should not be used
4. Rabies may develop following inadequate immunization.

Anti-Snake Venom

Polyvalent anti-snake venom serum should be given to neutralize the poison.

- Serum should be injected soon after the bite
- 20 ml is given IV after test dose

Repeated after one hour or even earlier

- If symptoms persist, further dose repeated every sixth hour—until symptoms disappear completely.

Prepared by

Hyper immunizing horse against—venom of four common poisonous snake, i.e. cobra, common krait, russels, viper (saw scaled viper).

Plasma obtained from hyperimmunized horses is concentrated and purified.

Serum is lyopolised by drying it from frozen state under high vaccum.

It is prepared in Haffkins Institute, Bombay and Kasauli—in India

Available in the form of lyopolized powder in an ampoule, dissolved in distilled water before being injected.

It is useful when given within 4 hours, doubtful value after—24 hours

- Serum will produce serum sickness and even acute anaphylaxis in sensitive persons
- To test the sensitivity
  0.05 to 0.1 ml in 1:10 dilution of serum is injected intradermally. +ve reaction—wheal 1 cm surrounded by erythema of same width develop in 5 to 20 minutes
  For desensitization—1/2 to 1 ml of antiserum is injected subcutaneously
- 40 ml of anti-venom is given IV and repeated as required. It is effective for cobra and russel
- In case of viper bite—inject anti-snake venom around to the site of bite
- If there are signs of neuroparalysis—give 1/2 mg neostigmine 1/2 hr before each injection 1/2 mg atropine should be given to block muscarinic side effects of neostigmine
  Heparin 1000 to 5000 IU if clotting abnormality is present
- Inject TT
- Broad spectrum antibiotics.

Newer Vaccines

HIV Vaccine

There are three different approaches to HIV vaccination:

Preventive vaccine: To prevent HIV-negative persons from being infected.

Perinatal vaccine: To vaccinate HIV-infected pregnant women, in order to protect the fetus or the newborn child from being infected.

"Therapeutic" or post-infectious vaccine: To delay the progression to AIDS in HIV-positive persons.

Leprosy Vaccine

Three leprosy vaccines are currently undergoing large scale human trials. The first is the WHO vaccine developed by Dr J Convict in Venezuela. It is a combined vaccine containing BCG and heat killed *M. leprae,* harvested from armadillo. The rationale for incorporating BCG in it is the fact that BCG has some protective action against leprosy. The other two are **Indian vaccines**—the ICRC vaccine developed by Dr MG Deo at Cancer Research Institute, Mumbai and the MW vaccine, developed by Dr GP Talwar at National Institute of Immunology, New Delhi from Mycobact. W, which is a nonpathological atypical *Mycobacterium* sharing antigens with *M. leprae.*

Chickenpox Vaccine

A live attenuated vaccine (OKA strain) developed by Takashasi in Japan has been extensively studied in field trials. The frequency of mild local reactions at the site of inoculation is about one percent. A general reaction to the vaccine, after vaccination, in healthy seronegative children is over 90 percent. The vaccine has proved safe and effective in preventing the disease.

Rubella Vaccines

In 1979, the RA 27/3 vaccine, produced in human diploid fibroblast has replaced all the other vaccines. This is because RA 27/3 vaccine induces higher antibody titers and produces an immune response more closely paralleling natural infection than the other vaccines. There is evidence that it largely prevents subclinical superinfection with wild virus.

RA 27/3 vaccine is administered in a single dose of 0.5ml subcutaneously. It may provoke mild reactions in some subjects such as malaise, fever, mild rash and transient arthralgia, but no serious disability. Seroconversion occurs in more than 95 percent vaccinees. Vaccine-induced immunity persists in most vaccinees for at least 14 to 16 years and probably is lifelong.

MMR: Rubella vaccine is also available as combined measles, mumps and rubella (MMR) vaccine. It is equally effective. It is given at 15 months of age in a dose of 0.5 ml intramuscularly/subcutaneously.

Influenza Vaccines

Split-virus vaccine: Also known as sub-virion vaccine. It is a highly purified vaccine, producing fewer side effects than the "whole virus" vaccine. Because of its lower antigenicity, it requires several injections instead of a single one. It is recommended for children.

Neuraminidase specific vaccine: It is a sub-unit vaccine containing only the N antigen, which induces antibodies only to the neuraminidase antigen of the prevailing influenza virus. Antibody to neuraminidase reduces both the amount of virus replicating in the respiratory tract and the ability to transmit virus to contacts. It significantly reduces clinical symptoms in the infected person, but permits subclinical infection that may give rise to lasting immunity.

Recombinant vaccine: By recombinant techniques, the desirable antigenic properties of a virulent strain can be transferred to another strain known to be of low virulence. Effort to improve influenza vaccine are continuing in several directions.

Hepatitis B Vaccines

Active immunization can be done using a vaccine prepared from plasma of HbsAg carriers. The whole virus is removed and inactivated with formalin. It is available as Hepativax-B (MSD) and Hevac-B (Pasteur) and is indicated only for high-risk groups.

A 3 ml vial of Hepativax-B contains 20 micrograms of the vaccine. Recent observations suggests as the routine higher dose and provides protection for 5 years. The use of this smaller 0.1 ml dose considerably lowers the cost of immunization (Table 8.6).

Table 8.6: Hepatitis B vaccine—immunization schedule

1st dose	1 ml	at selected date
2nd dose	1 ml	1 month later
3rd dose (booster)	1 ml	6 months after the first dose

Note: Children under 10 years of age should be given half of above dosage at the same time intervals.

rDNA-yeast derived vaccine: A subunit HbsAg containing vaccine made by recombinant DNA (rDNA) technology is also available. It is costlier but safer. The reason is that the plasma derived vaccine carries the risk of infection, especially AIDS. A combination of DPT with HB vaccine is also available.

Malaria Vaccines

Asexual blood-stage vaccines based on antigens derived from the blood states of *P. falciparum* present in man. These vaccines are designed to reduce severe and complicated manifestations of the disease.

A synthetic " cocktail" vaccine for *P. falciparum,* called SPf 66 is developed by Dr M Patarroyo in Colombia. It reduces the risk of developing clinical malaria by about 30 percent.

Pfs25 vaccine: As far as transmission blocking vaccines are concerned, Pfs25 is a leading candidate and a preparation based on it has gone into clinical trials in the USA and Africa during 1995.

Meningococcal Vaccines

Effective vaccines prepared from purified Group A, Group C, Group Y, and/or Group W135 meningococcal polysaccharides are now available. They may be monovalent (A or C) or polyvalent (A-C; A-C-Y, etc). Recent field trails have indicated that immunity lasts for about three years, and boosters every three years would be reasonable. High-risk population should be identified and vaccinated. The vaccine is not recommended for use in infants and children under two years. The vaccine is contraindicated in pregnant women.

BIBLIOGRAPHY

1. Ann Rev of PH 1988; 209.
2. Desai HG. Prevention and Control of Hepatitis B virus. Medical times (sandoz)1984;14:4.
3. Jawetz E, et al. Review of Medical Microbiology, 14th edn, Lang Med Pabl California, 1980.
4. Kallings LO. CARC Calling 1993; 6:(1) 3-5.
5. Ministry of Health and Family Welfare Govt. of India New Delhi. Conduct immunisation, 1989.
6. National Health Programmes of India, J Kishore 4th edn, 2002.
7. Pan American Health Organisation. Bull PAHO 1978;12(2):162.
8. Park's Textbook of PSM, 16th edn, 2000.
9. Peckham CS. Med Int 1988;51:2107.
10. Textbook of PSM, MC Gupta and BK Mahajan, 3rd edn, 2003.
11. Wahdan MH, et al. Bull WHO 1973;48:667-73.
12. Wahdan MH, et al. Bull WHO 1977;55:645-51.
13. WHO. Tech RCP Ser No. 693,1983.
14. WHO. Tech RCP Ser No. 771,1988.
15. WHO. The World Health Report 1995 Bridging the gaps, Report of the Director General WHO,1995.

Chapter 9

Nutrition

CHAPTER OUTLINE

- BALANCED DIETS

INTRODUCTION

The importance of nutritional support was realized in the late 1970's. Nutritional support is not merely administering calories and proteins, it also includes the provision of all nutritional substrates to facilitate the biological processes of inflammation and healing.

Dietetics

Dietetics is the practical application of principles of nutrition for the well and sick persons.

Balanced Diet

A balanced diet is defined as one which contains a variety of foods in such quantities and proportions that the need for energy, amino acids, vitamins, minerals, fats, carbohydrate and other nutrients is adequately met for maintaining health, vitality, and general well-being and also makes a small provision for extra nutrients to withstand short duration of leanness.

An Indian Reference Man

An Indian reference man is between 20 and 39 years of age and weighs 60 kg (Tables 9.1 and 9.2). He is free from disease and physically fit for active work. On each working day he is employed for eight hours in occupation that usually involves moderate activity, while not at work he spends eight hours in bed, four to six hours sitting and moving around and two hours in walking and in active recreation or household duties.

An Indian Reference Woman

An Indian reference woman is between 20 and 39 years of age, healthy and weighs 50 kg (Tables 9.1 and 9.2). She may be engaged for eight hours in general house hold work, in light industry or in other moderately active work. Apart from eight hours in bed, she spends four to six hours sitting or moving around only through light activity and two hours in walking or in active recreation or in household duties.

Table 9.1: Indian reference men and women

Reference man	*Reference woman*
1. Age 20-39 years	20-39 years
2. Weight 60 kg	50 kg
3. Household works 8 hours	8 hours
4. Sleep 8 hours	8 hours
5. Light activity 4-6 hours	4-6 hours
6. Active recreation (walking) 2 hours	2 hours

Table 9.2: Appropriate body weights for men and women

	Men		*Women*	
Height (cm)	*Average (kg)*	*Acceptable range (kg)*	*Average range (kg)*	*Acceptable range (kg)*
145	—	—	46.0	37.53
148	—	—	46.5	37.54
150	—	39.58	47.0	38.55
152	—	40.59	48.5	39.57
156	—	43.62	49.5	39.58
158	55.8	44.64	50.4	40.58
160	57.6	44.65	51.3	41.59
162	58.6	46.66	52.6	42.61
164	59.6	47.67	54.0	43.62
166	60.6	48.69	55.4	44.61
168	61.7	41.71	56.8	45.65
170	63.5	51.73	58.1	45.66
172	65.0	52.74	60.0	46.67
174	66.5	53.75	61.3	48.69
176	68.0	54.77	62.6	49.70
178	69.4	55.79	64.0	51.72
180	71.0	58.80	65.3	52.74
182	72.6	59.82		
184	74.2	60.84		
186	75.8	62.86		
188	77.6	64.88		
190	79.3	66.90		
192	81.0	68.93		

The dietary sources of energy are:

Protein	4 kcal/gm
Fat	9 kcal/gm
Carbohydrate	4 kcal/gm

Macronutrients: These are proteins, fats and carbohydrates. These are also called as "proximate principles" which form the major bulk of food.

Micronutrients: These are vitamins and minerals. They are required in very small quantities.

Energy expenditure for work:

Persons require energy for daily activities—sitting, standing, walking, talking.

Male: 1250 kcal for 8 hours of work

Female: 820 kcal for 8 hours of work

Energy requirements: Energy requirements for persons doing

1. Light work	1.7 kcal/kg/hr
2. Moderate work	2.5 kcal/kg/hr
3. Heavy work	5 kcal/kg/hr

Energy requirement decreases as age advances, after 40 years, there is 5 percent decrease per decade up to 60 years, another 10 percent decrease during 60-70 years and further 10 percent decrease after 70 years of age.

Nutrition: Nutrition signifies a dynamic process in which the food that is consumed is utilized in the human body for nourishment.

Nutrient: Chemical compounds found in food which are needed for the body.

Meal: It is sum of the total food ingested at one feeding.

Diet: It is sum of the meals per day.

Dietary: It is the prescription of course of diet.

Food: It is composite mixture of various substances in various quantities.

Foodstuff: Anything which can be used as food is foodstuff.

Assessment of Nutritional Status

The assessment of nutritional status involves various techniques. Proper evaluation demands many angled approach.

The assessment method includes:

1. Clinical examination
2. Anthropometry
3. Biochemical evaluation
4. Functional assessment
5. Assessment of dietary intake
6. Vital and health statistics
7. Ecological studies
8. Weighment of raw food

9. Weighment of cooked food
10. Oral questionnaire method
11. Mortality data
12. Morbidity
13. Food balance sheet
14. Socioeconomic factors
15. Health and educational services
16. Conditioning influences.

Assessment of the Energy Requirement for Family

The recommendation co-efficients for calculating energy need of different members of the family are given in Table 9.3.

Table 9.3: Assessment of the energy requirements of a group of family

Category	*Co-efficient (for calculating energy requirements)*
Adult male (sedentary worker)	1.0
Adult male (moderate worker)	1.2
Adult male (heavy work)	1.6
Adult female (sedentary)	0.8
Adult female (moderate worker)	0.9
Adult female (heavy worker)	1.2
Adolescents—12 to 21 years	1.0
Children—9 to 12 years	0.8
Children—7 to 9 years	0.7
Children—5 to 7 years	0.6
Children—3 to 5 years	0.5
Children—1 to 3 years	0.4

Cereals and Millets

In India, cereals like wheat, rice and maize form the staple food of people. Millets (smaller grains that are eaten without removing the outer layer) are also used to fair extent by same segment of the population. More common among the millets are jawar and bajra.

Cereals and millets are rich in carbohydrates and sources of dietary protein. They are a good source of minerals and several B complex vitamins (Table 9.4).

Milling Process Deprives

Thiamine—15 percent
Riboflavine—75 percent
Protein—60 percent
Washing and cooking—60 percent loss of water soluble vitamins.

Table 9.4: Food value per 100 g

Cereals name of foodstuff	*Carb-ohyd-rates* (gm)	*Fat (gm)*	*Protein (gm)*	*Calcium (mg)*	*Iron (mg)*	*Energy* (kcal)	*Limiting amino acid*
Jawar	72.6	1.9	10.4%	25	4.1	349	Lysine and threonine
Bajra	67.5	5	11.9	42	8	361	
Ragi	72	1.3	7.3	344	3.9	328	
Maize (dry)	66.2	3.6	11.1	50	3.8	342	Tryptophan and lysine
Wheat (whole)	71.2	1.5	11.8	50	5.3	346	Lysine and threonine
Rice (row, milled)	78.2	0.5	6.8	23	6.6	345	Poor source of A_1, C and D vitamins

Parboiling

Process starts with soaking the paddy in hot water at 65 to 70°C for three to four hours which swells the grain. This is followed by draining of water and steaming the soaked paddy in same container for 5 to 10 minute. The paddy is then dried and home pounded or milled. During steaming, greater part of vitamins and minerals present in outer aleurone layer of rice grain are driven into the inner endosperm. With subsequent drying process the germ get attached more firmly to the grain. It results in the grains becoming resistant to insect invasion and more suitable for storage than raw rice. The starch also get gelatinized which improves keeping qualities of rice.

Pellagra

It is a nutritional deficiency disease. High leucine content in jawar and maize interferes in the conversion of tryptophan into niacin and thus aggravates the pellagragenic action of maize and jawar.

- Pellagra manifestations—3D's
- Diarrhea
- Dementia
- Dermatitis

Pulses (Legumes)

Pulses are called "poor man's meat". In fact pulses contain more protein than egg, fish and flesh food, but in regards to the quality, pulse's protein is inferior to animal protein. Pulses are poor in methionine and to a lesser extent in cystein and are rich in lysine (Table 9.5).

Soyabean is exceptionally rich in protein, containing up to 40 percent.

Table 9.5: Nutritive value of pulses

Food stuff	*Energy (kcal)*	*Protein (gm)*	*Fat (gm)*	*Carbo-hydrate*	*Iron (mg)*	*Thia-mine*	*Ribo-flavin*	*Niacin mg*	*Vit 'C'*
Bengal gram (whole)	360	17.1	5.3	202	4.6	0.30	0.15	2.9	0
Black gram (dhal)	347	24.0	1.4	154	3.8	0.42	0.20	2.0	0
Red gram (dhal)	335	22.3	1.7	73	2.7	0.45	0.19	2.9	0
Soya bean	432	43.2	19.5	240	10.4	0.73	0.39	3.2	0

Germination and Fermentation

The simple measures of soaking pulses in water for 2 to 3 hours improves their nutritive value and vitamin 'A' and vitamin 'C' content.
Germination increases the content of folic acid and other vitamin 'B' group by a factor of two or three. Pulses contain an antidigestive factor (trypsin inhibitor) which is destroyed by cooking.

Anti-nutritional factors: In the raw state, pulses have some anti-nutritional factors such as phytate and tannins most of anti-nutritional factors destroyed by heat.

Presence of certain sugar known as oligosaccharides is known to be associated with flatulence.

Lathyrism

Lathyrism is a paralyzing disease of human and animal, occuring mostly in adults consuming the pulse, lathyrus sativus in large quantity (more than 30% of this dhal over a period of 2-6 months).

In humans it is referred to as neurolethyrism.

In animals it is referred to as osteolethyrism.

Toxin present in lathyrus seeds has been known as (Beta-oxalyl amino alanine) BOAA .

Manifestation (in Different Stages)

1. Latent stage
2. No stick stage
3. One stick stage
4. Two stick stage
5. Crawler stage.

Intervention

1. Vitamin "C" prophylaxis
2. Banning the crop

3. Removal of toxin
   a. Steeping method
   b. Parboiling
4. Education
5. Genetic approach.

Vegetables

Vegetables are classed as "protective foods"
Vegetables are divided into:
1. Green leaves
2. Roots and tubers
3. Other vegetables.

Leafy vegetables are high in water content and dietary fiber. These vegetable contain a high proportion of cellulose, which human intestinal juices (unlike those of herbivorous animals) can not digest. It thus remains unabsorbed and increase bulk of the intestinal contents.

The bioavailability of calcium and iron from green vegetables is rather poor because of the presence of high amount of oxalates.

Don't soak cut leaves for a long time, by doing so water soluble vitamins "B" and "C" will be dissolved in water and are wasted.

Addition of baking powder will not only destroy the flavor and texture but vitamin "B" will also be lost.

Don't cook in excess water, avoid over cooking and reheating to avoid vitamin "C" loss.

The recommended daily intake of green leafy vegetables is about 40 gm for an adult.

Fruits (Fructua—to Enjoy)

Fruits are protective foods.

The costly fruits are not necessarily the best one. Banana is the cheapest when considered as a food rather than a fruit. Grape and apple are not of high nutritional value.

Composition of Fruits per 100 gm (Table 9.6)

Clinical use

Banana
a. Acts as a mild laxative

Table 9.6: Composition of fruits per 100 gm

Fruits	*Protein (gm)*	*Fat (gm)*	*Carbohydrate*	*Vit "A"*	*Vit "C"*	*Caloric value*
Apple	0.2	0.5	13.4	Trace	2	59
Banana	1.2	0.3	27.2	Trace	1	116
Grapes (pellagra)	0.5	0.3	16.5	15	31	71
Mango	0.6	0.4	16.9	800	13	74
Papaya (ripe)	0.6	0.1	7.2	2020	46	32
Jack fruit	1.9	0.1	19.8	540	10	88
Lemon	1.0	0.9	11.1	0	39	57

b. A high-banana diet probably increases the butyric acid concentration in intestine and this may control diarrhea.
c. Steamed banana leaves are effectively used for dressing burn wounds.

Mango
a. Eating mangoes in season may provide a store of vitamin "A" in the liver, sufficient to last for the rest of the year.

Papaya
a. Papaya can be prescribed for dyspeptic patients as the pepsin may help in the digestion of proteins.
b. Papaya seeds have an antihelminthic action.
c. A protein digestive enzyme chymopapain derived from papaya is used as injection into herniated intervertebral lumbar disks to relieve pain caused by pressure on nerves.

Nuts and Oil Seeds

The common nuts consumed in the tropics are coconut, groundnut, cashew nut, almonds and pista.

They are rich in proteins, fat, carbohydrates, minerals, and factors of vitamin "B" complex. Nuts approach on ideal food by supplying high calories in a palatable form. Groundnut is palatable and cheap—used in multipurpose food Balahar, used as balanced malt food due to high fat content and partly cellulose content.

Aflatoxin: Stored groundnut may be contaminated with the fungus *Aspergillus flavors* which produce toxins known collectively as aflatoxins.

Sweet Food and Sweetening Agents

Sugar is almost pure sucrose—A diasaccharides made up of glucose and fructose (levulose). One gm of sugar supplies—4 kcal.

One teaspoonful (5 g) gives—20 kcal.

The average consumption of sugar is well over 100 gm a day per person.

Honey: Golden colored syrup made by bees from the nectar of flowers which contains mixture of glucose and fructose which gives it a particular sweetness.

Composition
- Glucose—25 to 37 percent
- Fructose—34 to 43 percent
- Sucrose—0.5 to 12 percent
- Maltose—5 to 12 percent
- 100 gm honey provides—288 Kcal

Honey may contain the bacteria *Clostridium botulinum* which may produce infant botulism.

1. Honey 50 mg/liter recommended instead of sugar in oral rehydration fluid.
2. Honey in warm water or milk can be a soothing drink for patients with pharyngitis and tracheitis.

Nutrient Requirements during Pregnancy (Tables 9.7 to 9.14)

Table 9.7: Daily allowances for nutrients for expectant and nursing mothers (ICM R Nutrition Export Group, 1998)

Nutrient	*Sedentary*	*Moderate work*	*Heavy work*	*Pregnancy*	*Lactation*
Calories (kcal)	1900	2200	3000	+300	+700
Proteins (g)	45	45	45	55	65
Calcium (g)	0.45-0.5	0.4-0.5	0.4-0.5	1.0	1.0
Iron (g)	30	30	30	40	30
Vitamin (A)					
as Retinol (μg)	750	750	750	750	1150
Or					
as Carotene (mg)	3000	3000	3000	3000	4600
Thiamine (mg)	1.0	1.1	1.5	+0.2	+0.4
Riboflavin (mg)	1.0	1.2	1.7	+0.2	+0.4
Nicotinic acid (mg)	13	15	20	+2	+5
Ascorbic acid (mg)	50	50	50	50	80
Folic acid (mg)	100	100	100	150-300	150
Vitamin B_{12} (mg)	1.0	1.0	1.0	1.5	1.5
Vitamin D (IU)	200	200	200	200	200

Table 9.8: Suggested substitution for nonvegetarians

Food item which can be deleted from non-vegetarian diets	*Substitution that can be suggested for deleted item or items*
1. 50% of pulses (20-30 g)	1. One egg or 30 g meat or fish 2. Additional 5 g fat or oil
2. 100% of pulses (40-60 g)	1. Two eggs or 50 g of meat or fish, one egg plus 30 g meat 2. 10 g of fat or oil

Table 9.9: Additional allowances during pregnancy and lactation

Food items	*During pregnancy*	*Calories (kcal)*	*During lactation*	*Calories (kcal)*
Cereals	35 g	118	60 g	203
Pulses	15 g	52	30 g	105
Milk	100 g	83	100 g	83
Fat	–	–	10 g	90
Sugar	10 g	– 40	10 g	40
Total		293		521

Diet: For a child suffering from protein calorie malnutrition and weighing 12 kg, the daily calorie intake should be about 12 × 140 = 1680 kal and protein intake should be 12 × 4 or 5 = 48 to 60 g.

Table 9.10: Diet for a child suffering from kwashiorkor or marasmus (Body wt 12.12 kg calories 1700 kcal protein 50-60 g)

Foodstuffs	*Diet for Ist to 10th day*	*Diet for 11th to 30th day*
Milk, skimmed (ml)	1000	–
Milk, skimmed (ml)	1000	2000
Cane sugar (g)	100	100
Dextrimaltose (g)	50	–
Ripe banana (two) (g)	150	150
Corn or wheat flour (g)	25	50
Bread and biscuit (g)	25	10-100
Vitamins	Daily requirements added to milk	

Table 9.11: Daily menu for a child suffering from kwashiorkor or marasmus

1st day to 10th day	*11th day to 30th day*
Morning 6.00 am	**Morning 6.00 am**
Milk (half fat)	Milk (full fat)
With sugar—1 cup	With sugar—1 cup
Breakfast 8.00 am	**Breakfast 8.00 am**
Corn flour milk pudding—1 serving	Bread (1 slice) with milk
Banana (one)	Banana (one)
Milk with sugar—1 cup	Corn flour milk pudding—1 serving
	Milk with sugar—1 cup
10.00 am	**10.00 am**
Milk with sugar—1 cup	Milk with sugar—1 cup
1.00 pm (lunch)	**1.00 pm (lunch)**
Bread soaked in milk—1 slice	Bread—2 slices (with milk)
Banana—1	Banana—1
Milk with sugar—1 cup	Milk pudding—1 serving
	Milk with sugar—1 cup
4.00 pm	**4.00 pm**
Milk with sugar—1 cup	Milk with sugar—1 cup
	Biscuit —2

Contd...

Contd...

1st day to 10th day	*11th day to 30th day*
7.00 pm (Dinner)	**7.00 pm (Dinner)**
Bread soaked in milk—1 slice	Same as lunch
Banana—1	
Milk with sugar—1 cup	
10.00 pm	**10.00 pm**
Milk with sugar—1 cup	Milk with sugar—1 cup

Table 9.12: Daily menu for adults suffering from tuberculosis

Vegetarian	*Nonvegetarian*
Early morning	
Milk with sugar—1 cup	Milk with sugar—1 cup
Breakfast	
Bread—4 slices or	Bread—4 slices or
Idli—4 or	Idli— 4 or
Dosa—2 or	Dosa—2 or
Poori—3	Poori—3
Cheese—1 slice	Boiled egg—1
Nuts—2 tablespoons	Nuts—2 tablespoons
Mid-morning	
Fruit juice—1 glass	Fruit juice—1 glass
Lunch	
Cooked rice or chappati—1 serving	Cooked rice or chappati—1 serving
Vegetable curry—1 serving	Mutton or fish curry—1 serving
Dal soup—1 cup	Vegetable curry—1 cup
Curd—1 cup	Dal soup—1 cup
Milk pudding—1 serving	Milk pudding—1 serving
Fruits—1 serving	Fruits—1 serving
Mid-afternoon	
Fruit juice—1 glass	Fruit juice—1 glass
Tea	
Biscuits—2	Biscuits—2
Nuts—2 tablespoons	Nuts—2 table spoons
Milk with sugar—1 cup	Milk with sugar—1 cup
Cheese—1 slice	Cheese—1 slice
Fruits—1 serving	Fruits—1 serving
Dinner	
	Same as lunch

Table 9.13: Diet in severe jaundice in viral hepatitis for an adult (g/caput/day)

Proteins, 40-45 g; Fats 25-30 g; Carbohydrates 300-340 g and Calories 1600-1700 Kcal	
Cereals	200
Skimmed milk	500
Potato	100
Leafy vegetables	50
Fruits (apple, mango, papaya or banana)	200
Fruit juice	600
Fat and oils	15
Sugar and Jam	60

One multivitamin tablet providing the daily requirements of all vitamins should be included along with the diet.

Table 9.14: Daily menu for severe jaundice

Morning	
Fruit juice	1 glass
Breakfast	
Corn flakes with skimmed milk and sugar	1 serving
Toast with a little butter and jam	2 slices
Fruits	1 serving
Tea or coffee	1 cup
Mid morning	
Fruit juice	1 glass
Lunch	
Cooked rice or bread or chappati	1 serving
Vegetable soup	1 cup
Cooked vegetables	1 serving
Fruits	1 serving
Skimmed milk pudding	1 serving
Tea	
Biscuits	2
Fruit juice	1 glass
Dinner	
Similar to Lunch	

Rich Sources of Essential Nutrients

- Richest source of poly unsaturated fatty acid: Safflower oil—75 percent.
- Richest source of saturated fatty acid is coconut oil—92 percent.
- Richest source of Linoleic acid (EFA) is safflower oil—73 percent.
- Richest source of vitamin A (retinol) is Halibut liver oil—(900,000 mcg/100 g) and cod liver oil (18000 mcg/100 g).
- Green leafy vegetable rich in vitamin A (Carotene) is Colocasia leaves—12000 mcg/100 g. Others are Amaranth, Spinach.

- Vegetable rich in vitamin A is carrot—1167 mcg/100g.
- Fruit rich in vitamin A is Ripe mango.
- Richest source of vitamin D is halibut liver oil (50-10,000 mcg/100 g) and cod liver oil.
- Thiamine rich foods—wheat, rice parboiled, bengal gram dhal, gingelly seeds.
- Rich source of riboflavin in sheep liver—1.70 mg/100 mg.
- Rich source of niacin-ground nut (22.1/100 g), sheep liver.
- Fruits rich in vitamin C—amla (600 mg/100 g), guava (212).
- Pulse with high vitamin C—content bengal gram.
- Vegetables rich in vitamin C—amaranth (99), cabbage (124).
- Rich source of calcium—ragi (344 g/100 g).

Protein Requirements

Men and women	1 gm/kg/day
Infants (0-6 mon)	1.8-2.3
Infants (6-9 mon)	1.65
Children (1-6 years)	1.52-1.83
Children (6-9 years)	1.48
Adolescent males	1.3-4.6
Adolescent females	1.21-1.45

Principles in Calculating Balanced Diet

India

- Energy from cereals not to be more than 75 percent.
- Cereal protein to pulse protein ratio to be kept at 4:1.
- Vegetables to constitute 80 gm.
- Inclusion of green leafy vegetables.
- Minimum milk intake of 100 ml needed.
- Fat not to contribute more than 15 percent of energy.
- Energy from refined carbohydrates kept around 5 percent and total calories from sugar not to exceed 20 percent.

BALANCED DIETS (TABLE 9.15)

Table 9.15: Balanced diets (The quantities are given in grams)

Food items	Adult man			Adult woman		
	Sedentary	Moderate worker	Heavy worker	Secondary worker	Moderate worker	Heavy worker
Cereals	460	520	670	410	440	575
Pulses	40	50	60	40	45	50
Leafy vegs	40	40	40	100	100	50
Other vegs	60	70	80	40	40	100
Roots and tubers	50	60	80	50	50	60
Milk	150	200	250	100	150	200
Oils and fats	40	45	65	20	25	40
Sugar	30	35	55	20	20	40

Balanced Diet for Children (Table 9.16)

Table 9.16: Balanced diet for children

Food items	*Children 1-3 years*	*Children 4-6 years*	*Boys 10-12 years*	*Girls 10-12 years*
Cereals	175	270	420	380
Pulses	35	35	45	45
Leafy vegs	40	50	50	50
Other vegs	20	30	50	50
Roots and tubers	10	20	30	30
Milk	300	250	250	250
Oil and fats	15	25	40	35
Sugar/jaggery	30	40	45	45

Food items	*Approx Quantity*	*Approx Weight (gm)*	*Protein (gm)*	*Calories*
Musambi	1 average	150	1.2	63
Watermelon		100	0.5	28
Strawberries	10 large	100	0.8	37
Almonds		100	20.8	655
Cashewnuts		100	20.2	596
Groundnut		100	26.7	559
Pista		100	19.8	626
Coconut		100	6.8	662
Butter		100	0.0	729
Cheese		100	24.1	348
Curds		100	3.1	60
Buffalo milk	1 cup	200	8	206
Cow's milk	1 cup	200	7	160
Goats milk	½ cup	100	3.3	75
Milk powdered	1 table spoon	7	1.9	35
Human milk		100	1.1	65
Ice cream	1 spoon	100	4.1	196
Ghee	1 table spoon	5	0.0	45
Chicken boiled	1 serving	100	17.0	132
Egg boiled	1 medium	48	6.1	77
Egg omlet	1	62	6.6	120
Mutton (Goat)	5-6 pieces	100	21.0	120
Beef boiled		100	25.4	242
Pork	1 serving	100	24.6	317
Fish	1 plate	100	18	81
Limbu juice	1 glass	240	0.0	73
Rice gangi	1 glass	193	8.7	312
Ragi ganji	1glass	280	6.9	263
Butter milk	1 glass	200	2.4	66
Biscuit	2 in number	16	1.6	64
Milk chocolate	1 piece	28	2.4	152
Bengal gram	1 cup	200	7	105
Chana Dal	1 cup	200	7	105

Contd...

Contd...

Food items	*Approx Quantity*	*Approx Weight (gm)*	*Protein (gm)*	*Calories*
Black gram, Green gram, Masor dal, Toor dal, Beans baked, Peas dried	1 cup	200	7	105
Cabbage cooked	½ cup	85	1.2	20
Carrot cooked	½ cup	75	0.5	23
Carrot raw	1 large	100	1.2	42
Cauliflower, Brinjal, Bhendi, Bitter guard Cooked		125	3.0	36
Cucumber	½ medium	50	0.4	06
Green leafy (palak, menthe)		125	3.0	32
Potato		100	1.6	97
Radish		99	0.7	17
Sweet potato		100	1.2	120
Beet root		85	1.7	43
Pumpkin		79	1.4	25
Tomato		150	1.5	30
Banana	1 big	100	1.2	99
Mango	1 in no.	100	1.0	54
Apple	1 medium	150	0.3	66
Grapes	22.24	100	1.4	70
Guava	1 medium	100	0.9	51
Orange	1 medium	150	1.4	68
Papaya	1 medium	100	0.6	32
Pineapple	1 slice	84	0.3	44
Whisky	1 peg	30 ml		91
Neera	1 glass	200 ml	0.8	90
Toddy	1 glass	200 ml	0.2	20
Beer	1 glass	240 ml		98
Brandy	1 peg	30 ml		98
Gin	1 peg	30 ml		84
Rum	1 peg	30 ml		98
Red wine	1 glass	100 ml		82
Champagne	1 glass	100 ml		78
Cola/Orange/ Lemon drink	1 bottle	300 ml		84
Soda	1 bottle	300 ml		00
Samosa	1		2.0	94
Kachori	1		3.0	152
Rasagolla	1		3.0	162
Burfi	1		4.0	74
Bournvita	1 cup	230 ml	10.2	625

Contd...

Contd...

Food items	*Approx Quantity*	*Approx Weight (gm)*	*Protein (gm)*	*Calories*
Horlicks	2 table spoon	30	4.1	113
Ovaltine	2 table spoon	30	3.8	109
Chapati	2	57	5	193
Poori	2	32	2.2	136
Jowar roti	2	150	7.5	232
Ragi roti	3	185	8.0	460
Ragi balls	1	336	8.0	446
Plain rice	1 plate	170	4.2	200
Wheat bread	1 slice	30	2.3	75
Wheat bread, butter and jam—1 tea spoon each	1 slice	40	2.6	130
Wheat bun	1 average	35	2.6	120
Wheat parota	1	60	4.8	256
Bajra roti	1	45	3.5	108
Mazia roti	1	45	3.3	102
Idli	1 no	68	2.3	65
Plain dosa	1 no	50	2.0	108
Masala dosa	1 no	101	4.6	212
Uppit/Upma	1 plate	128	3.8	163
Uttappa(onion dosa)	1 no	132	7.3	337
Rava Idli	2 in no	114	5.0	212
Shira(Kesari bath)	1 plate	180	4.0	564
Uddin wada	2 in no	50	5.1	138
Bajji	6 in no	40	2.3	132
Chakli	3 in no	44	8.6	408
Dahi wada	2 in no	99	6.5	177
Tomato omelette	1 in no	56	3.2	100
Poha	1 plate	30	1.8	114
Mysorepak	1 piece	56	2.6	345
Bundi laddu	1 no	34	1.8	150
Rava laddu	1 in no	57	2.9	285
Halva	2 pieces	109	2.6	342
Jalabi	2 in no	41	1.4	313
Cake plain	1 piece	75	3.5	218
Custard	½ cup	130	7.1	164

Preparation	*Weight (g)*	*Measure*	*Calories (kcal)*	*Proteins (g)*	*Fats (g)*	*Carbo-hydrates (g)*
Chutneys						
Coconut chutney	55	2 tbsp	125	2	10	6
Coriander chutney	20	1 tbsp	45	1	4	2

Contd...

Contd...

Preparation	*Weight (g)*	*Measure*	*Calories (kcal)*	*Proteins (g)*	*Fats (g)*	*Carbo-hydrates (g)*
Groundnut chutney	20	1 tbsp	65	3	5	3
Mint chutney	18	1 tbsp	7	-	-	2
Tomato chutney	50	½ k	32	1	1	5
Nonvegetarian						
Dam ka chicken	125	1 k	260	26	15	4
Fish cutlet	80	Two	190	14	9	12
Fish fried	85	Two	220	18	12	6
Fish jhol	110	1 k	140	18	3	12
Liver do-pyaza	140	1 k	330	22	22	11
Mutton ball curry	145	1 k	240	10	18	10
Prawn curry	145	1 k	220	18	7	22

Average Weight of Vegetables (Table 9.17)

Table 9.17: Average weight of vegetables

Vegetable	*Weight per piece*
Ash gourd	1000
Beans	3
Brinjal (small)	20
Brinjal (long)	50
Brinjal (big)	250
Cabbage	500
Capsicum	30
Carrot	40
Cauliflower	200
Drumstick	30
Fenugreek leaves (bundle)	12
Ladies' finger	10
Onion (medium)	50
Pumpkin	1100
Radish	150
Raw banana	60
Ridge guard	50
Spinach (bundle)	20
Tomato	40

Approximate Weight of Foods Equal to 1 Level Katori (Bowl) of 150 ml Volume (Table 9.18)

Table 9.18: Approximate weight of foods

Item	*Weight 1 katori (gm)*
Cereals	
Rice	150
Rice flour	90
Semolina	120
Wheat flour	90
White flour (maida)	80
Pulses	
Bengal gram dhal	130
Bengal gram dhal flout	80
Black gram dhal	130
Green gram dhal	140
Lentil dhal	130
Red gram dhal	140
Whole pulses and legumes	
Black-eye beans	130
Green gram whole	140
Kabuli chana	130
Kidney beans	120
Lentil whole	125

Source: Pasricha-count what you eat. National Institute of Nutrition Hyderabad,1989

Average Weight of Nuts and Spices (Table 9.19)

Table 9.19: Average weight of nuts and spices

Nuts	*Measure/number*	*Weight (gm)*
Almonds (small)	15	20
Cashewnut	15	25
Coconut (dry)	1	160
Coconut (fresh)	1	150
Groundnuts	20	6
Poppy seeds	1 tsp	4
Raisins	15	5
Sesame seeds	1 tsp	3
Spices		
Asafoetida	1 tsp	6
Black pepper	1 tsp	5
Cardamom	10	1
Chilli powder	1 tsp	7
Cinnamom	1 piece	0.5

Contd...

Contd...

Nuts	*Measure/number*	*Weight (gm)*
Cloves	12	1
Coriander leaves	1 bundle	3
Coriander powder	1 tsp	7
Curry leaves	1 bundle	5
Cumin	1 tsp	5
Fenugreek seeds	1 tsp	6
Garlic	1 pod	0.5
Green chillies	5	5
Mint	1 bundle	5
Mustard seeds	1 tsp	10
Salt	1 tsp	10
Sugar	1 tsp	7
Turmeric	1 tsp	8

Recommended Dietary Allowances for Indians (Table 9.20)

Table 9.20: Recommended dietary allowances for Indians

Group	Particulars	Body wt kg	Net energy kcal/d	Protein g/d	Fat g/d	Calcium mg/d	Iron** mg/d	Vit μg/d retinol	B-carotene	Thiamin mg/d	Riboflavin	Nicotinic acid mg/d	Pyridoxin mg/d	Ascorbic acid mg/d	Folic acid mg/d	Vit B_{12} μg/d mg/d
Men	Secondary work		2425							1.2	1.4	16				
	Moderate work	60	2875	60	20	400	28	600	2400	1.4	1.6	18	2.0	40	100	1
	Heavy work		3800							1.6	1.9	21				
Women	Sedentary work		1875							0.9	1.1	12				
	Moderate work	50	2225	50	20	400	30	600	2400	1.1	1.3	14	2.0	40	100	1
	Heavy work		2925							1.2	1.5	16				
	Pregnant women	50	+300	+15	30	1000	38	600	2400	+0.2	+0.2	+2	2.5	40	400	1
	Lactation									+0.3	+0.3	+4				
	0-6 months		+550	+25	45	1000	30	950	3800				2.5	80	150	1.5
	0-12 months	+400	+18						+0.2	+0.2	+0.3					
Infants	0-6 months	5.4	108/kg	2.05/kg		500				55 μg/kg	65 μg/kg	710 μg/kg	0.1	25	25	0.2
	6-12 months	8.6	98 kg	1.65 kg			350	1200	50 μg/kg	60 μg/kg	650 μg/kg	0.4				
Children	1-3 years	12.2	1240	22	25	400	12	400	1600	0.6	0.7	8	0.9		30	
	4-6 years	19.0	1690	30			18	400	2400	0.9	1.0	11	0.9		40	
	7-9 years	26.9	1950	41			26	600	2400	1.0	1.2	13	1.6		60	
Boys	10-12 years	35.4	2190	54	22	600	34	600	2400	1.1	1.3	15	1.6		70	

Contd...

Contd...

Group	Particulars	Body wt kg	Net energy kcal/d	Protein g/d	Fat g/d	Calcium mg/d	Iron** mg/d	Vit µg/d retinol	B-carotene	Thiami mg/d	Riboflavin	Nicotinic acid mg/d	Pyridoxin mg/d	Asorbic acid mg/d	Folic acid mg/d	Vit B_{12} µg/d mg/d
Girls	10-12 years	31.5	1970	57			19			1.0	1.2	13	1.6	40	70	0.2-1.0
Boys	13-15 years	47.8	2450	70	22	600	41	600	2400	1.2	1.5	16			100	
Girls	13-15 years	46.7	2060	65			28			1.0	1.2	14			100	0.2-1.0
Boys	16-18 years	57.1	2640	78	22	500	50	600	2400	1.3	1.6	17	2.0		100	
Girls	16-18 years	49.9	2060	63	22		30			1.0	1.2	14			100	0.2-1.0

** On mixed cereal diet with absorption of 3% in man, 5% in woman 8% in pregnant woman.

Approximate Nutritive Value of Some Common Food Preparations (Table 9.21)

Table 9.21: Approximate nutritive value of some common food preparations (per serving and per 100 g)

Food preparations	*Qty (per serving)*	*Wt. (per serving)*	*Calories (Kcal)*	*Protein (g)*	*Fat (g)*	*Carbohydrate (g)*	*Calcium (g)*	*Phosphorus (g)*	*Iron (mg)*	*Vitamin A value (IU)*	*Thiamin (mg)*	*Nicotinic acid (mg)*	*Riboflavin (mg)*	*Vitmin C (mg)*
Ragiputtu	1 plate	146	422	4.4	7.4	2.0	0.20	0.20	3.0	280	0.20	0.6	0.06	–
"	-	100	289	3.3	5.1	57.7	0.14	0.14	5.5	193	0.14	0.4	0.4	–
Pulse preparations, Bengal gram dal cooked	1½ cup	151	284	9.0	16.4	25.2	0.07	0.13	3.8	366	0.14	2.4	0.10	2.0
"	–	100	188	6.0	10.9	16.7	0.05	0.9	2.5	242	0.10	1.6	0.7	1.2
Green gram dal cooked	1½ cup	142	171	7.0	7.7	18.4	0.08	0.9	2.7	33	0.14	2.4	0.11	1.6
"	–	100	120	4.9	5.4	12.9	0.06	0.06	1.9	23	0.10	1.7	0.08	1.1
Red gram dal cooked	½ cup	96	110	6.4	2.0	16.4	0.05	0.07	2.6	64	0.13	0.7	0.7	–
"	–	100	115	6.7	2.1	17.1	0.05	0.07	2.7	67	0.14	0.73	0.73	–
Dal rasam	1½ cup	196	29	1.5	0.9	3.8	0.03	0.03	0.9	72	0.03	0.2	0.2	1.5
"	–	100	15	0.8	0.5	1.9	0.02	0.02	0.5	37	0.02	0.1	0.1	0.8
Amaranth sambar	1½ cup	140	97	5.1	2.7	13.0	0.50	0.08	8.0	2009	0.07	0.7	0.03	53.0
"	–	100	69	3.6	1.9	9.3	0.36	0.06	5.7	1435	0.05	0.5	0.02	37.9
Radish sambar	1½ cup	196	101	4.1	3.6	13.1	0.04	0.07	2.2	73	0.07	0.05	0.03	3.0

Contd...

Contd...

Food preparations	*Qty (per serving)*	*Wt. (per serving)*	*Calories (Kcal)*	*Protein (g)*	*Fat (g)*	*Carbohydrate (g)*	*Calcium (g)*	*Phosphorus (g)*	*Iron (mg)*	*Vitamin A value (I.U.)*	*Thiamin (mg)*	*Nicotinic acid (mg)*	*Riboflavin (mg)*	*Vitmin C (mg)*
"	–	100	52	2.1	1.8	6.7	0.02	0.04	1.1	37	0.04	0.26	0.02	1.5
Green gram Sundal	1 plate	142	259	13.1	9.2	30.9	0.08	0.20	4.8	120	0.24	1.2	0.10	1.1
"	–	100	182	9.2	6.5	21.8	0.06	0.14	3.4	85	0.17	0.9	0.07	0.8
Bangal gram Sundal	1 plate	142	272	13.2	11.1	29.7	0.11	0.15	5.5	198	0.16	1.4	0.08	1.1
"	–	100	192	9.2	7.8	20.1	0.08	0.11	3.9	140	0.11	0.98	0.06	0.8
Cowpea Sundal	1 plate	142	255	13.5	8.8	30.3	0.05	0.20	2.5	71	0.30	0.9	0.15	1.1
"	–	100	180	9.5	6.2	21.4	0.03	0.14	1.8	50	0.21	0.6	0.11	0.8
Vegetable preparations amaranth curry	½ plate	28	47	1.4	2.3	5.1	0.04	0.04	6.6	1942	0.03	0.4	0.03	51.0
"	–	100	168	5.6	8.2	17.6	0.14	0.14	23.6	6934	0.11	1.4	0.11	182.2
Brinjal curry	½ plate	45	122	1.4	10.7	4.9	0.02	0.05	0.9	9	0.03	0.5	0.06	10.1
"	–	100	266	3.1	23.8	10.9	0.04	0.11	2.0	20	0.07	1.1	0.13	22.5
Amaranth maseal	½ plate	42	46	1.2	2.6	4.4	0.05	0.05	6.8	1946	0.02	0.4	0.02	55.0
"	–	100	110	3.0	6.2	10.3	1.2	0.12	16.2	4634	0.05	0.95	0.05	119.1
Cabbage and carrot curry	½ plate	56	81	1.5	5.6	6.1	0.04	0.12	0.9	1028	0.04	0.3	0.03	38.0
"	–	100	145	2.7	10.0	10.9	0.07	0.21	1.6	1835	0.07	0.05	0.05	67.9

Contd...

Contd...

Food preparations	*Qty (per serving)*	*Wt. (per serving)*	*Calories (Kcal)*	*Protein (g)*	*Fat (g)*	*Carbohydrate (g)*	*Calcium (g)*	*Phosphorus (g)*	*Iron (mg)*	*Vitamin A value (IU)*	*Thiamin (mg)*	*Nicotinic acid (mg)*	*Riboflavin (mg)*	*Vitmin C (mg)*
Preparations containing milk:coffee	–	100	52	1.9	1.7	7.2	0.05	0.05	0.10	77	0.02	0.09	0.09	0.7
"	1 cup	200	104	3.8	3.4	14.4	0.10	0.10	1.20	154	0.04	0.18	0.18	1.4
Tea	–	100	36	0.7	0.8	6.5	0.03	0.02	–	38	0.01	0.05	0.05	0.3
"	1 cup	200	72	1.4	1.6	13.0	0.06	0.0.4	–	76	0.02	0.10	0.10	0.6
Cocoa	1 cup	200	174	7.5	7.0	20.2	0.20	0.15	0.30	306	0.08	0.2	0.34	2.7
"	–	100	87	3.8	3.5	10.1	0.10	0.08	0.15	153	0.04	0.1	0.17	1.35
Wheat Payasam	1 cup	154	178	3.4	4.3	31.5	0.09	0.08	0.40	160	0.05	0.1	0.12	–
"	–	100	116	4.2	2.8	20.5	0.06	0.05	0.26	104	0.03	0.06	0.08	–
Rice Payasam	1 cup	154	178	3.2	4.2	31.7	0.09	0.08	0.40	160	0.05	0.1	0.26	–
"	–	100	116	2.1	2.7	20.6	0.06	0.05	0.26	104	0.03	0.06	0.17	–
Bengal gram dal Payasam	1 cup	140	221	7.7	5.1	35.9	0.07	0.14	4.7	197	0.05	0.2	0.40	–
"	–	100	158	5.5	3.6	25.5	0.05	0.10	3.4	141	0.04	0.14	0.28	–
Sago porridge	1 cup	266	227	3.7	4.0	44.0	0.14	0.10	0.17	204	0.06	–	0.23	2.0
"	–	100	85	1.4	1.5	16.5	0.05	0.04	0.26	77	0.02	–	0.09	0.8
Rice porridge	1 cup	280	263	7.6	6.2	44.3	0.30	0.20	0.7	306	0.10	0.3	0.34	2.0
"	–	100	94	2.7	2.2	15.2	0.11	0.07	0.25	109	0.04	0.11	0.123	0.8

Contd...

Contd...

Food preparations	*Qty (per serving)*	*Wt. (per serving)*	*Calories (Kcal)*	*Protein (g)*	*Fat (g)*	*Carbohydrate (g)*	*Calcium (g)*	*Phosphorus (g)*	*Iron (mg)*	*Vitamin A value (I.U.)*	*Thiamin (mg)*	*Nicotinic acid (mg)*	*Riboflavin (mg)*	*Vitmin C (mg)*
Wheat porridge+	1 cup	193	317	8.7	8.0	52.7	0.24	0.22	1.0	408	0.13	0.2	0.28	1.6
"	–	100	164	4.5	4.1	27.3	0.12	0.11	0.52	211	0.07	0.1	0.13	0.8
Ragi porridge	1 cup	280	263	6.9	6.3	44.7	0.30	0.20	1.7	321	0.20	0.2	0.34	2.0
"	–	100	94	2.5	2.2	16.0	0.11	0.07	1.61	115	0.07	0.07	0.12	0.7
Milk (cow's)	1 cup	200	130	7.0	7.4	9.8	0.24	0.20	0.8	280	0.06	0.2	0.34	4.0
"	–	100	65	3.5	3.7	4.9	0.12	0.10	0.4	140	0.03	0.1	0.17	2.0
Milk (buffalo)	1 cup	200	216	8.4	16.0	9.2	0.42	0.30	0.8	368	0.06	0.2	0.42	3.4
"	–	100	108	4.2	8.0	4.6	0.21	0.15	0.4	184	0.03	0.1	0.21	1.7
Butter milk (curd from cow's milk)	1 cup	200	36	1.8	2.8	2.0	0.07	0.07	0.2	102	0.03	0.10	0.11	0.9
"	–	100	18	0.9	1.4	1.4	0.04	0.04	0.1	51	0.02	0.05	0.06	0.45
Butter-milk (curd from Buffalo milk)	1cup	200	66	2.4	5.4	2.8	0.07	0.07	0.2	92	0.02	0.10	0.10	0.9
"	–	100	33	1.2	2.5	1.4	0.04	0.04	0.1	46	0.06	0.05	0.05	0.45
Egg, Fish and Meat Preparations: Omelette	1 cup	39	77	5.8	5.7	0.5	0.03	0.10	1.0	940	0.06	0.1	0.15	–
Omelette	–	100	187	14.9	14.6	1.3	0.08	0.26	2.6	2410	0.15	0.26	0.38	–

Contd...

Contd...

Food preparations	*Qty (per serving)*	*Wt. (per serving)*	*Calories (Kcal)*	*Protein (g)*	*Fat (g)*	*Carbohydrate (g)*	*Calcium (g)*	*Phosphorus (g)*	*Iron (mg)*	*Vitamin A value (IU)*	*Thiamin (mg)*	*Nicotinic acid (mg)*	*Riboflavin (mg)*	*Vitmin C (mg)*
Meat curry	1 serving	128	220	11.6	18.0	2.7	0.10	0.07	2.1	227	0.10	0.9	2.20	2.4
"	–	100	172	9.1	14.1	2.1	0.08	0.08	1.6	2.16	0.08	0.7	0.16	1.9
Meat fry	1 serving	142	339	21.8	26.0	4.5	0.23	0.20	3.3	294	0.23	7.8	0.30	7.6
"	–	100	239	15.4	18.8	3.2	0.16	0.14	2.3	207	0.16	5.5	0.21	5.4
Fish fry	1 serving	100	220	17.5	16.2	1.4	0.05	0.45	1.2	216	0.11	1.3	0.02	1.0
"	–	–	–	–	–	–	–	–	–	–	–	–	–	–
Rice Mutton Pulav	2 servings	341	686	20.4	39.0	63.6	0.10	0.22	3.5	100	0.20	6.0	0.20	1.1
"	–	100	201	6.0	11.4	18.7	0.03	0.06	1.03	29	0.06	1.8	0.06	0.32

BIBLIOGRAPHY

1. Behar M. In: Nutrition in Preventive Medicine, WHO Monograph Ser No 62, 1976.
2. Clinical Dietetics and Nutrition, 4th edn, Second impression, FP Antia and Philip Abraham, 2001.
3. Food and nutrition facts and figures. Kusum Gupta and others, 5th edn, 2000.
4. Gopalan C, et al. Nutritive Value of Indian Foods, National Institute of Nutrition, Hyderabad, 1989.
5. ICMR. Recommended Dietary Intakes for Indians, New Delhi, 1990.
6. Narsinga Rao BS. Nutrition, 1986;20(1)14.
7. Nutritive value of Indian foods. Gopalan C and others. NIN (ICMR) Hyderabad, Revised Edition-1989.
8. Ramachandran LK. Science Reporter, Feb 1978, Council of Scientific and Industrial Research, New Delhi, 1978.
9. Swaminathan MC. Nutrition Oct. 1970 NIN.
10. Swaminathan M. Handbook of Food and Nutrition, Ganesh & Co, Madras, 1977.
11. Taber's Cyclopedic Medic al Dictionary, 17th edn, 1993; vol. 2:2222.

Chapter 10 Medical Entomology and Worm Infestations

CHAPTER OUTLINE

- ARTHROPODS
- PUBLIC HEALTH IMPORTANCE OF WORM INFESTATION

ARTHROPODS

Arthropods comprise the most numerous and varied of the living things in the environment of man. Some of them are man's allies helping in the fertilization of flowers, but the majority of arthropods, in general, are either of no use to man or his most dangerous enemies. They destroy man's crops and his food reserves; and some which live close to man act as vectors or carriers of disease. A study of the arthropods of medical importance is known as medical entomology which is an important branch of preventive medicine.

Arthropods of Medical Importance

The arthropods of medical importance are given below.

Class: Insecta (Flow chart 10.1)

Flow chart 10.1: Class: Insecta

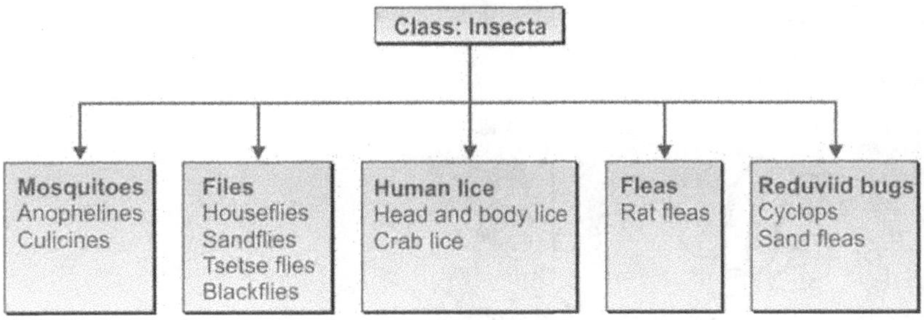

Distinctive Characters

Distinctive characters of class: Insecta (Fig. 10.1)

Body divisions—head, thorax, abdomen

1. Three pairs of legs
2. One pair of antennae
3. One or two pairs of wings, some are wingless
4. They are found on land

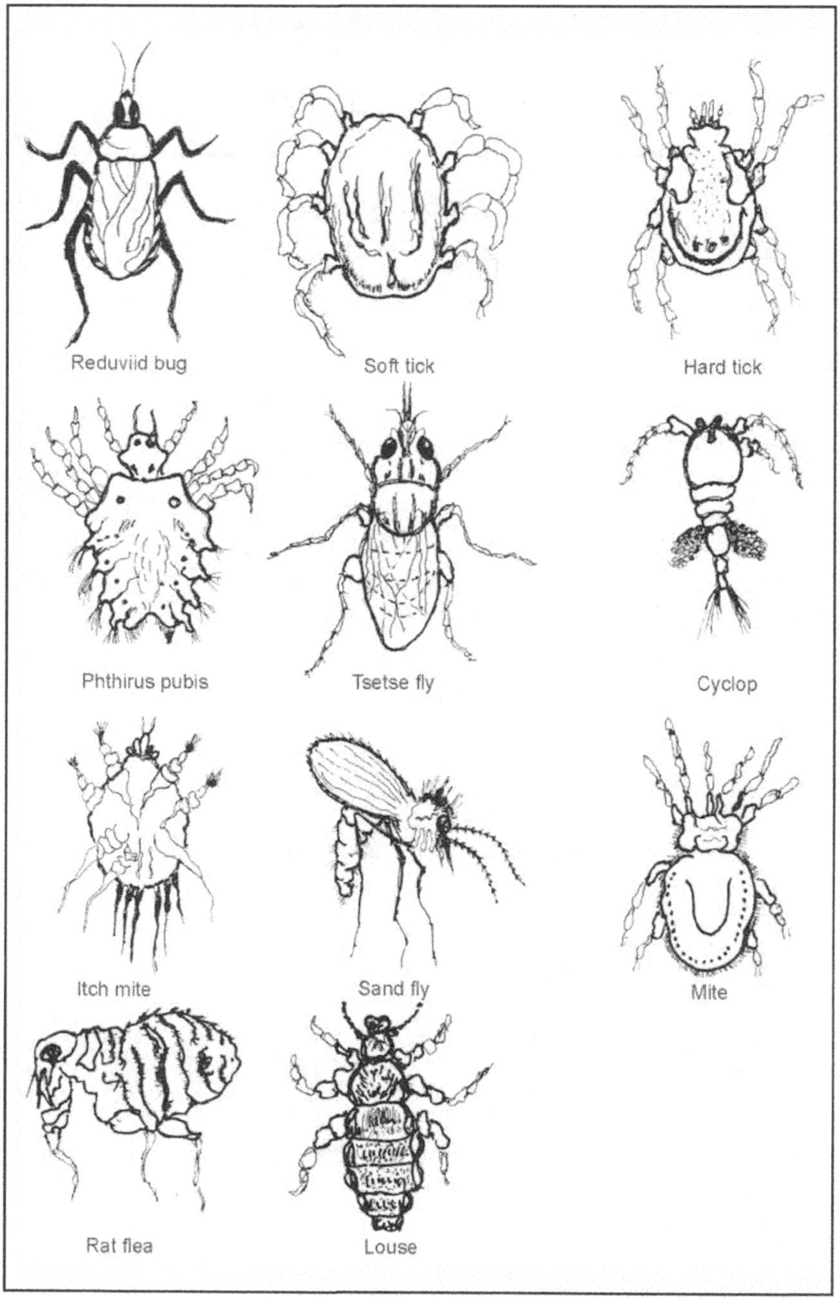

Fig. 10.1: Characteristics of insecta

Class: Archnida (Flow chart 10.2)

Flow chart 10.2: Class: Archnida

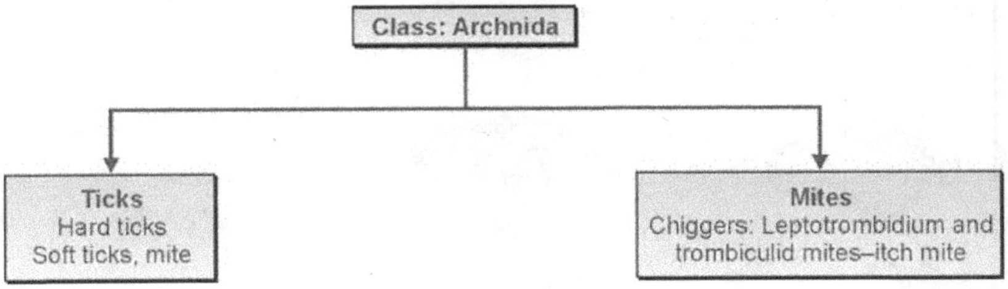

Distinctive Characters

Distinctive characters of class: Archnida

1. Body divisions—cephalothorax and abdomen (no division) in some cases
2. Four pairs of legs
3. No antennae, no wings
4. Found on land.

Class: Crustacea (Flow chart 10.3)

Flow chart 10.3: Class: Crustacea

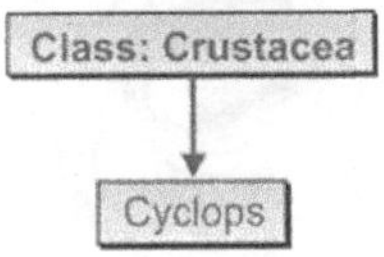

Distinctive Characters

Distinctive characters of class: Crustacea

1. Body divisions—cephalothorax and abdomen
2. Five pairs of legs
3. Two pairs of antennae
4. Found in water.

Mosquito

General Description

Mosquitoes constitute the most important single family of insects from the standpoint of human health. They are found all over the world. The four important groups of mosquitoes in India which are related to disease transmission are the Anopheles, Culex, Aedes and Mansonia (Fig. 10.2 and Table 10.1).

Mosquito-borne Diseases

Apart from their pestiferous nature, mosquitoes play an important role in the transmission of human disease. They act as vectors of many diseases in India (Flow chart 10.4).

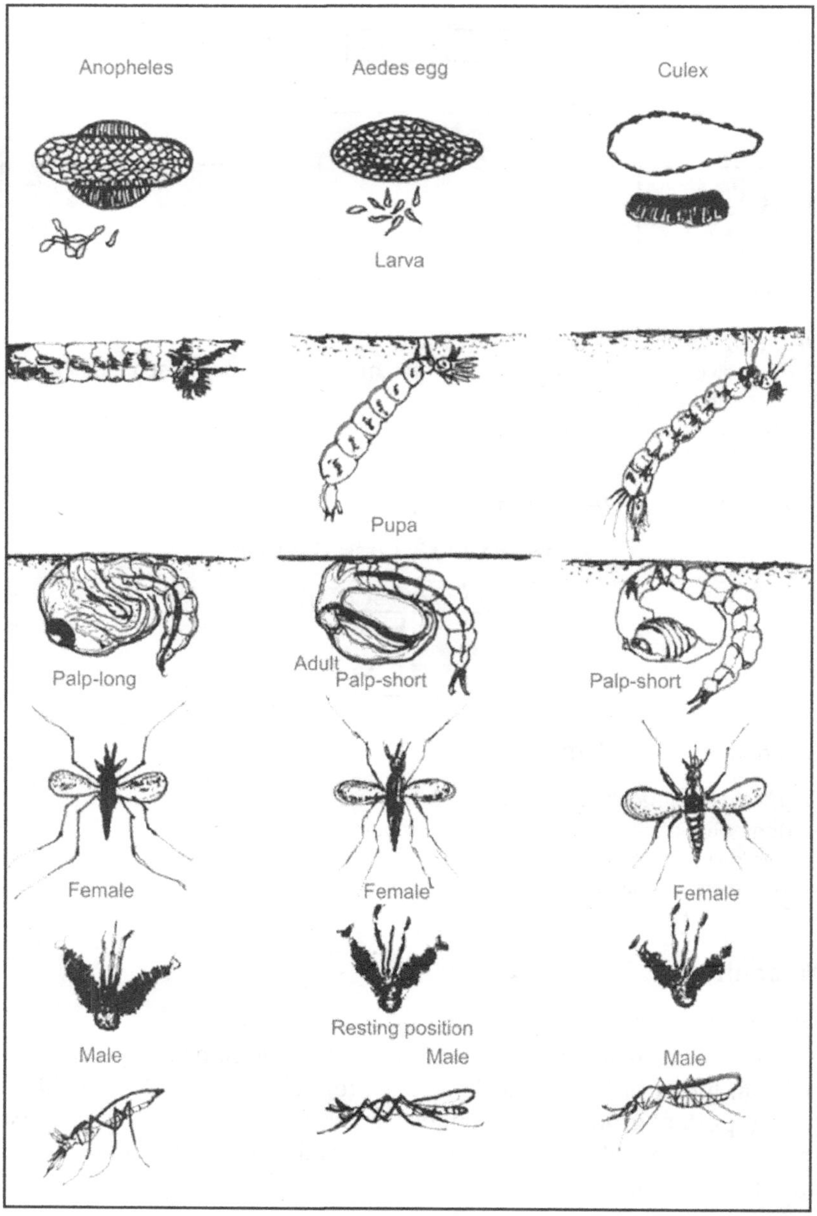

Fig. 10.2: Characteristics of mosquitoes

Table 10.1: Differentiation between anopheline and culicine

Tribe genus mansonia	*Anopheline—Anopheles*	*Culicine—Culex, Aedes*
Eggs	A. Laid singly B. Eggs are boat-shaped, and provided with lateral floats	A. Laid in clusters or rafts, each raft containing 100-250 eggs (except-Aedes) B. Eggs are oval-shaped, and not provided with lateral floats
Larva	A. It has segmented body consisting of head and rest parallel to water surface B. No siphon tube C. Palmate hairs present on abdominal segments	A. Suspended with head downwards at an angle to water surface B. Siphon tube is long and slender C. No palmate hairs
Pupae	A. Siphon tube is broad and short	A. Siphon tube is long and narrow
Adults	A. When at rest, inclined at an angle to surface B. Wings spotted C. Palpi long in both sexes D. In male 1. Proboscis not adopted for piercing and suckling blood 2. No public health importance E. In female 1. Proboscis specially adopted for piercing skin and suckling blood 2. Public health importance—vector of malaria 3. Proboscis in straight line with body F. Breeds in clear water and slow—running streams	A. When at rest, the body exhibits a hunch back B. Wings unspotted C. Palpi short in female, long and tapering in male D. In male 1. Proboscis bent at an angle with the body 2. No public health importance E. In female 1. Proboscis specially adopted for piercing skin and suckling blood F. Breeds in dirty water like cesspools, stagnant drains containing organic materials and polluted water

Flow chart 10.4: Mosquito-borne diseases

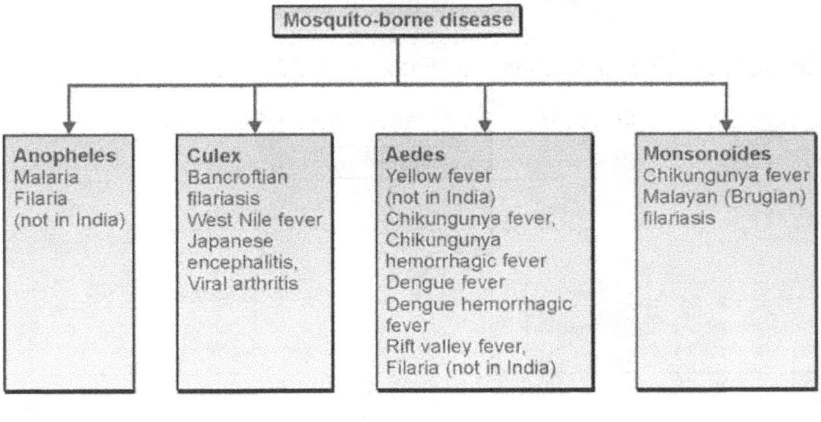

Mosquito Control Measures

While there are many methods of mosquito control, experts now recommend an "integrated approach", that is, an approach which avoids the excessive use of any one method (e.g. insecticides) but tries to combine one or more methods with a view to obtain maximum results with minimum inputs and also to prevent environmental pollution with toxic chemicals and development of insecticide resistance. The various methods of mosquito control may be classified as below:

Anti-larval Measures

a. Environmental control
b. Chemical control
c. Biological control.

Anti-adult Measures

a. Residual sprays
b. Space sprays
c. Genetic control.

Protection against Mosquito Bites

a. Mosquito net
b. Screening
c. Repellents.

Ticks

- Ticks are blood sucking parasites.
- They are found in warm climate, and are nocturnal in habits.
- Natural hosts for ticks are domestic animals like dogs, cats, and cattle. They attack man only accidentally.
- They can live without food for two to three years.

Families of Medical Importance (Flow chart 10.5)

Flow chart 10.5: Families of medical importance

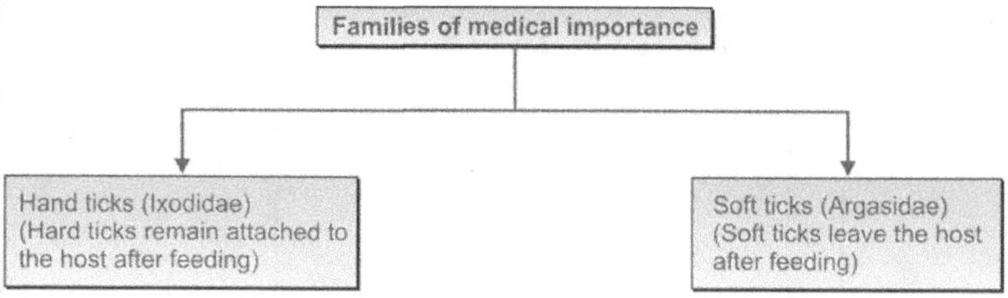

Public Health Importance of Ticks (Flow chart 10.6)

Flow chart 10.6: Public health importance of ticks

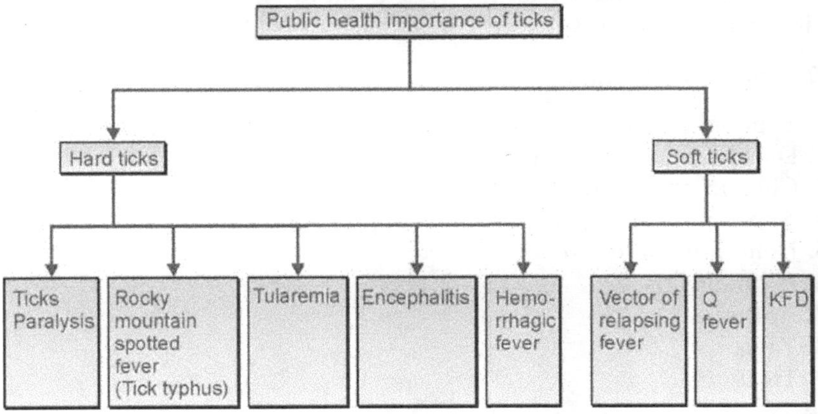

Control Measures (Flow chart 10.7)

Flow chart 10.7: Control measures for ticks

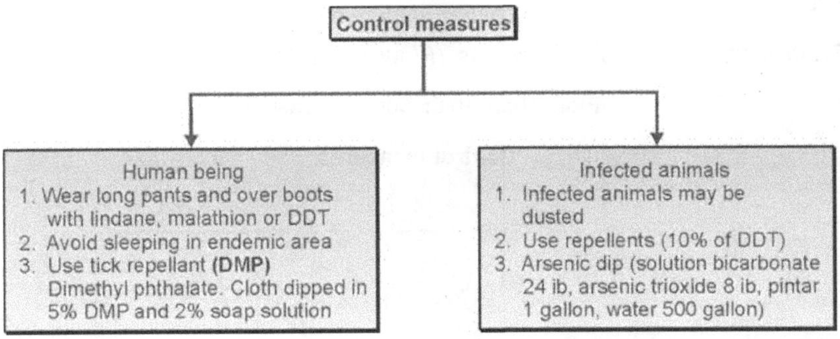

Houseflies

Houseflies are the commonest and most familiar of all insects which live close to man.

The most important of these are:

- Musca domestica
- Musca vicinia
- Musca nebulo
- Musca sorbens.

Life History

Egg: The female lays about 120 to 150 eggs at one sitting. The fly lays from 600 to 900 eggs during lifetime.

Larva: Measures about 12 mm, larval period lasts for two-seven days.

Pupa: Dark brown barrel shaped, measures about quarter of an inch, Pupal stage lasts for three to six days.

Adult: Complete life cycle from egg to adult lasts for five to six days. Life span 15 days in summer and 25 days in winter.

Diseases Transmitted

1. Typhoid and paratyphoid
2. Diarrheas and dysenteries
3. Cholera and gastroenteritis
4. Amoebiasis and giardiasis
5. Helminthic infestations
6. Poliomyelitis
7. Anthrax
8. Yaws
9. Trachoma.

Routes of Transmission

1. Mechanical transmission
2. Through vomit drop
3. Defecation.

Control Measures for Houseflies (Flow chart 10.8)

Flow chart 10.8: Control measures

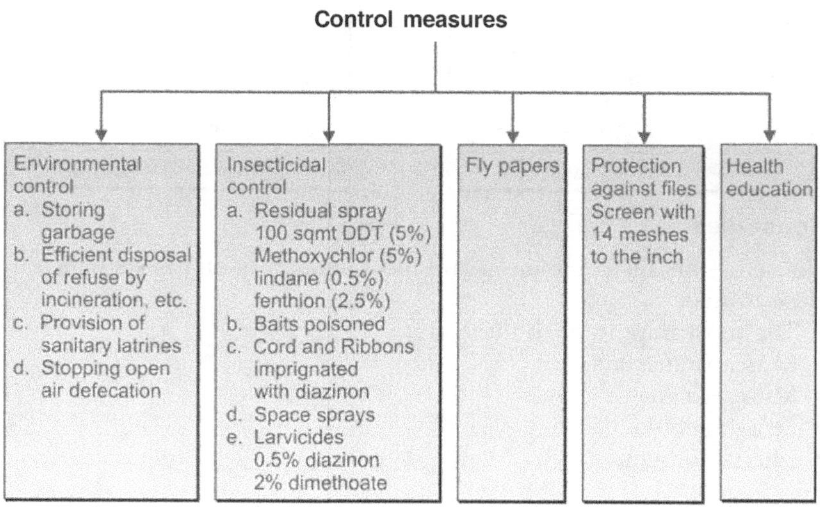

Spread of Diseases (Flow chart 10.9)

1. Sandfly
2. Lice
3. Cyclops
4. Rat flea

Flow chart 10.9: Spread of diseases

Disease spread by

Sandy
1. Kala-azar Systermic and Dermal Leishmaniasis
2. Sandifly fever
3. Oriental sore

Lice
1. Rickettsia Prowazekii
2. Borrelia recurrentiis
3. Rickettsia quintana

Cyclops
1. Dracontiasis Guinea worm disease
2. Diphyllobo-trium latum infestation

Rat flea
1. Plague
2. Endemic or marine typhus
3. Chiggerosis
4. Hymenolepsis diminuta

Control Measures

Sandfly (Flow chart 10.10)

Flow chart 10.10: Control measures for sandfly

Sandfly

Insecticides
1. DDT 1-2 gm/m^2
2. Lindane 0.25 gm/m^2

Sanitation
1. Removal of shrubs and vegetation within 50 years of human dwelling
2. Filling up of crack and crevices in walls and floors
3. Location of cattle sheds and poultry houses at a fair distance from human habitation

Lice (Flow chart 10.11)

Flow chart 10.11: Control measures for lice

Lice

Insecticidal control
0.5% malathion for head and crab lices, 1% for body lice, 50 gm powder/person
Single application-eradicate and ifestation
Second application (after 7 days)–
To kill late hatching lice

Personal hygiene
A daily bath with soap and water wash and clean their hair frequently

Cyclops (Flow chart 10.12)

Flow chart 10.12: Control measures for cyclops

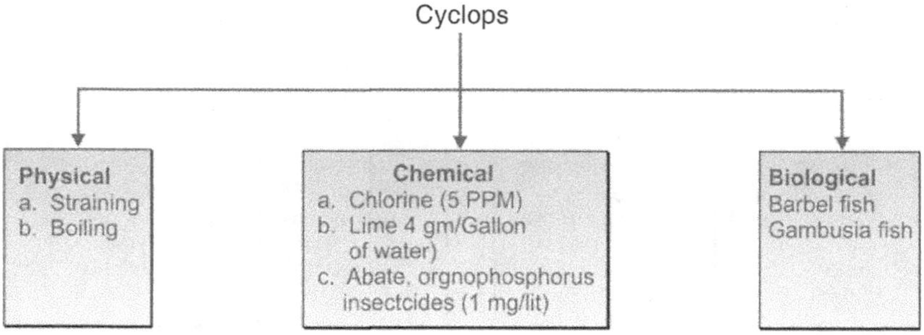

Ratflea (Flow chart 10.13)

Flow chart 10.13: Control measures for ratflea

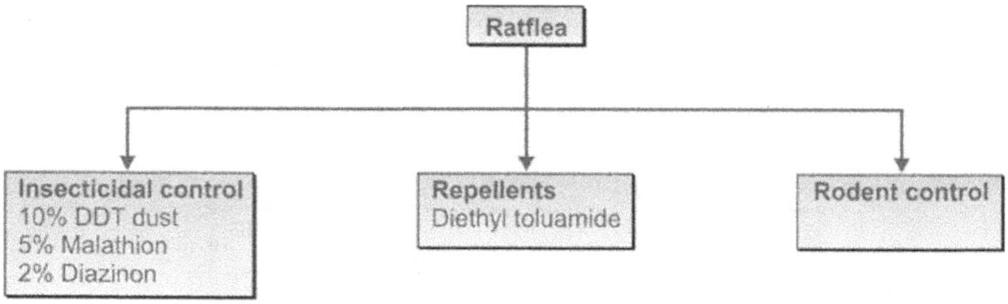

Itch mite (Flow chart 10.14)

Flow chart 10.14: Control measures for itch mite

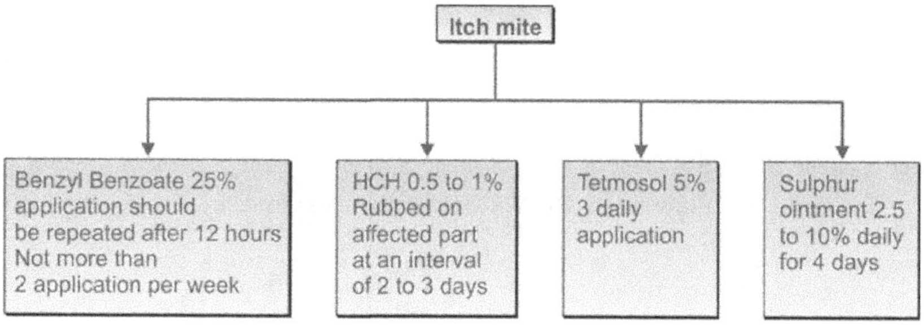

PUBLIC HEALTH IMPORTANCE OF WORM INFESTATION

Ascariasis (Table 10.2)

Table 10.2: *Ascariasis* treatment

Infestation	*Drug*	*Dose*
Ascariasis (round worm)	Mebendazole or pyrentel pamoate	100 mg bd x 3 days 10 mg/kg single dose

Symptoms of Ascariasis

1. Passage of worm in stool or vomitus
2. Vomiting, diarrhea, abdominal distention, flatulence
3. Cough
4. Skin rashes
5. Encephalopathy.

Prevention

1. Personal hygiene
2. Untreated sewage should not be used as fertilizer
3. Proper disposal of sewage.

Enterobius vermicularis (Table 10.3)

Table 10.3: *Enterobius vermicularis* treatment

Infestation	*Drug*	*Dose*
Enterobius vermicularis (pin worm)	Pyrentel pamoate or Albendazole	10 mg/kg single dose 100 mg once (repeated after 4 weeks)

Symptoms

1. Irritability
2. Perianal itching
3. Loss of appetite
4. Symptoms of appendicitis.

Prevention

1. Personal hygiene
2. Nails to be cut and trimmed
3. Washing of nails and perianal area with soap and water.

Trichuris trichiura (Table 10.4)

Table 10.4: *Trichuris trichiura* treatment

Infestation	*Drug*	*Dose*
Trichuris trichiura	Mebendazole Albendazole	100 mg bd x 3 days 400 mg/kg once

Symptoms

1. Asymptomatic, if light infection
2. Vague abdominal pain
3. Mild diarrhea
4. Blood in stool
5. Tenesmus
6. Loss of weight

7. Failure to grow if heavy infection
8. Rectal prolapse
9. Volvulus.

Prevention

1. Personal hygiene
2. Untreated sewage should not be used as fertilizer
3. Proper disposal of sewage.

Wuchereria bancrofti (Table 10.5)

Table 10.5: *Wuchereria bancrofti* treatment

Infestation	*Drug*	*Dose*
Wuchereria bancrofti	Diethyl carbamazine (DEC)	6 mg /kg body weight in divided doses × 12 days
Brugia malayi	DEC	3-6 mg/kg × 6-12 days
Loa loa	DEC	1mg/kg as a single dose initially double on second day then 2-3 mg /kg tds daily for 18 days
Onchocerciasis	Ivermectin	Single dose 200-400 μg/kg annually or biannually

Symptoms

1. Lymphangitis
2. Lymphadenitis
3. Elephantiasis
4. Hydrocole
5. Chyluria.

Prevention

1. Protection against mosquito bite
2. Destruction of mosquitoes
   a. Antilarval measures
   b. Antiadult measures.

Ancylostoma duodenale (Table 10.6)

Table 10.6: *Ancylostoma duodenale* treatment

Infestation	*Drug*	*Dose*
Ancylostoma duodenale, Necator americanus (Hook worm)	Mebendazole or Pyrentel pamoate	100 mg bd × 3 days 10 mg/kg single dose and second dose after 2-4 weeks needed in North American

Symptoms

1. Abdominal pain
2. Diarrhea
3. Anemia
4. Dyspnea
5. Swelling of feet.

Prevention

1. Avoid walking bare foot
2. Proper disposal of feces

Strongyloides stercoralis (Table 10.7)

Table 10.7: *Strongyloides stercoralis* treatment

Infestation	*Drug*	*Dose*
Strongyloides stercoralis	Thiabendazole	25 mg/kg bd 5-7 days

Symptoms

1. Abdominal pain
2. Diarrhea
3. Malabsorption.

Prevention

1. Avoid walking barefoot
2. Proper disposal of feces.

BIBLIOGRAPHY

1. Chatterji KD. Human Parasites and Parasitic Diseases, Calcutta, 1952.
2. Orkin M. JAMA 1971;217:593.
3. Park's Textbook of Preventive and Social Medicine, 17th edn, 2002.
4. Puri IM. The House-Frequenting Flies, their relation to Disease and their control. Health Bulletin No. 31 Manager of Publications, Govt of India Press Delhi, 1948.
5. Puri IM. Synoptic Table for the identification of the Anopheline Mosquitoes in India, Health Bulletin No. 10, Manager of Publications, Govt of India Press, Delhi,1955.
6. Roy DN, Brown AWA. Entomology, Medical and Veterinary, Excelsior Press, Calcutta, 1954.
7. Sharma MID. J. Com. Dis, 1974;6, 136.
8. WHO. Control Control of Arthropods of Public Health Importance. WHO Training Leaflet No. 1 Vector Control Series Geneva, 1966.
9. WHO. Techn. Rep Ser, No.443,1970.
10. WHO. Techn Rep Ser, No.561,1975.

Chapter 11 Disinfection

CHAPTER OUTLINE

- DEFINITIONS (DISINFECTANT OR GERMICIDE)

Semmelweis (1818-1865) demonstrated the value of handwashing with antiseptic solutions.

DEFINITIONS (DISINFECTANT OR GERMICIDE)

Disinfectant

It is a substance which destroys harmful microbes (not usually spores) with object of preventing transmission of disease. Disinfectants are suitable for application of only to inanimate objects.

Antiseptic

Antiseptic is a substance which destroys or inhibits the growth of microorganisms.

Antiseptic are suitable for application to living tissues. A disinfectant in low concentrations or dilutions can act as an antiseptic.

Deodorant

It is a substance which suppresses or neutralizes bad odours, e.g. lime and bleaching powder.

Detergent

It is a surface cleaning agent which acts by lowering surface tension, e.g. soap which remove bacteria along with dirt.

Sterilization

It is a process of destroying all life including spores. This is widely used in medical practice.

Disinfection

Refers to the killing of infectious agents outside the body by direct exposure to chemical or physical agents.

It can refer to the action of antiseptic as well as disinfectants.

Types of Disinfection

1. Concurrent disinfection
2. Terminal disinfection
3. Precurrent (Prophylactic) disinfection.

Concurrent Disinfection

The disease agent is destroyed as soon as it is released from the body, and in this way further spread of the agent is stopped, e.g. urine, feces vomit, contaminated linen, clothes, hands, dressings, aprons, gloves, etc. throughout the course of illness.

Terminal Disinfection

Application of disinfective measures after the patient has been removed by death or to a hospital, or has ceased to be a source of infection, terminal cleaning is considered adequate, along with airing and sunning of rooms, furniture and bedding.

Precurrent Disinfection

For example, disinfection of water by chlorination, pasteurization of milk and handwashing.

Disinfecting Agents

They are classified as:
1. Natural agent
2. Chemical agent
3. Physical agent.

Natural Agents

1. Sunlight
2. Air.

Physical Agents

1. Burning
2. Hot air
3. Boiling
4. Autoclaving
5. Radiation.

Chemical Agents

1. Phenol and related compounds
2. Quaternary ammonia compounds
3. Halogens and their compounds
4. Alcohols
5. Formaldehyde
6. Miscellaneous.

Natural Agents

Sunlight

The ultraviolet rays of sunlight are particularly lethal to bacteria and some viruses, e.g. bedding, linen and furniture.

Air

Acts by drying or evaporation of moisture which is lethal to most bacteria.

Physical Agents

Burning

Burning should not be done in open air. It is best done in incinerator.

Hot Air

For sterlizing articles such as glassware, syringes, swabs, dressings, vaseline, oils and sharp instruments.

Hot air sterilization is done at hot air oven maintained at 160 to 180°C at least for one hour to kill spores.

Boiling

Boilers provide temperature above 90°C. Boiling for 5 to 10 minutes will kill the bacteria.

The destruction of spores which require 100°C temperature which can not be achieved in boilers. Boiling is suitable for disinfection of small instruments which are not used for subcutaneous insertion. Addition of 1 percent soap and 0.3 percent of washing soda enhances the effect of boiling, e.g. linens, rubber goods such as gloves.

Autoclaving

Sterilizers, which operate at high temperatures (in excess of 100°C) and pressure are called autoclaves.

Two types: 1 Single chambered 2 double chambered autoclaves.

It attains temp 122°C under 15 lbs/sq inch pressure.

Absolute sterility can be obtained only by raising the temperatures of articles to over 135°C, e.g. linen, dressing, gloves, syringes, certain instruments and culture media.

Radiation

Ionizing radiation is being increasingly used for sterilization of bandages, dressings, catgut, surgical instruments.

Chemical Disinfectants

Articles which can not be sterilized by boiling or autoclaving may be immersed in chemical disinfectants.

Phenol and Related Compounds

Phenol

- Pure phenol or carbolic acid is the best known member of this group.
- On exposure to air, the colorless crystals of phenol become pinkish and on long exposure to air, the color deepens to dark-red.
- Pure phenol is not an effective disinfectant.

Crude phenol: It is mixture of phenol and cresol

- It is dark oily liquid.
- It is effective against gram-positive and gram-negative bacteria.
- It is slowly effective against spores and acid-fast bacteria.
- It is also effective against certain viruses.
- Its effect is weakened by dilution. So it should not be used in less than 10 percent strength for disinfection of fecal matter.
- In 5 percent strength, it may be used for mopping floors and cleaning drains.
- Aqueous solutions of 0.2 to 1 percent are bacteriostatic.

Cresol: It is an excellent coal-tar disinfectant. It is 3 to 10 times as powerful as phenol.

- Cresol is best used in 5 to 10 percent strength for disinfection of feces and urine
- A 5 percent solution is prepared by adding eight ounces of cresol to one gallon of water (or 50 ml to one liter of water)
- Cresol is an all purpose general disinfectant.

Cresol emulsions

- Cresol emulsified with soap is known as "Saponified cresol". Lysol contain 50 to 60 percent cresol.
- A two percent solution of lysol may be used for disinfection of feces.

Chlorhexidine : It is most useful skin antiseptic

- Highly effective against vegetative gram +ve organisms and moderately active against gram +ve microbes
- It is soluble in water and alcohol
- It is inactivated by soap and detergents.
- Creams and lotions containing one percent chlorhexidine are recommended for burns and hand disinfection.

Hexachlorphane: Highly active against gram +ve organisms, less active against gram –ve organisms.

Dettol : Nontoxic antiseptic. Can be used safely in high concentrations. Dettol 5 percent is suitable for disinfection of instruments and plastic equipment, a contact of at least 15 minutes will be required.

Quaternary Ammonia Compounds

Cetrimide: It is manufactured under trade name "cetavlon".
- Active against gram +ve organisms
- Less effective against gram –ve organisms
- It is soluble in water
- It is used in one o two percent strength.

Savlon: It is a combination of cetavlon and hibitane.
Savlon one in six in spirit is more effective than savlon 1 in 20 aqueous solution.

For example, clinical thermometer may be best disinfected in savlon one in six in spirit in just under three minutes.

Halogens and their Compounds

Halogens are actively bactericidal agents, and are the only useful antiseptics with a sporocidal action.

Bleaching powder
- It is chlorinated lime.
- It is white amorphous powder with pungent smell of chlorine.
- A good sample of bleaching powder contains about 33 percent of available chlorine.
- It kills organisms when used in the strength of one to three percent.
- It is widely used for disinfection of water, feces and urine and as a deodorant.

Drawbacks: It is an unstable compound and loses its chlorine content on storage. Its action is rapid but brief.

Sodium hypochlorite
- A five percent solution is suitable for disinfection of feces and urine allowing a period of one hour for disinfection.
- Freshly prepared hypo-solution containing 100-200 ppm of available chlorine has been recommended for sterilizing infants feeding bottles.

Halazone tablet: One tablet of halazone containing 4 mg of halazone is sufficient to disinfect about one liter of water in about half to one hour.

The taste of residual chlorine may be removed by adding sodium thiosulphate normally in the form of tablets containing about 5.5 mg.

*Iodine:*Iodine in an alcoholic solution of one to two percent is still one of the most effective skin antiseptics available. Iodine is cheap, readily available and quick in action.

A drop of tincture of iodine may be added to a one liter of drinking water for disinfection in an emergency.

Iodophors: These are complexes of iodine and 'solubilizers'.
For example, Povidine-iodine (Betadin)

It is nonirritant and does not stain the skin.

Alcohols: Seventy percent alcohol is lethal in a period of seconds to all types of non-sporing bacteria. It has no action against spores, but will inactivate viruses. Below 50 percent concentration activity decreases rapidly.

Formaldehyde: It is highly toxic and irritant gas which precipitates and destroys protein. It is effective against vegetative bacteria, fungi, and many viruses. Slow effective against bacterial spores (e.g. tetanus spores). It is used as two to three percent solution (20-30 ml of 40% formalin in 1 liter of water) for spraying rooms, walls and furniture.

Formaldehyde gas: Gas is most effective at a high temperature and at a relative humidity of 80 to 90 percent.

It is used for disinfection of blankets, beds, books and other valuable articles which cannot be boiled.

Miscellaneous

Lime: About 10 to 20 percent aqueous suspension of lime is known as "milk of lime". Feces and urine can be disinfected by mixing 10 to 20 percent aqueous suspension of lime and allowing the disinfectant to act for two hours. It is used as a deodorant in public urinals and latrines.

Ethylene oxide: Heat sensitive articles may be sterilized at 55 to 60°C by ethylene oxide which kills bacteria, spores (e.g. tetanus spores) and viruses.

BIBLIOGRAPHY

1. Bres P. Public Health action in Emergencies caused by Epidemics, WHO, Geneva, 1986.
2. Park's Textbook of Preventive and Social Medicine, 17th edn, 2002.
3. Report by the Public Health Laboratory Service Committee, Brit Med J 1965; 1:408-13.
4. Today's Drugs Brit. Med J 1964;2:1513-15.
5. WHO. Techn. Rep Ser, 1972; No. 493, p. 58.

Chapter 12 Insecticides and Rodenticides

CHAPTER OUTLINE

INSECTICIDES AND PESTICIDES

Insecticides are used to kill the insects.

Pesticides—insecticides, herbicides, rodenticides (Table 12.1), repellents, fungicides all come under pesticides which are used for control of pests.

Table 12.1: Characteristics actions and doses of various rodenticides

Rodenticide	*Characteristics*	*Mode of action*	*Dose*
1. Barium Carbonate	White tasteless powder	It is a single dose rodenticide but it is a weak rodenticide as compared to others. On eating the bait, rats are killed in 2 to 4 hours	It is mixed with wheat or rice flour in the proportion of 1 to 4 parts of flour. The mixed material is moistened with water and made into small round marbles
2. Zinc phosphide	1. It is a grayish powder 2. It has a garlic odour	It is a single dose rodenticide. Rats are killed in about 3 hours	1 part of Zinc phosphide to 10 parts of wheat or rice flour mixed with a few drops of edible oil in order to render it more attractive to the rats
3. Warfarin	White crystalline powder, turns brownish yellow on keeping	It is a multiple dose (cumulative) poison, which causes internal hemorrhage and slow death in 4 to 10 days	Mixed with wheat or rice flour 1 : 10 parts and moistened with oil.
4. Cyanogas Powder	White/brownish amorphous powder	It gives off hydrogen cyanide gas when moistened, which is	It is prepared in powder form and is pumped into the

Contd...

Contd...

	lethal to both rats and their fleas. The gas is very toxic to other animals and humans also.	rat burrow by a special foot pump (cyanogas pump). About 2 ounces of poison are pumped into each burrow after moistening it and closing the exit openings.

Classification

- Contact poisons—DDT, HCH, pyrethrum
- Stomach poisons
- Fumigants.

Class I — Organochlorine compounds,
DDT, HCH, chlordane, methoxychlor dieldrin,

Class II — Organophosphorous compounds
1. Malathion
2. Fenthion
3. Abate, etc.

Class III — Carbamates
1. Propoxur
2. Carbaryl.

DDT (Dichloro-diphenyl-trichloroethane)

DDT synthesized in 1874, by Ziedler.

Insecticidal properties were discovered by Swiss scientist—Paul Muller in 1939.

Properties

- It is white amorphous powder
- It is insoluble in water
- Active ingredient of DDT is para-para-isomer (70-80%)
- Soluble in oil and organic solvents.

Action

It is primarily a contact poison.

- It acts on nervous system of insects and permeates into the insect body through cuticle, after dissolving in the waxy coverings of feet and it paralyses the legs and wings of insect and finally leads to death.
- It does not cause immediate death.

- Residual action lasts up to 18 months.
- It has no repellent action on insects.

Application

It is applied at a dosage of 100 to 200 mg/sq foot area. A five percent of suspension of DDT is sprayed, at a rate of 1 gallon over an area of 1000 sq feet.

- Two percent strength used for — mosquito control
- Five percent strength used for — housefly control and
- Ten percent strength used for — flea control

  It should be applied every six months.

HCH (BHC) Hexachlorocyclohexane

Benzene hexachloride or hexachlorocyclohexane or hexidol or gammexane

- Synthesized earlier than DDT in 1825 by Michael Faraday.
- It is white chocolate powder. The active ingredient is 13 to 16 percent of gamma isomer.

Pure HCH containing 99 percent of gamma isomer is called lindane.

Action

By direct contact with insects.

Application

Every three months. A dose of 25 to 50 mg/sq foot of gamma HCH is recommended for residual treatment.

Malathion

- It is yellow or clear-brown liquid with unpleasant smell.
- It is water dispersible.

Dosage

It is 100 to 200 mg/sq foot every three months. It has been used for killing adult mosquitoes to prevent or interrupt dengue hemorrhagic fever and mosquito-borne encephalitis epidemic.

Mineral Oil

Kerosene, fuel oil, crude oil, (mosquito larvicidal oil).

- Kills larvae and pupae within short time after application
- When applied on water, mineral oil spreads and forms thin film, which cuts off air supply.

Dosage

It is 40 to 90 lit/hectare applied once a week.

The killing power of oil is increased by the addition of 1 percent DDT.

Paris Green (Copper aceto-arsenite)

It is emerald green—microcrystalline powder and it is insoluble in water. A good sample of paris green contains over 50 percent arsenious oxide.

- It is stomach poison.
- It kills surface feeder Anopheline larvae.
- When applied in granular formulation—it kills bottom feeder.
- It is applied as two percent dust which is prepared by mixing 2 kg paris green and 98 kg of diluent such as soapstone powder or slaked lime in a 'rotary mixture'.

Dosage

1 kg of paris green/hectare of water surface.

BIBLIOGRAPHY

1. Dhir SL. Swasth Hind 1970;14:269.
2. Park's Textbook of Preventive and Social Medicine, 16th edn, Nov 2000.
3. WHO. Techn Rep Ser, No. 125, 1957.
4. WHO. Manual on Larval Control Operations in Malaria, Geneva, 1973.
5. WHO. Techn Rep Ser, No. 553, 1974.
6. WHO. Techn Rep Ser, No. 561, 1975.

Chapter

13 Environmental Models

CHAPTER OUTLINE

CHLOROSCOPE/CHLORINOMETER

It is used to determine the amount of excess/residual chlorine in water after chlorination.

It consists of:

1. Orthotolidine reagent
2. Standard test tubes or disks.
3. Empty test tube.
4. Plastic or metal container.

Procedure

1. Take the water to be tested and add it up to the mark in the empty test tube.
2. Add drops orthotolidine reagent 1:10 parts of water.
3. Shake slowly and match the yellow color formed with the standard tubes/disks. This gives directly the amount of residual chlorine in the water if read quickly (within 10 seconds of adding the reagent). After 15 to 20 minutes the color developed is due to free plus combined chlorine.
4. Orthotolidine arsenite (OTA) test is a modification of the OT test which avoids the errors due to the presence of other elements like, manganese, iron and nitrites. It also allows the reading of free and combined chlorine separately.

DRY AND WET BULB THERMOMETER (HYGROMETER)

This is used for measuring the relative humidity.

It consists of:

1. Ordinary mercury thermometer, which measures the room temperature.
2. Another ordinary mercury thermometer, whose mercury bulb is kept moist by covering it with a muslin cloth, whose end is dipping in a small water container.

Procedure

1. The continuous evaporation of water through the muslin cloth, causes reduction in the temperature in that thermometer (with a cloth) hence it shows a lower reading than the other thermometer (without a cloth).
2. The drier the air, more rapid will be the evaporation and hence lower will be the temperature in that thermometer.
3. The difference in the temperatures of the two thermometers varies inversely with the amount of moisture in the air.
4. The humidity can be read from available charts or slide scale.
5. At 100 percent humidity, both thermometers will show the same temperature. Since, then there would be no evaporation.
6. The thermometers should be protected from radiant heat, direct sunlight and rain.

MAXIMUM AND MINIMUM THERMOMETER

This is used for measuring the maximum and minimum temperatures of a place on a given day (Fig. 13.1).

It consists of:

1. A mercury thermometer with a constriction at the neck of the mercury bulb.
2. A spirit thermometer with a dumb-bell shaped rider or index.

Procedure

1. When the temperature rises the mercury in the mercury thermometer expands.
2. When the temperature falls, the mercury cannot fall back into the bulb, due to the constriction, hence the mercury column will remain at the maximum temperature.
3. After taking the maximum reading, the mercury thermometer is shaken briskly to push the mercury back into the bulb (like in a clinical thermometer).
4. When the temperature falls, the spirit in the spirit thermometer contracts and drags the rider down along with it, due to surface tension.

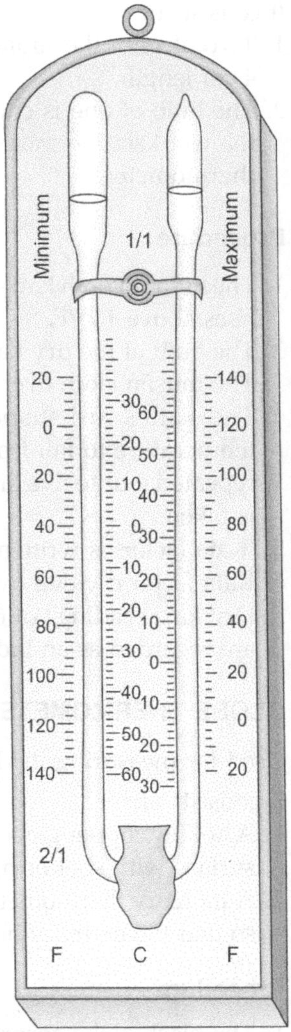

Fig. 13.1: Maximum and minimum thermometer

5. When the temperature rises, the spirit expands and runs past the rider, hence the rider remains stuck at the minimum temperature.
6. After taking the minimum temperature reading, the rider can be moved to the surface of the spirit column by gently tapping with fingers.

KATA THERMOMETER (FIG. 13.2A)

Used for Measuring

a. Cooling power of air.
b. Velocity of air.

It consists of:

1. Two alcohol thermometers each with a bulb of 1.8 cm diameter and 4 cm length.
2. The bulb of one is covered with a wet muslin cloth. This is known as the wet kata thermometer and the other one is known as the dry kata thermometer.

Procedure

1. The bulbs of both katas are immersed in warm water till the temperature rises above 130°F.
2. The bulb of the dry kata is wiped dry.
3. The muslin cloth over the wet kata is moistened.
4. The kata's are suspended in air and the time required for the temperature to fall from 100°F to 95°F is noted for both kata's. This is repeated four to five times and the mean of the last three to four readings is taken.
5. 'Kata factor' is written on the thermometer or the instruction leaflet.
6. Kata factor divided by the mean cooling time gives the cooling power.
7. Dry kata readings of 6 or more, and wet kata readings of 20 or more, are regarded as an index of thermal comfort.

GLOBE THERMOMETER (FIG. 13.2B)

Used for measuring the Mean radiant heat.

It consists of:

1. A hollow copper globe, 15 cm in diameter, which is coated on its external surface with soot or black paint.
2. A mercury thermometer, is inserted into the globe through an opening, so that the mercury bulb lies exactly at the center of the globe.

Procedure

1. The black globe absorbs the radiant heat from the surroundings.
2. The mercury thermometer registers the room temperature plus the radiant heat.

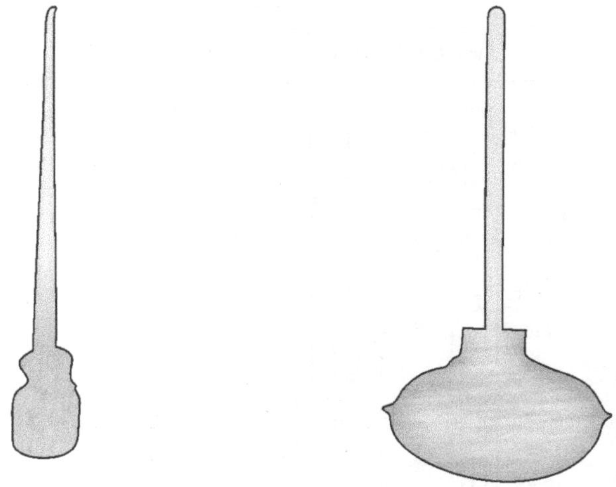

(A) (B)

Figs 13.2A and B: (A) Kata thermometer; (B) Globe thermometer

3. The difference between the readings of a globe thermometer and an ordinary thermometer kept side by side is equal to the mean radiant heat.
4. The globe thermometer is also influenced by the air velocity.

Note: A wet globe thermometer is a globe thermometer whose globe is covered with a wet black cloth. This thermometer exchanges heat with the surroundings by evaporation, radiation, convection and conduction, like a human being. Hence, a wet globe thermometer is considered to provide the most comprehensive measure of the cooling capacity of the environment and is used extensively to measure the thermal comfort in industries.

Sling Psychrometer (Fig. 13.3)

This is used to measure the relative humidity.

It consists of:

One dry and one wet bulb thermometer mounted side by side on a rotating wooden frame.

Procedure

1. The cloth over the wet bulb is moistened and the wooden frame is rotated for about 15 seconds at a rate of 4 revolutions per second so as to achieve a rotational speed of 5 meters per second. Note the wet bulb thermometer reading.
2. The psychrometer is again rotated for 10 seconds and the wet bulb thermometer reading is noted.
3. This is repeated several times, till the wet bulb thermometer temperature remains constant, with no further fall. Now note the dry bulb thermometer reading.
4. Relative humidity can be read directly from available charts.

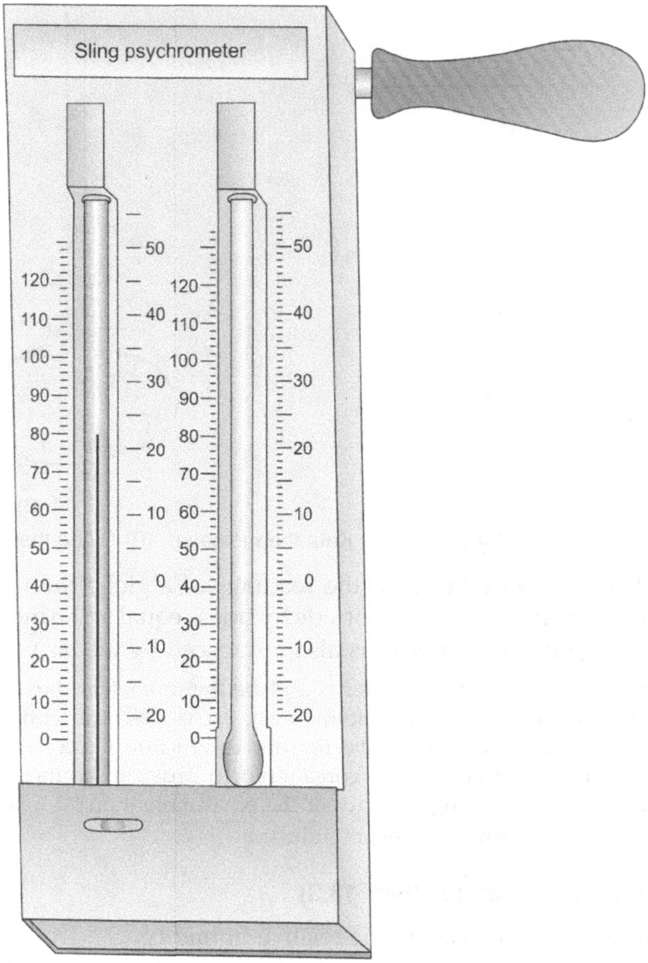

Fig. 13.3: Sling psychrometer

Gully Trap

Three types of pipes are usually seen on the outer wall of sanitary blocks in a building. The largest is the storm or rain water pipe which drains rain water from the roof into the gully trap. The medium sized is the soil pipe while the small sized pipe is the sullage water pipe draining bathrooms and sinks (Fig. 13.4).

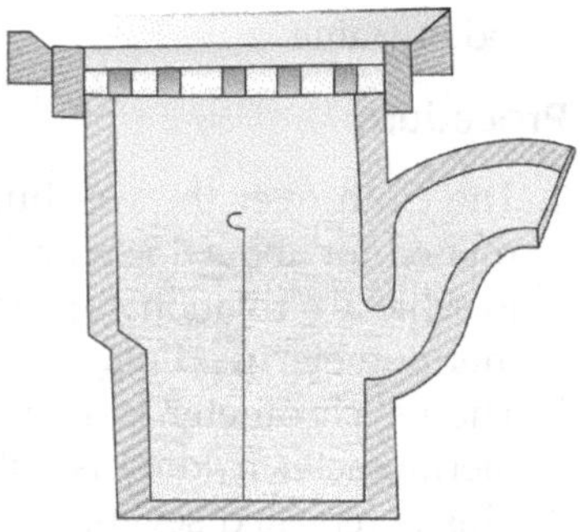

Fig. 13.4: Gully trap

SOAK PIT

In the absence of a drainage system in rural areas, sullage water spills and stagnates along open streets, leading to nuisance an unhygienic conditions, apart from acting as breeding source for mosquitoes. The soak pit is a cheap, simple and sanitary method of disposing sullage water. Besides acting as a sanitary sullage disposal system, the soak pit also acts as a device for recharging of ground water. Improvements in soak pit have been suggested by the Safai Vidyalaya, the Central Building Research Institute, Roorkee, and the Consortium on Rural Technology, Delhi. The steps in constructing an improved soak pit as suggested by the latter are given below:

1. Choose a proper site which should be away from a house wall and at least 10 m distant from any well. The water table should not be very high. Its water is present three to four meter below ground level, this technology may not be appropriate.
2. Dig a pit about one meter long, broad and deep. The bottom of the pit must have a slope of about 15 cm, the direction of the slope being away from the house.
3. Divide the depth of the pit into roughly four equal parts. Fill the low,ermost part with stones or bricks the size of a coconut. Fill the second part with stones or bricks the size of a big apple. The third part is to be filled with stones of the size of an average lemon. The fourth or uppermost part is for the inlet chamber.
4. The inlet chamber is constructed as follows:
    a. At the center, lay the foundation of the chamber in the form of 4 bricks arranged as shown laid with a gap of 5 cm between the bricks, leaving a central space of 12.5 × 12.5 cm (5″× 5″).
    b. Lay over these bricks a second layer of bricks without leaving any space between the joints.
    c. If necessary, similarly lay a third or fourth layer of bricks. This will depend upon the slope of the drain from the source outlet of waste water to the inlet chamber of the soak pit.
5. Take a 1 sq m gunny cloth with a hole in the center about the size of the inlet chamber. Cover the stone layer of the pit with this gunny cloth.
6. Cover the gunny cloth with a similar sized polythene sheet having a similar hole in the center.
7. Cover the polythene sheet with soil and fill the pit. Compact the soil properly. The soak pit is now ready.
8. Make a pucca drain 7 cm (3″) wide and 10 cm (4″) deep from the water outlet to the soak pit inlet. It should have a slope of about 8 cm per meter, i.e. about 1″ per foot. The drain should be covered by bricks or flat stones without joining them. This helps in checking the entry or solid waste and rain water.
9. Provide a trap near the middle of the drain to check the entry of suspended solid wastes from entering the pit. Dimensions of the trap are: length 35 cm (14″), breadth 25 cm (10″) and height, progressively sloping along the flow of water, so as to be 25 cm (10″) in beginning,

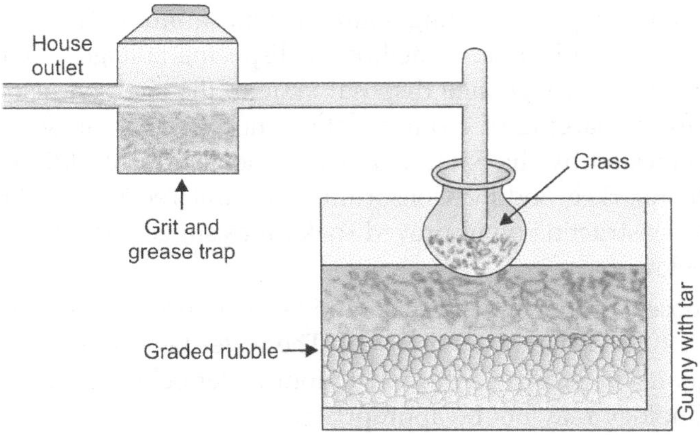

Fig. 13.5: Soak pit

22.5 cm (9″) in the middle and 20 cm (8″) at end. At the middle provided a partition with a 7.5 cm × 7.5 cm (3″ × 3″) hole at the bottom as shown in Figure 13.5.

10. Cover the trap and the inlet chamber of the pit with a flat stone.
11. Cover the top surface of the soak pit with soil so as to raise it 5 cm above the surrounding ground level.

SLOW SAND FILTER (FIG. 13.6)

1. Slow sand filter requires ½ to 1½ acre area. So the initial cost is much more (about 20-30 times) than rapid filter, maintenance cost is however low.

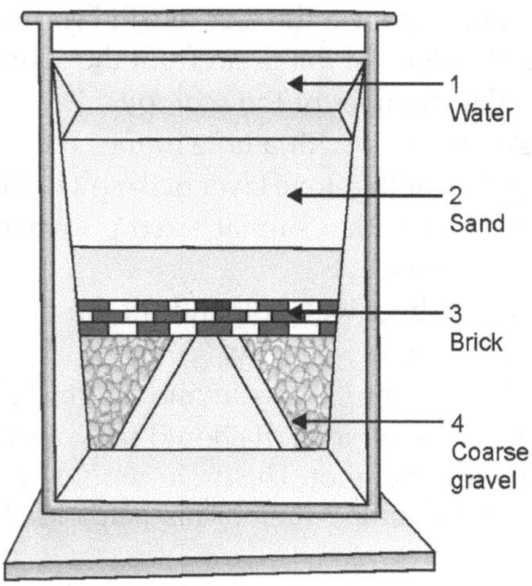

Fig. 13.6: Slow sand filter

2. Total depth of filter is about 3.6 meters and various layers from below upward are as follows:

Underdrain	Two layered bricks
Gravel	15-30 cm
Coarse sand	15-30 cm
Fine sand	0.6 meter
Water on top	1.5 to 1.8 meter

3. Dust free sand insoluble in dilute HCL and having effective size of 0.25 to 0.35 mm is used in slow sand filter.
4. Heart of slow sand filter vital layer, which formed by algae, bacteria, plankton and diatoms. The development of vital layer is called ripening of filter, which removes organic matter, holds bacteria and oxidises organic material.
5. Loss of head—when vital layer increases in thickness, loss of head occurs. If this is above 4 feet "Scraping the filter" is needed.
6. Quality of work—it removes 99.9 to 99.99% bacteria.

Rapid Sand Filter (Fig. 13.7)

This is introduced to the world after 80 years after the discovery of slow sand filter.

1. It occupies very little space.
2. Vital layer is not required. Alum block bring about changes in surface tension which help to clear out the impurities.
3. Quality of work—it removes 98 to 99 percent bacteria. Washing is easy (back-wash).

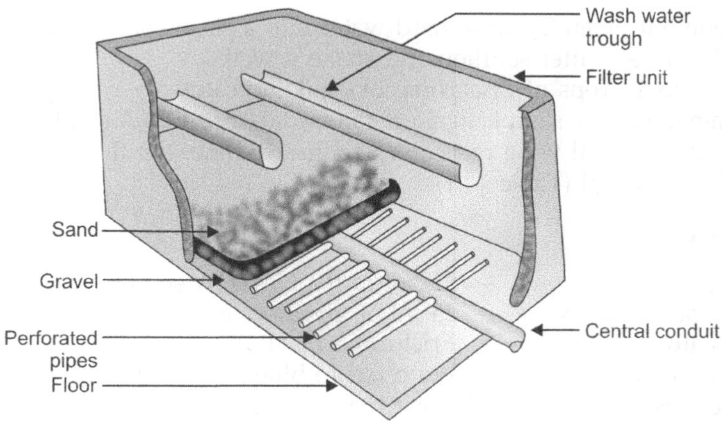

Fig. 13.7: A rapid sand filter

Chapter 14 Water Analysis

CHAPTER OUTLINE

- DETERMINATION OF TOTAL HARDNESS
- BACTERIOLOGY OF WATER
- STEPS IN WELL DISINFECTION

DETERMINATION OF TOTAL HARDNESS

Determination of total hardness of water by ethylenediaminetetraacetic acid (EDTA) method.

Theory

The characteristic of water that prevents the lathering of soap is called hardness. EDTA is an excellent complexing agent, which forms insoluble complexes with divalent ions (Ca^{++} Mg^{++}) present in water. Therefore, hardness causing salts of calcium and magnesium present in water can be estimated by titrating the given water sample against standard EDTA solution using Erichrome Black-T as an indicator. The indicator is effective in the PH range of about 8 to 11, so while performing the experiment it is essential to maintain the PH of water sample in between 8 and 11 by adding a suitable buffer solution.

Procedure

1. Pipette out given 25 ml of hard water into a clean conical flask.
2. Add 2 ml of buffer solution and shake it well.
3. Add 1 to 2 drops of Erichrome Black–T indicator.
4. Titrate the above sample against standard 0.02 M EDTA solution from the burette until wine red color changes to blue. Let this volume of EDTA be V_2 ml (Table 14.1).

Example

1. In burette – Standard 0.2 N EDTA solution.
2. By pipette – 25 ml of given water solution.
3. Indicator – Erichrome Black–T
4. Color change – Wine red to blue.
5. Reactions – Wine red to blue.

i. Ca^{++} + EDTA - - - - $(Ca_{Mg}\ EDTA)$

Stable colorless sample

ii. Ca^{++} + EBT - - - - $(Ca_{Mg}\ EBT)$
Mg^{++}

Unstable wine red color complex

iii. $(Ca_{Mg}\ EBT)$ + EDTA - - - - $(Ca_{Mg}\ EDTA)$ + EBT

Stable complex

Table 14.1: Burette readings

Burette	*Pilot*	*I*	*II*	*III*	*Mean*
Final reading	6.0	11.7	17.7	23.6	
Initial reading	0.0	6.0	11.7	17.7	
Difference	6.0	5.7	6.0	5.9	5.9

Calculations

1000 ml of 1 M EDTA = 100 gm of $CaCO_3$
1 ml of 1 M EDTA = 0.1 gm of $CaCO_3$
1 ml of 0.02 M EDTA = 0.01 × 0.02 gm of $CaCO_3$
5.9 ml of 0.02 M EDTA = 0.1 × 0.02 × 5.9 gm of $CaCO_3$
i.e. 25 ml of water sample contains = 0.002 × 5.9 gm of $CaCO_3$
1000 ml of sample contains = 0.002 × 5.9 × 40 gm of $CaCO_3$
Total hardness of water = 0.02 × 5.9 × 1000 mg of $CaCO_3$
= 475.2 ppm of $CaCO_3$

BACTERIOLOGY OF WATER

Drinking water has to be visually acceptable, being clear and colorless, and without disagreeable taste or odor. It should also be safe, being free from chemical toxins and pathogenic microorganisms. Many more human diseases, for example, typhoid fever, cholera and other diarrheal diseases, poliomyelitis and viral hepatitis A and B are waterborne. These pathogens reach water sources through fecal or sewage pollution. It is essential to prevent such contamination, treat the water suitably to remove or destroymicroorganisms, and also to ensure the safety of such protected water supplies by regular bacteriological surveillance.

Bacteriological Examination of Water

Bacteriological analysis of water supplies should be a regular periodical procedure and not a random exercise.

Plate Count

This consists of counting the numbers of colonies formed in pourplate cultures of the water samples, on nutrient agar incubated aerobically, in parallel, at 37°C for 1 to 2 days and at 22°C for 3 days. Those that grow at 37°C are those most likely to be associated with organic material of human or animal origin, whereas those growing at a lower temperature are mainly saprophytes that normally inhabit water are derived from soil and vegetables.

The agar count at 22°C gives an indication of the amount of decomposing organic matter in the water available for bacterial nutrition. Though most bacteria growing at 22°C are nonpathogenic to human beings, on general grounds, the greater the amount of organic matter present, the more likely is the water to be contaminated with parasitic and potentially pathogenic organisms. The agar count at 37°C is a more important index of dangerous pollution. A rise in colony count is the usual signal of some defect in filter beds demanding immediate attention.

Detection of Coliform Bacteria and E. coli

Presumptive coliform count (Multiple tube technique): The test is called presumptive because the reaction observed may occasionally be due to the presence of some other organisms and the presumption that the reaction is due to coliform organisms has to be confirmed.

An estimate of the number of coliform organisms is usually made by adding varying quantities of water (0.1-50 ml) to bile salt lactose peptone water (with an indicator for acidity) and incubating at appropriate temperatures. Acid and gas formations indicate the growth of coliform bacilli. Thus, it is possible to state the smallest quantity of water containing a coliform bacillus and to express the degree of contamination with this group of organisms.

The following ranges are put up:

- One 50 ml quantity of water added to 50 ml double strength medium.
- Five 10 ml quantities each to 10 ml double strength medium.
- Five 1 ml quantities each to 5 ml single strength medium.
- Five 0.1 ml quantities each to 5 ml single strength medium.

MacConkey's fluid medium (modified) is used. The range of quantities depends on the likely strength of contamination. For highly contaminated waters, smaller volumes are tested. The bottles are incubated at 37°C and examined after 18 to 24 hours. The 'presumptive positives' are read off and the remaining negative bottles are reincubated for another 24 hours. Any further positives are added to the previous figures. The probable number of coliforms per 100 ml are read off from the probability tables of McCrady. This is known as the 'presumptive coliform count' or the most probable number of coliforms (MPN).

Differential coliform test: The Eijkman's test is usually employed to find out whether the coliform bacilli detected in the presumptive test are *E. coli*. After the usual presumptive test, subcultures are made from all the bottles showing acid and gas to fresh tubes of single strength MacConkey's medium already warmed to 37°C. They are incubated at 44°C and examined after 24 hours. Incubation at 44°C should be carried out in thermostatically controlled water baths that do not deviate more than 0.5°C from 44°C. Those showing gas in Durham's tubes contain *E. coli*. From the number of positive tubes obtained, results are read off the probability tables. Further confirmation of the presence of *E. coli* can be obtained by testing for indole production and citrate utilization (Table 14.2).

Table 14.2: Bacteriological quality of drinking water [a]

Organisms	*Guideline value*
All water intended for drinking	
E. coli or thermotolerant coliform bacteria [b,c]	Must not be detectable in any 100 ml sample
Treated water entering the distribution system	
E. coli or thermotolerant coliform bacteria [b]	
Total coliform bacteria	Must not be detectable in any 100 ml sample
Treated water entering the distribution system	Must not be detectable in any 100 ml sample
E. coli or thermotolerant coliform bacteria [b]	Must not be detectable in any 100 ml sample
Total coliform bacteria	In the case of large supplies where sufficient samples are examined, must not be present in 95% of samples taken throughout any 12-month period.

a. Immediate investigative action must be taken if either *E. coli* or total coliform bacteria are detected. The minimum action in the case of total coliform bacteria is repeat sampling: if these bacteria are detected in the repeat sample, the cause must be determined by immediate further investigation.

b. Although *E. coli* is the more precise indicator of fecal pollution, the count of thermotolerant coliform bacteria is an acceptable alternative necessary, proper confirmatory tests must be carried out. Total coliform bacteria are not acceptable indicators of the sanitary quality of rural water supplies, particularly in tropical areas where many bacteria of no sanitary significance occur in almost all untreated supplies.

c. It is recognized that, in the great majority of rural water supplies in developing countries, fecal contamination is widespread. Under the conditions, the national surveillance agency should set medium term targets for progressive improvement of water supplies.

Membrane filtration method: A measured volume of water is filtered through a millipore filter. All the bacteria present are retained on its surface. It is placed on suitable media face upwards and incubated at the appropriate temperature, and the colonies that develop on the surface of the membrane are counted. After 18 hours of incubation the presumptive coliform counts and *E. coli* counts can be directly made.

Detection of Fecal Streptococci

Subcultures are made from all the positive bottles in the presumptive coliform test into tubes containing 5 ml of glucose azide broth. The presence of *Streptococcus faecalis* is indicated by the production of acid in the medium within 18 hours at 45°C. The positive tubes should be plated onto **MacConkey's** agar for confirmation.

Millipore membrane technique can also be adopted for this purpose.

Examination for Clostridium perfringens

This is tested by incubating varying quantities of the water in litmus milk medium (anaerobically) at 37°C for five days and looking for stormy fermentation.

Tests for Pathogenic Bacteria

Under special circumstances, specific pathogens such as typhoid bacilli or cholera vibrios may have to be looked for in water. This used to be done by adding the water samples to ten-fold concentrated liquid media, incubating and subculturing onto appropriate solid media. A simpler and more sensitive method is to filter the water, sample through membrane filters and incubate the filters on appropriate solid media.

STEPS IN WELL DISINFECTION

Find the Volume of Water in a Well

a. Measure the depth of water column (h) meters
b. Measure the diameter of well (d) meters

Take the average of several readings of the above measurements

c. Substitute h and d in:

$$\text{Volume (liters)} = \frac{3.14 \times d^2 \times h \times 1000}{4}$$

d. 1 cubic meter = 1000 liters of water.

Find the Amount of Bleaching Powder Required for Disinfection

Estimate the chlorine demand of the well water by "Harrock's apparatus (for water testing) which contains six white cups (200 ml capacity). One black cup with a circular mark on inside, two metal spoons (each holds 2 g of bleaching powder) seven glass stirring rods, one special pipette, two droppers, starch iodide indicator solution, instruction folder and calculate the amount of bleaching powder require to disinfect the well.

= 2.5 gm bleaching powder is required to disinfect 1000 liters of water

= 0.7 mg applied chlorine per liter of water.

Procedure

Take one level spoonful (2 g) of bleaching powder in the black cup and make it into a thin paste with a little water. Add more water to the paste and make up the volume up to the circular mark with vigorous stirring. Allow to settle. This is the stock solution.

- Fill the 6 white cup with water to be tested up to about a cm below the brim.
- With the special pipette provided add one drop of the stock solution to the 1st cup, 2 drops to 2nd cup, 3 drops to 3rd cup and so on.
- Stir the water in each cup using a separate rod.
- Wait for half hour for the action of chlorine.
- Add 3 drops of starch iodide indicator to each of the white cups and stir again. Development of blue color indicates the presence of free residual chlorine.
- Note the first cup which shows distinct blue color, supposing 3rd cup shows blue color then 3 level spoonfull, 6 gm of bleaching powder would be required to disinfect 4.55 liters of water.

Dissolve Bleaching Powder in Water

The bleaching powder required for disinfecting the well is placed in a bucket (< 100 g in one bucket of water) and made into a thin paste. More water is added till the bucket is nearly ¾ full. The content is stirred well and allowed to sediment for 5 to 10 minute then lime settle down. The supernatant solution which is chlorine solution, it is transferred to another bucket and the chalk or lime is discarded (Since lime hardens well water, it should not be poured into the well).

Delivery of Chlorine Solution into the Well

The bucket containing the chlorine solution is lowered some distance below the water surface, and the well water is agitated by moving the bucket violently but vertically and laterally. This should be done several time and so that the chlorine is mixed intimately to the water inside the well.

Contact Period

A contact period of one hour is allowed before the water is drawn for use.

Orthotolidine Arsenite Test

To test for residual chlorine at the end of one hour contact. If the residual chlorine itself is < 0.5 mg/lit, the chlorination procedure should be repeated before any water is drawn. Wells are best disinfected at night after the days drawn off. During epidemics of cholera, wells should be disinfected every day.

National Water Supply and Sanitation Program (1972): The stipulated norm of water supply is 40 liters of safe drinking water per capita per day and at least one hand pump/spot source for every 250 persons. Provide safe drinking water to all the villages by the turn of century as available to about 85 percent of the total population and 16 percent population has access to adequate sanitation.

Chapter 15 Bacteriology of Milk

CHAPTER OUTLINE

BACTERIA IN MILK

Types of Bacteria in Milk

1. Acid forming bacteria
2. Alkali forming bacteria
3. Gas-forming bacteria
4. Proteolytic bacteria
5. Inert bacteria.

Bacteriological Examination

The routine bacteriological examination of milk consists of the following:

Viable Count

This is estimated by doing plate counts with serial dilutions of the milk sample. Raw milk always contains bacteria, varying in number from about 500 to several million per ml.

Test for Coliform Bacteria

This is tested by inoculating varying dilutions of milk into MacConkey's fluid medium noting the production of acid and gas after incubation. Contamination with coliforms comes mainly from dust, dirty utensils and dairy workers.

Methylene Blue Reduction Test

This is a simple substitute for the viable count. It depends on the reduction of methylene blue by bacteria in milk when incubated at 37°C in complete darkness. The rate of reduction is related to the degree of bacterial contamination. Raw milk is considered satisfactory if it fails to reduce the dye in 30 minutes under standard conditions.

The Resazurin test is similar but the dye resazurin, on reduction, passes through a series of color changes—from blue to pink to colorless—the shade of color after incubation with milk for a particular period of time, depending on the degree of contamination. Generally, the 10 minute resazurin test is done, in which the shade of color is noted after incubation with the milk for 10 minutes.

Phosphatase Test

This is a check on the pasteurization of milk. The enzyme phosphatase normally present in milk is inactivated if pasteurization has been carried out properly. Residual phosphatase activity indicates that pasteurization has not been adequate.

Turbidity Test

This is a check on the 'sterilization' of milk. If milk has been boiled or heated to the temperature prescribed for 'sterilization', all heat coagulable proteins are precipitated. If ammonium sulphate is then added to the milk, filtered and boiled for five minutes, no turbidity results. This test can distinguish between pasteurized and 'sterilized' milk.

Examination for Specific Pathogens

Tubercle bacillus: The milk is centrifuged at 3000 rpm for 30 minutes and the sediment inoculated into two guineapigs. The animals are observed for a period of three months for tuberculosis. Tubercle bacilli may also be isolated in culture. Microscopic examination for tubercle bacilli is unsatisfactory.

Brucella: Isolation of brucella may be attempted by inoculating cream heavily on serum dextrose agar or by injecting centrifuged deposit of the milk sample intramuscularly into guineapigs. The animals are sacrificed after six weeks and the serum tested for agglutinins and the spleen inoculated in culture media.

Brucellosis in animals can be detected also by demonstrating the antibodies in milk, by the milk-ring or the whey agglutination tests.

Chapter 16 Staining, Culture Media and Microscopy of Slides of Public Health Importance

Chapter Outline

- GRAM STAIN
- ALBERT STAIN
- MICROSCOPIC SLIDES
- ZIEHL-NEELSEN STAIN
- CULTURE MEDIA

GRAM STAIN

Aim

To study the morphology and arrangement of bacteria and to classify the bacteria into gram +ve and gram –ve. Gram stain is a differential stain.

Requirement

1. Methylviolet	—	5 gm
2. Grams iodine	—	10 gm
Potassium iodide	—	20 gm
Distill water	—	1 liter
3. Counterstain	—	0.5% Safarin
Safarin	—	5 gm
Distill water	—	2 liter

Procedure

1. Cover the smear with methylviolet solution and allow to act for one minute, wash with water.
2. Cover the smear with Gram's iodine, keep it for 1 minute.
3. Decolorize with absolute alcohol for 10 to 30 seconds with gentle agitation till no more stain comes off. Again wash with water.
4. Apply the counter stain (Safarin) for one to two minutes. Wash with water and dry between blotting paper. Observe under oil immersion objective.

Result

Gram +ve bacteria take violet color and gram –ve bacteria are stained pink.

ZIEHL-NEELSEN STAIN

Aim

To demonstrate acid fast bacteria

a. Ziehl-Neelsen carbol fuschin
   i. Basic fuschin—10 gm
   ii. Absolute alcohol—100 gm
   iii. Solution of phenol (5%)—1000 ml in water
b. Twenty percent sulfuric acid solution
c. Counter stain—Loeffler's methylene blue.

Procedure

1. Smear should be prepared from the thick purulent part of the sputum.
2. Smears are dried, heat fixed and stained by Ziehl-Neelsen technique. The smear is covered with strong carbol fuschin and gently heated to steaming for five to seven minutes, without letting the stain boil and become dry.
3. The slide is then washed with water and decolorized with 20 percent sulphuric acid till the stain become faint pink and then decolorize with ethanol for two minutes.
4. After washing, the smear is counter-stained with Loeffler's methylene blue or 1 percent picric acid or 0.2 percent malachite green for one minute. Dry with bloting paper.
5. Under the oil immersion objective, AFB are seen as bright red rods while the background is blue, yellow or green depending on the counterstain used.

Result

Acid fast bacilli stain bright red while the tissue cell and other organisms are stained blue.

ALBERT STAIN

Aim

To demonstrate *Corynebacterium diphtheriae*, it is a special stain to demonstrate intracytoplasmic granules.

Requirement

Toludine blue	— 15 gm	Albert A
Malachite green	— 20 gm	
Glacial acetic acid	— 100 ml	
Alcohol (95%) ethenol	— 200 ml	
Distilled water	— 1000 ml	

Alberts iodine (iodine)	—	60 gm	Albert B
Potassium iodide	—	90 gm	
Distilled water	—	900 ml	

Procedure

1. Make smear dry and fix by heat.
2. Cover the slide with Albert A and allow to act for two to three minutes.
3. Cover the slide with Albert B, allow to act for one minute
4. Wash and blot dry.

Result

By this method intracytoplasmic granules stain bluish black, the protoplasm green and other organisms lightly green.

CULTURE MEDIA

Types of Media

1. Solid media, liquid media.
2. Simple media, complex media, special media.
3. Aerobic media, anaerobic media.

Simple Media

Nutrient broth consists of peptone, meat extract, sodium chloride and water. Nutrient agar is made by adding two percent agar to nutrient broth.

Complex Media

In complex media ingredients are added for growth of special bacteria.

Synthetic or Defined Media

Prepared from pure chemical substances and exact composition of the medium is known, e.g. simple peptone water medium, one percent peptone with 0.5 percent sodium chloride in water.

Enrichment Media (Liquid Media)

In mixed culture wanted bacteria is over grown as compared to unwanted bacteria, e.g. *E. coli* overgrow than salmonellae in fecal culture tetrathionate broth—which inhibits the coliforms while allowing typhoid and paratyphoid bacteria to grow freely, e.g. Selinate 'F' broth for dysentery bacilli.

Selective Media

The inhibiting substance is added to solid media, it enables a greater number of required bacterium to form colonies than the other bacteria, e.g. desoxycholate citrate medium for dysentery bacilli.

Indicator Media

This media contain indicator which changes color when a bacterium grows in them, e.g. incorporation of sulphite in Wilson and Blair medium.

MICROSCOPIC SLIDES

Microorganisms which cause diseases of public health magnitude should be identified and certain important characteristics related to their identification, special stains and special media are expected to be known by the students (Fig. 16.1). The diseases caused by these microorganisms, their signs and symptoms,their management as well as prevention and control should also be known to the student. Important aspects related to the identification, stains and media are mentioned here. For the disease aspects the student is advised to refer back to the description of these diseases in the chapter related to case examination.

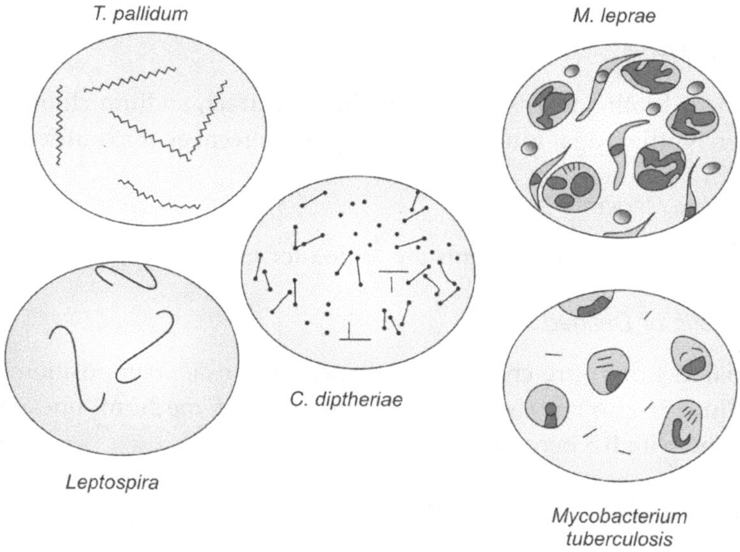

Fig. 16.1: Microscopy of slides of public health importance

Mycobacterium tuberculosis

Identification

Mycobacteria means 'fungus like bacteria'

1. It is an acid fast bacillus (AFB).
2. They are slender rod shaped that sometimes show branching filamentous forms resembling fungal mycelium.
3. AFB appear pink against a blue background in the Ziehl-Neelsen stain.
4. They are aerobic, nonmotile, noncapsulated and nonsporing.
5. They are straight or slightly curved rods occurring singly, in pairs or in small clumps.
6. Solid media for growth includes:
   a. Löwenstein-Jensen media
   b. Löeffler's serum slope
   c. Dorset's egg media.

Mycobacterium leprae

Identification

1. They are acid fast bacilli seen singly and in bundles, intracellularly or lying free outside the cells.
2. They frequently appear as conglomerates the bacilli being bound together by a lipid like substance, the glia. These masses are known as "globi".
3. The parallel rows of bacilli in the globi present a 'cigar bundle' appearance.
4. *Mycobacterium leprae* appear pink against a blue background in the Ziehl-Neelsen (5% sulfuric acid) stain.

Treponema pallidum

Identification

1. 'Trepos' meaning to turn and 'nema' meaning thread.
2. They are slender spirochaetes with fine spirals and pointed or rounded ends.
3. They are thin, delicate, spirochaete with tapering ends, and have about ten regular spirals which are sharp and regular at an interval of about 1μ (1 micron).

4. They are motile, exhibiting rotation round the long axis, backward and forward movements and flexion of the whole body.
5. It stains light rose red with Giemsa's stain and can be stained by silver impregnation.

Neisseria meningitidis

Identification

1. They are Gram-negative, aerobic, nonsporing, nonmotile cocci, which are both intra- and extracellular.
2. They are spherical cocci arranged in pairs, with the adjacent sides flattened.
3. Culture media are:
   a. Blood agar.
   b. Chocolate agar.
   c. Müeller-Hinton media.

Clinical Features

1. Meningococcemia
   a. Sudden onset.
   b. Prodromal symptoms like cough, bodyache, headache, myalgia.
   c. Fever with chills, tachycardia, tachypnea and shock.
   d. Petechial rash.
2. Meningitis
   a. Fever, headache and vomiting.
   b. Altered sensorium and convulsions.
   c. Neck stiffness with other meningeal signs.

Complications

a. Addison's crisis (Waterhouse-Friderichsen syndrome)
b. Deafness and other neurological damage.
c. Disseminated intravascular coagulation (DIC).

Treatment

1. Antibiotics
   a. Benzylpenicillin 10 to 20 lacs units intravenously 2 hourly.
   b. Chloramphenicol 500 mg intravenously, 6 hourly.
   c. Third generation cephalosporins like cefatoxime.
2. Treatment of raised intracranial tension with mannitol.
3. Treatment of shock:
   a. IV fluids
   b. Steroids
   c. Electrolyte imbalance correction.

4. Treatment of Addison's crisis
   a. Saline infusion.
   b. Hydrocortisone.

Corynebacterium diphtheriae

Identification

1. They are Gram-positive, nonacid fast, nonmotile rods with irregularly stained segments and metachromatic granules and polar bodies.
2. They are nonsporing, and noncapsulated.
3. They show club-shaped swelling, (coryne meaning club), arranged in pairs or small groups and form various angles with each other so as to resemble 'V' or 'L' letter (Chinese letter arrangement).
4. Culture media are:
   - Löeffler's serum slope
   - McLeod's and Hoyle's media
   - Potassium tellurite blood agar.

Neisseria gonorrhoeae

Identifications

1. They are gram-negative, aerobic, nonsporing, nonmotile cocci.
2. They are diplococci with adjacent sides concave, the cocci are reniform or bean shaped.
3. They are found predominantly within the polymorphs, some cells may contain as many as hundred cocci. Extracellular forms are also seen.
4. Culture media are:
   a. Blood agar.
   b. Chocolate agar.
   c. Thayer-Martin medium.

Clostridium tetani

Identification

1. They are gram-positive, motile, anaerobic, spore-forming bacilli.
2. Spores are spherical and placed terminally giving a 'drumstick appearance'.
3. The spores are wider than the bacillary bodies, giving the bacillus a swollen appearance resembling a spindle (Closter means a spindle) hence the name *Clostridium*.
4. Grown in anaerobic conditions only. Special medium used is Robertson's cooked meat broth.

Clinical Features

1. Inability to open the mouth (Trismus).
2. Inability to swallow.
3. Repeated fall in case of children due to stiffness of muscles.
4. Risus sardonicus (facial muscle contraction giving the appearance of a smile).
5. Spatula test becomes positive, i.e. on touching the spatula to the soft palate, patient forcefully closes the mouth.

Complications

1. Laryngeal spasm.
2. Secretions and chest infection.
3. Autonomic nervous system disturbance like cardiac arrhythmia, hypotension.

Treatment

1. Anti-tetanus serum (ATS) is given intravenously, dose 5000 to 10,000 units.
2. Antibiotic: Benzathine penicillin is given 0.6 to 1.2 megaunit intramuscularly.
3. Muscle relaxants:
   a. Diazepam
   b. Chlorpromazine
   c. Barbiturate.
   d. Baclofen
4. Ryles tube feeding.
5. Local wound or infection site should be cleaned and antiseptic applied.

Leptospira

Identification

1. They are elongated, motile, flexible bacteria, they are twisted spirally round the long axis and stained with Giemsa stain.
2. They possess numerous coils, set so close together that they can be distinguished only under dark ground illumination in the living state or by electron microscopy.
3. Culture media are:
   a. Stuart's medium
   b. Fletcher's medium.

Clinical Features

1. Leptospirosis
   a. Primary phase: Fever, headache and joint pain.
   b. Secondary phase:
      i. Signs and symptoms of meningeal irritation occurs.
      ii. Optic neuritis.
      iii. Myelitis.
      iv. Peripheral neuropathy.
2. Weil's syndrome
   a. Fever.
   b. Jaundice.
   c. Hepatorenal failure.
   d. Subconjunctival hemorrhages.

Treatment

1. Benzylpenicillin 20 lacs units Intravenous, 6 hourly.
2. Fluid and electrolyte imbalance to be corrected.
3. Blood transfusion if required.
4. Renal dialysis if required.

Note: Leptospirosis is transmitted by rats and is an occupational hazard of sewage drainage workers.

BIBLIOGRAPHY

1. Difco Manual of Dehydrated Culture Media and Reagents, 9th edn, Michigan: Difco Laboratories, 1977.
2. Oxoid Manual, 3rd edn. Baringstoke, R Ananthanarayan, CKJ Paniker, 6th edn. 2000.

Chapter

17 Hospital Waste Management

CHAPTER OUTLINE

- HOSPITAL WASTE DISPOSAL
- PLANNING AND ORGANIZATION
- INCINERATORS

INTRODUCTION

The following estimates for an average distribution of health care wastes useful for preliminary planning of waste management. Eighty percent general health care waste, which may be dealt by the normal domestic and urban waste management system:

- Fifteen percent pathological and infectious waste;
- One percent sharps waste;
- Three percent chemical and pharmacological waste.
- Less than one percent special waste, such as radioactive or cytotoxic waste, pressurized containers or broken thermometers and used batteries.

The wastes generated by the hospitals add to the community waste, thereby putting the load on the already scarce resources. Most of the hospital-generated waste is potentially infectious and therefore, spreads infections amongst the community causing a major health problem (Fig. 17.1).

Fig. 17.1: International infectious substance symbol

Type of Hospital Waste

The waste generated by the hospitals is of two types:
1. High-risk waste (which requires special handling)
2. Non-risk waste (general wastes).

The High-risk Waste

Chemical wastes: Which comprises of materials discarded from diagnostic and experimental works, cleaning, housekeeping and disinfecting work.

Pathological wastes: Consists of tissues, organic body parts and human fetuses, which may be infectious.

Highly infectious wastes: Contain pathogens in sufficient quantity, so that exposure could result in diseases. This category includes cultures and stocks of infectious agents from laboratory work, wastes from surgery and autopsies of patients with infectious diseases, waste from infectious patients in isolation wards, etc.

Sharp: Include needles, syringes, scalpels, blades, broken glasses, nails and any other material which can cause puncture.

Pressurized containers: Include those containers used for demonstration or instrumental purposes containing innocuous or inert gas and aerosol cans which may explode, if incinerated or accidentally punctured.

Laboratory wastes: Include pharmaceutical products, drugs and chemicals that have been returned from wards, outdated, contaminated or discarded for any other reason.

General Wastes

General wastes includes domestic wastes, packing material, noninfectious bleeding from animals, garbage from hospital kitchens and other waste materials that are not infectious or hazardous to the human health or environment.

In view of the large number of government hospitals and the rapidly increasing number of nursing homes and clinics in the private sector, in the urban as well as in the rural areas, proper training and awareness is essential for the safe and efficient management of hospital wastes. It is highly desirable that the wastes disposed should be free from disease organisms, the disposal system should prevent re-entry of the disease organisms in the community, there should be no contamination of the surface soil, water and a check on air pollution (including odors).

Getting rid of the hospital wastes in a proper manner plays a major role in prevention of emergence and re-emergence of infectious diseases and also other nosocomial infections and iatrogenic infections.

Hazards and Risks from Hospital Waste Exposure

Indiscriminate Disposal of Infectious Hospital Waste is Hazardous in Many Ways

1. Occupational hazard to persons who are constantly exposed to these wastes, like patients and hospital workers and contact personnel such as milkmen, laundry staff, cleaners, etc.
2. Inappropriately handled waste can be a public health nuisance as it can spread fatal diseases like Hepatitis B and C and HIV through injuries caused by contaminated needles or sharps picked by rag—pickers, children, etc. The people who visit hospital to see patients also are at risk.
3. Impact of badly disposed infectious hospital waste like blood soaked bandages, used needles and gloves, syringes and linen is great. When these wastes are indiscriminately thrown in backyards of hospitals or into open municipal pits, they become breeding sources for disease producing mosquitoes, flies, rodents and microbes. Besides being an environmental pollutant, this poses additional health risk to health workers and rag pickers. The ugly sight and stench of these biomedical wastes can be highly discouraging for the users of hospital services. Epidemics can result from the contamination of drinking water and food sources with these infectious wastes, which can be washed by rains. Indiscriminate open burning of infectious waste, especially plastics will result in emission of noxious gases which may produce cancer.

HOSPITAL WASTE DISPOSAL

Disposal strategies form a critical part of total waste management in hospitals, as any failure in this aspect will have hazardous consequences. The basic principle is that wastes are disposed in most hygienic and cost-effective manner, by methods which at all stages, minimize risk to health environment. Any strategy adopted should have a scientific bases. The Government of India has prescribed strict procedures and guidelines for each step in waste management leading to waste disposal in hospitals (Fig. 17.2).

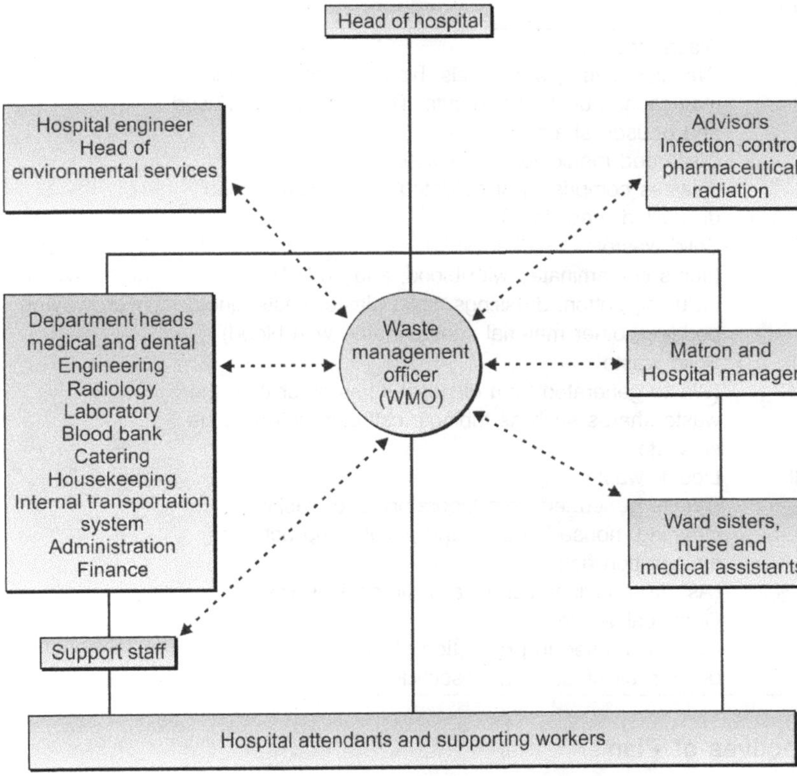

Fig. 17.2: Hospital waste management structure

Categories of Biomedical Waste (Table 17.1)

Table 17.1: Categories of biomedical waste

Category	*Waste category*	
I	Human anatomical waste (Human tissues, organs, body parts)	
II	Animal waste (Animal tissues, organs, body parts carcasses, bleeding parts, fluid, blood and experimental animals used in research, waste generated by veterinary hospitals colleges, discharge from hospitals, animal houses)	
III	Microbiology and biotechnology waste (Wastes from laboratory cultures, stocks or specimens of microorganisms live or attenuated vaccines, human and animal cell culture used in research and infectious agents from research and industrial laboratories, wastes from production of biological, toxins, dishes and devices used for transfer of cultures)	Local autoclaving/microwaving/incineration

Contd...

Contd...

IV	Waste sharps (Needles, syringes, scalpels, blades, glass, etc. that may cause puncture and cuts. This includes both used and unused sharps)	
V	Discarded medicines and cytotoxic drugs (Wastes comprising of outdated, contaminated and discarded medicines)	
VI	Solid waste (Items contaminated with blood, and body fluids including cotton, dressings, solid plaster casts, lines, bedding, other material contaminated with blood)	Incineration @ autoclaving/ microwaving
VII	Solid waste (Waste generated from disposal items other than the waste sharps such as tubings, catheters intravenous sets, etc.	
VIII	Liquid waste (Waste generated from laboratory and washing, cleaning, house keeping and disinfecting activities)	
IX	Incineration ash (Ash from incineration of any biomedical waste)	
X	Chemical waste (Chemical used in production of biological, chemicals used in disinfection, as insecticides, etc.)	

Objectives of Plan

The objectives of this plan are:

Immediate Objectives

a. To ensure safe, efficient, cost-effective disposal of hospital waste by developing a waste disposal plan.
b. To train hospital workers on waste management.

Long-term Objectives

a. To develop strategies for reduction of waste generation in the hospital.
b. To create awareness among workers about healthy hospital surroundings.
c. To create community awareness on environment issues in hospital surrounding.

PLANNING AND ORGANIZATION

The medical officer incharge of the hospital prepares a strategy on the following aspects.

Organization

Medical officer incharge will be the overall supervisor of the waste management program, and composes his team as follows:

- Team leader
  - Waste management co-ordinator (Medical officer incharge of the hospital)
- Members
  - The second medical officer
  - Senior staff nurse
  - FDA
  - SDA
  - Senior Group 'D' worker.

Responsibilities

The team will be responsible for:

1. Implementing effective waste disposal procedures—collection, transport, storage and final disposal and continuously monitoring them.
2. Designating Group 'D' workers for daily collection of waste, transport and disposal and monitoring their works.
3. Ensuring that adequate and correct waste containers are kept and maintained in all strategic areas of the hospital and used appropriately.
4. Supply and monitor use of protective—clothing, gloves, footwear, etc. by workers.
5. Arranging training of all staff on waste management through workshops, demonstrations and talks.
6. Creating environmental awareness among hospital patients, visitors and community leaders.
7. Developing waste reduction, reuse and recycling strategies.
8. Arranging periodic health check-up of involved personnel and immunization for all workers.

The team leader will delegate responsibilities to subgroups within the team to supervise and coordinate all activities.

Staff Appraisal on Hospital Waste Management

The well motivated and committed Medical Officer incharge of the hospital adopts an effective strategy for proper disposal of the waste. Entire staff of the hospital will be involved in a dialogue which will make them understand the mission of the hospital, present status with regard to hospital waste generation and implications of improper disposal to patients, workers and to community at large.

Waste Disposal Strategy

Different types of wastes are generated in different quantities by different sections of the hospital. To achieve the immediate objective of effective and scientific disposal of hospital waste, the following strategy will be adopted.

Collection of Waste with Source Segregation

Personnel in each department/section will collect wastes generated in their areas of responsibility into appropriate plastic bags kept inside hard, plastic containers which are coded with suitable colors which indicate nature and type of waste that should be put inside them, e.g. waste receptacle coded yellow and labeled as "put infectious wastes only" with a biohazard sign will receive all infectious waste materials, blue waste receptacle will receive only sharp waste and plastic/rubber waste and so on. This process of segregating wastes into their respective types at the point where they are generated is called segregation at source. This is a very critical step in proper waste management as this will facilitate correct disposal strategy and prevent mixing and cross contamination which can create a serious health risk. Hence, it is essential that all hospital workers are trained well on color coding and collection techniques. The table below gives details of color coding for different kinds of hospital wastes.

Plastic bags should be collected preferably on a daily basis to reduce spread of infection by flies or spillage by dongs. They should be allowed to fill to a maximum of three quarters of their capacity to prevent the bag from tearing and also to facilitate the ease of transport by workers.

Storage

Daily hospital waste from different facilities of the hospital awaiting final disposal are stored in a store-room meant for the purpose. The store-room should be away from the service areas and should be dry and well secured to prevent rodent nuisance.

Transportation

The waste segregated and collected in each point of generation will be transported daily in a trolley to a central store-room. The transport will be done in an orderly way according to stipulated rules:

1. Only designated hospital workers will transport the waste.
2. Only one waste receptacle at a time be transported on a trolley to the store-room where the plastic bag containing the waste is left in store and the plastic container washed with disinfectant brought back and kept in the designated place.

3. The wastes will be transported at specified time of the day and through specified routes which the waste management coordinator will decide and draw.
4. Before removing from the waste receptacle the transported should ensure that the mouth of the bag is well secured by tying to prevent pilferage.
5. Waste from white receptacles will be sorted out for recyclable waste which are bundled and transported to the store-room separately.

Temporary Storage

The wastes collected daily will be stored in a temporary store-room which is specially designated for the purpose. The store-room should be away from all patient care areas and offices as well as residences and well secured and locked. Recyclable materials are all stored separately away from other infectious categories of wastes.

Final Disposal of Waste

Recyclable waste: Waste in white containers which may be marketed for recycling, e.g. all kinds of papers—typing, computer prints, drafts, etc. corrugated card board packing materials, books, news papers, magazines, empty metal cans, bottles of aerated water are disposed off periodically by trading for going rates. Hyposolution used for developing films can also be marketed for its silver content. Mutilated and treated wastes of category 4 and category 7, viz. used disposable needles and syringes, blades, broken glassware, intravenous infusion and blood bags, tubing's, catheters collected in blue containers will be transported and stored until they are disposed to the market for recycling.

Chemical disinfection: Chemical disinfection involves destruction of most of the pathogenic microorganisms from inanimate body surface or material by using chemicals. Instruments and equipment in contact with patients, infected sharps contaminated floor, beds, etc. may be disinfected by using neutral disinfectants. Liquid waste from laboratories may be decontaminated chemically. Bleaching powder, glutaraldehyde, alcohol's or quaternary ammonium compounds may be used. Factors like concentration and stability of chemicals, surface contact time determines effectiveness of a chemical disinfectant. The main disadvantage of chemical disinfectants is that there is no disinfectant which attains the desirable level III disinfection and there is no easy but accurate post-treatment test to judge whether the wastes have been effectively decontaminated. Chemically disinfected medical wastes should continue to be treated hazardous, unless bacterial testing shows completed disinfection (Managing medical wastes in developing countries, WHO,

1994). Hence, this type of treatment option may be used only to decontaminate liquid infection waste from laboratories.

Autoclaves: In autoclaving technology wastes are steam-heated in a special autoclave meant for waste treatment at specified temperature and pressure for specific period of time. Decontamination occurs when steam penetrates the waste. The equipment requires supply of high temperature and pressurized steam from a boiler unit. Equipment should conform to standards, mentioned in rules. A gravity flow autoclave or a vaccum autoclave which functions within specified range of internal waste load temperature (121°C-149°C), pressure (15-51 psi) and residence time (30 to 60 min) should be used. Vaccum autoclaves are more efficient as absence of air ensures uniform and total penetration of waste by steam and thus total disinfection. The equipment should have computerized recording devices to monitor operational parameters and should answer specified validation tests such as spore testing for Bacillus subtilis at concentration of 10^4 spores/mm. Treated waste from an autoclave remains wet and disinfected to level III, with no volume change. The emission is likely to give emits foul odour and may be infectious. Autoclaves can decontaminate most categories of waste except biodegradable organic waste and toxic waste. Autoclaves with superior technology conforming to regulations of Central Pollution Control Board (CPCB) are efficient and offer advantages of volume reduction and odourless and nontoxic emission. But they may cause more occupational hazard and are not cost-effective, besides, requiring special elaborate infrastructure.

INCINERATORS

The Central Pollution Control Board has recommended two types of incinerators:

1. Incinerators for individual hospital/nursing homes/medical establishments.
2. Common incinerator to handle waste from a number of hospital/ nursing homes/pathological laboratories, etc.

Site for Incinerator

Incinerators should be installed at appropriate location to avoid nuisance to patients and neighborhood.

Standards for Incinerators

All incinerators shall meet the following operating and emission standards:

Operating Standards

- Combustion efficiency (CE) shall be at least 99.0 percent
- The combustion efficiency is computed as follows:

$$CE = \frac{\% CO_2}{\% CO_2 + \% CO} \times 100$$

1. The temperature of the primary chamber shall be 800 ± 50°C.
2. The secondary chamber gas residence time shall be at least 1 (one) second at 1050° ± 50°C, with a minimum % CO_2 oxygen in the stack gas.

Emission Standards

Parameters	Concentration mg/Nm 3 at (12% CO_2 correction)
1. Particulate matter	150
2. Nitrogen oxides	450
3. HCl	50
4. Minimum stack height shall be 30 meters above ground	
5. Volatile organic compounds in ash shall not be more than 0.01%	

Incineration or mass burn technology: The technique of incineration involves conversion of solids into ash and harmless gas by subjecting to high temperature. Incineration, as a simple technique known as burning, has been used to dispose off all types of wastes from hospitals. When unsorted waste is burnt in simple kilns incinerators, the high temperature (1000°C) in them converts the solid waste into bottom ash (noncombustible matter) and fly ash which may contain particulate matters and some environmentally hazardous noxious gases. Adverse publicity has resulted in innovation of technically superior, state of the art models equipped with pollution control components such as scrubbers, gravity settlers, condenses and deodorants that take care of the possible environmental hazards due to their emissions. Global/local environmental benefits, consumption of landfull space, disposal of harmful substances into environment are factors which are addressed favorably by incinerators. Incineration offers a direct disposal technology with zero occupational hazard (from cradle to grave) and a volume reduction of 85 to 95 percent.

Incinerable hospital waste categories include organic waste from surgery, autopsy and delivery, blood and body fluids from dialysis and transfusion, microbial and pathological waste from laboratories and general wastes like papers, cardboard, etc. Heavy metals like mercury, cadmium and chloride based plastics (PVC) cannot be incinerated as at low temperatures (800°C) they produce hazardous particulate matter and gases like Hydrogen Chloride dioxins and furons. Reports on PVC usage in India indicate that hospitals use only two percent of the total PVC products. Heavy metals are not present in most of the materials used for patient care in hospitals. Proper source segregation and installing multi-chambered electrical incinerators with pollution control technology are key points to ensure environmental safe use of this technology. The environment protection agency (EPA) recommends use of electrical incinerator with adequate control devices to ensure safe emission standards. Regular monitoring and recording of flue gas temperature, periodic checking of emission gases, annual check-up for wear and tear and importantly ensuring source segregation and recycling of plastics are EPA guidelines. With these measures taken, incineration represents the best practical environmental option (Royal Commission on Environmental Pollution).

As source segregation can identify the actual quantity of incinerable waste, hospitals can decide on the capacity of the incinerator they would like to invest in. Incinerators of different capacities to burn waste beginning with 3 to 40 kg/hr are available at competitive costs. Incineration as a process involves waste preparation (segregation) waste charging and combustion, treatment of emission (through controls) and handling of incinerator ash. The ash may be collected in thick puncture proof bags and stored for periodic dumping into a community landfull. Factors which help the hospital management to decide on characteristics of their incinerator system are:

i. Air distribution to combustion chambers (stored excess air combustion).
ii. Mode of operation (batch/continuous).
iii. Method of removal of ash (batch/continuous).

Microwave: In microwaving technique, the heat generated inside the equipment during bombardment of electromagnetic waves into the rotating molecules of the waste, disinfects the waste. The waste should have some water content to enhance molecular mobility and thus the heat generated. Shredded waste is more efficiently disinfected than bully materials, microwaving attains level III disinfection of all categories of biomedical waste except those of category 1 and 2, viz. human body parts and blood-soaked tissues and large metal items. Any microwave equipment installed must comply with efficacy tests stipulated under the biomedical rules and have performance guarantee. At the maximum design capacity, microwave unit should show total destruction of Bacillus subtilis spores at a concentration of 10^4 spores per min. Main advantage of this treatment technology are high efficiency, 30 to 40 percent volume reduction. Minimal environmental pollution and occupational risk, compact nature of equipment and cost-effectiveness. Simple and computerized operation enable semiskilled hospital staff to operate the equipment. Microwave system has made good advance years. Available data on microwave system suggest that it satisfies more selection criteria for choosing suitable technology for waste disposal than any other acceptable option.

Landfill: Sites are specially constructed areas used as one of the options for disposal of nonbiodegradable infectious hospital wastes. Hospitals with large surrounding land may choose this mode of disposal as it is comparatively simple and cost-effective. The area chosen should be away from service areas and residential localities. A hospital with bed strength of 100 may require a landfill site of about 500 to 600 cft. Basic features of an engineered landfill are:

i. An impermeable clay and pebble base liner to present uncontrolled release of leachate, a toxic liquid that is released by decomposition of waste.
ii. Graded base create leachate collection.
iii. Stored earth for covering at the end of each disposal operation.

Essential features of a correct landfill operation are:

i. That all the waste bags are completely pushed into landfill without getting opened up.
ii. Enough earth and hay cover is put to cover the entire waste so that stray animals do not pick the waste.
iii. Frequent spray of insecticides is done
iv. Personnel use proper protection like boots, gloves, aprons.

Deep burial: Wastes belonging to category 1, 3 and 6 collected in yellow containers are disposed by deep burial. The waste coordinator identifies a suitable place for digging a deep pit or trench within the premises of the hospital but at a fair distance from the hospital and houses. The place should not be prone for flooding or erosion and should be away from shallow wells. The pit may be a 4 feet square with a depth of 6 feet covered with wire mesh to deny access to animals and prevent accidents. Each time the waste (human tissues—placenta, amputated parts, blood soaked tissues, etc.) is disposed into the pit, should be covered completely with a thick layer of soil to ensure biodegradation.

Land fill: General wastes from white containers and waste from black containers will be disposed into an 'engineered landfill' (8 ft × 8 ft × 4 ft depth) constructed at a distant corner of the hospital within its premises. In order to prevent contamination with subsoil water, the base of the landfill should be made impermeable by putting a stone masonry. Scattering by stray animals and rag-pickers should be prevented by covering with a metallic mesh of the size of the landfill which is fixed at one margin and can be locked at the other margin. The medical officer in-charge will liase with the engineer in-charge of the hospital to construct this landfill.

Disposal of biodegradable kitchen waste: The non-infectious, but biodegradable waste from kitchen, dining areas and wards such as food waste, vegetable and fruit peals, etc. will be disposed into a vermicompost, which will be constructed adjacent to the land filling site.

Inertization

The process of "inertization" involves mixing waste with cement and other substances before disposal, in order to minimize the risk of toxic substances contained in the wastes migrating into the surface waste or ground water. A typical proportion of the mixture is: 65 percent pharmaceutical waste, 15 percent lime, 15 percent cement and 5 percent water. A homogeneous mass is formed and cubes or pellets are produced on site and then transported to suitable storage sites.

Legislative Framework

The Government of India has, under Environment Protection Act (1986), passed the Biomedical Waste (Management and Handling) Rules in July 1998. The rules define the Administrative Medical Officers of health care facilities as biomedical waste 'generators' and fix responsibility on them for developing an effective waste disposal mechanism for the waste their facilities generate. While the rules spell out treatment and disposal options for the various categories of biomedical wastes that are generated in healthcare facilities, they leave the option of handling the general or domestic type of waste to the generator. Standards for various treatment and disposal technologies that may be employed have been stipulated. The rules have also fixed time scale for implementing a treatment and disposal technology (incinerator technology) in hospitals of different bed strengths. At state level the State Pollution Control Board is the regulatory body, which monitors the proper implementation of the rules.

Standards have been fixed for different technology options giving consideration to international standards accepted by environment protection agencies in developed countries.

Summary of Biomedical Waste Rules

This notification was issued on 20th July 1998 by the Ministry of Environment and Forests under Section 6, 8 and 25 of Environment (Protection) Act, 1986.

1. The rules apply to all persons who generate, collect, receive, store, transport, treat, dispose and handle biomedical waste in any form.
2. "Biomedical waste" is any waste generated during diagnosis, treatment, immunization and research activities involving human beings and animals.
3. "Authorized person" is an "occupier" or "operator" of any health care facility who has control over the facility and has been authorized by the prescribed authority to deal with all aspects of biomedical waste in accordance with rules.
4. Biomedical waste treatment facility is one where treatment and disposal of biomedical wastes is carried out.

5. Every "generator/occupier" of a health care facility has the duty to take steps to ensure that waste generated is handled without any adverse effect on human health and environment.
6. Biomedical waste shall be segregated from other wastes at the source, collected in color coded containers and transported for treatment and disposal within 48 hours of its generation (Table 17.2).

Table 17.2: Color coding and type of container for disposal of biomedical wastes

Color coding	*Type of container*	*Waste category*	*Treatment options as per schedule*
Yellow	Plastic bag	Cat 1, Cat 2, Cat 3 and Cat 6	Incineration/deep burial
Red	Disinfected container/ plastic bag	Cat 3, Cat 6, and Cat 7	Autoclaving/ microwaving/chemical treatment
Blue/ White translu-cent	Plastic bag/puncture proof container	Cat 4, Cat 7	Autoclaving/ Microwaving/Chemical treatment and destruction/shredding
Black	Plastic bag	Cat 5, Cat 9 and Cat 10 (solid)	Disposal in secured landfill

What You should Know and Do

Plastics

Plastics are a heterogenous family.

Plastic are polymers of hydrocarbons typically derived from petroleum of natural gas.

Plastic by not being biodegradable remain in the soil for more then one thousand years, contaminating the soil and the surrounding water bodies.

Plastics constitute a major chunk of Health Care Waste. More so, with the increase in use of disposable items like syringes, IV bags, blood bags, catheters, etc.

There is four times more plastic in Health Care Waste than in Municipal Waste.

Problems

Collection and reuse or resale of the single-use (disposable) products without adequate treatment result in possible spread of infections.

Infection to the waste handlers, especially the rag-pickers and pourakarmikas.

Improper burning or sub-standard incineration of these plastics release toxic gases like—dioxins and furans and also other harmful gases like—sulphur dioxide, oxides of nitrogen, hydrochlorides, etc. The dioxins and furans are said to be potent carcinogens.

Improper landfilling or dumping them results in leaching and contamination of soil and surrounding water bodies.

Proposed Method for Disinfection of Commonly Used Articles, Materials/Surfaces in Order of Preference (Table 17.3)

Table 17.3: Proposed method for disinfection of commonly used articles, materials/surfaces in order of preferences

Material	*Methods*
Ampoules	Disinfectant with alcohol/methylated spirit/Iodine (PVI) before cutting.
Skin	Handwashing is an effective method for preventing the infection between health professionals. Some microbial agents are always present in the skin, which passes from the hands of the health staff to the patients. Handwashing is a very effective method of decontamination of hands.
	Social handwashing: With soap and water removes microorganisms. This method should be practiced before handling food, eating and feeding the patient after visiting the toilet. In this method, mechanical friction is applied to all the surfaces of the hands using soap and water for 10 seconds and hands are rinsed under a stream of water and dried with sterilized paper towel.
	Hygienic handwashing: A procedure where an antiseptic detergent preparation is used for washing or is disinfected with alcohol. It is performed before any invasive procedure, before and after use of gloves and after contact with blood products. The agents used are 4% chlorhexidine gluconate solution, solution containing 0.75% available chlorine.
	Surgical handwashing: A procedure to kill the bacterial flora and to decrease the organisms present to prevent wound contamination. This is done before surgical procedures and any interventions. Only soap is used, but scrubbing of hands, fingers and nails is very important.
Thermometer	Keeping in gluteraldehyde/PVI/Hexachlorophenes/Chlorhexidine + cetrimide (salvon) for at least 10 minutes before next use.
Articles/Ware: Stainless steel/ Enamel plated/ Plastics, e.g. Bedpan/urine bottles/bowls	Wash with warm detergent, disinfect with chlorine releasing compound/PVI/Formaldehyde/Phenolic compounds/Chloroxylenols/ Hexachlorophenes/Chlorhexidine
Surfaces like: Floor/walls/ trolleys/ furnitures/sink/ wash basin	Wash with detergent disinfect with chlorine releasing compound/ Carbolic acid/PVI/Hexachlorophenes

Contd...

Contd ...

Material	*Methods*
Humidifiers and incubators	Fill daily humidifiers with sterile distilled water containing 0.1% silver nitrate. Clean and disinfect with chlorine releasing compounds/activated glutaraldehyde/alcohol or carbolic acid.
Crockery/ Cutlery disinfectant	Wash with warm detergent solution, keep in boiling water for 10 minutes/expose to steam. No chemical should be used.
Laboratory Discarding jar	Phenolic compounds (carbolic acid)/Chlorine releasing compounds/Chloroxylenols and Hexachlorophenes
Syringes and needles	Chemical disinfectant must not be used for needle and syringes.
Instruments Cheatle forceps	Keep in concentrations recommended for grossly contaminated articles of PVI/Chlorhexidine + cetrimides/Chloroxylenols, gluteradehyde. Change the disinfectant daily.
Sharp instruments —Skin piercing and invasive instruments (not sterilizable by heat)	All articles and surfaces to be disinfected must first be cleaned and washed with warm water preferable containing detergent chemical disinfection only as last resort, if sterilization by heat is not possible, activated gluteraldehyde/carbolic acid for at least 10 hours for sterilization.
Equipment: Catheters, Cystoscope Endoscope, Laproscope	Chemical disinfection only at last resort, if sterilization by heat is not possible. Immerse in activated solution of gluteraldehyde/ Carbolic acid for 4 to 10 hours or more. Only vegetative bacteria, fungi and viruses are killed by immersing in surface disinfectants for 30 minutes.

BIBLIOGRAPHY

1. Achary DB, Singh M. The Book of Hospital Waste Management, 2000.
2. Mannual for control of hospital associated infections, NACO, Ministry of Health and Family Welfare Government of India.
3. Pruss A, Cirouit E, Rushbrook P. Safe management of wastes from health-care actives, WHO, 1999.

Chapter 18

National Rural Health Mission (2005-2012)

CHAPTER OUTLINE

- GOALS
- PLAN OF ACTION
- TECHNICAL SUPPORT
- FOCUS ON THE NORTH EASTERN STATES
- ROLE OF NGOs IN THE MISSION
- FUNDING ARRANGEMENTS
- OUTCOMES
- NATIONAL URBAN HEALTH MISSION
- STRATEGIES
- INSTITUTIONAL MECHANISMS
- ROLE OF STATE GOVERNMENTS UNDER NRHM
- ROLE OF PANCHAYATI RAJ INSTITUTIONS
- MAINSTREAMING AYUSH
- TIMELINES (FOR MAJOR COMPONENTS)
- MONITORING AND EVALUATION

INTRODUCTION

Health is fundamental to national progress in any sphere. In terms of resources for economic development, nothing can be considered of higher importance than the health of the people. Recognizing the importance of health in the process of economic and social development and improving the quality of life of our citizens, the Government of India has resolved to launch the National Rural Health Mission (NRHM) to carry our necessary architectural correction in the basic health care delivery system.

In India, 12th April 2005 was a historic day, when our honorable Prime Minister, Dr Manmohan Singh launched "the National Rural Health Mission." With a budget outlay of Rs.6500 crores for 2005 to 2006 and a commitment of the government to raise public health expenditure from 0.9 to 2-3 percent of GDP, the goal of the Mission is to improve the availability of and access to quality health care by people, especially for those residing in rural areas, the poor, women and children, with initial focus on 18 "high focus" states.

Any successful development program stands on four pillars, i.e. political will, financial resources, administrative infrastructure and scientific leadership.

The National Rural Health Mission seeks to provide effective health care to the rural population, especially the disadvantaged groups improving access, enabling community ownership and demand for services, strengthening public health systems for efficient service delivery, enhancing equity and accountability and promoting decentralization.

The National Rural Health Mission subsumes key national programs, the Reproductive and Child Health II project (RCH II), the National Disease

Control Programs (NDCP) and the National Disease Surveillance Project (NDSP). The National Rural Health Mission will also enable the mainstreaming of AYUSH, i.e. Ayurvedic, Yoga, Unani, Siddha and Homeopathy Systems of Health.

The Mission covers the country, with special focus on 18 states where the challenge of strengthening poor public health systems and there by improve key health indicators is the greatest. These are Uttar Pradesh, Uttaranchal, Madhya Pradesh, Chhattisgarh, Bihar, Jharkhand, Orissa, Rajasthan, Himachal Pradesh, Jammu and Kashmir, Assam, Arunachal Pradesh, Manipur, Meghalaya, Nagaland, Mizoram, Sikkim and Tripura. NRHM lists a set of core and supplementary strategies to meet its goals.

GOALS

- Reduction in infant mortality rate (IMR) and maternal mortality ratio (MMR).
- Universal access to public health services such as Women's health, child health, water, sanitation and hygiene, immunization, and Nutrition.
- Prevention and control of communicable and noncommunicable disease, including locally endemic diseases.
- Access to integrated comprehensive primary health care.
- Population stabilization, gender and demographic balance.
- Revitalize local health traditions and mainstream AYUSH.
- Promotion of healthy lifestyles.

STRATEGIES

Core Strategies

- Train and enhance capacity of Panchayati Raj Institutions (PRIs) to own, control and manage public health services.
- Promote access to improved health care at household level through the female health activist (ASHA).
- Health plan for each village through Village Health Committee of the Panchayat.
- Strengthen sub-center through an united fund to enable local planning and action and more multi-purpose workers (MPWs).
- Strengthening existing PHCs and CHC per lakh population for improved curative care to a normative standard (Indian public Health standards defining personnel, equipment and management standards).
- Preparation and Implementation of an intersect oral District Health Plan prepared by the District Health Mission, including drinking water, sanitation and hygiene and nutrition.
- Integrating vertical Health and Family Welfare programs at National, State, block and District levels.

- Technical support to National, State, and District Health Mission, for Public Health Management.
- Strengthening capacities for data collection, assessment and review for evidence based planning. Monitoring and supervision.
- Formulation of transport policies for deployment and career development of human resources for health.
- Developing capacities for preventive health care at all levels for promoting healthy lifestyles, reduction in consumption of tobacco and alcohol, etc.
- Promoting nonprofit sector particularly in underserved areas.

Supplementary Strategies

- Regulation of private sector including the informal rural practioners to ensure availability of quality services to citizen at reasonable cost.
- Promotion of public private partnerships for achieving public health goals.
- Mainstreaming AYUSH—revitalizing local health traditions.
- Reorienting medical education to support rural health issues including regulation of medical care and medical ethics.
- Effective and viable risk pooling and social health security to the poor by ensuring accessible, affordable, accountable and good quality hospital care.

PLAN OF ACTION

Component (A): Accredited Social Health Activists

- Every village/large habitat will have a female Accredited Social Health Activist (ASHA)—chosen by and accountable to the panchayat to act as the interface between the community and the public health system.
- ASHA would act as a bridge between the ANM and the village and be accountable to the panchayat.
- She will be an honorary volunteer, receiving performance-based compensation for promoting universal immunization, referral and escort services for RCH, construction of household toilets, and other health care delivery programs.
- She will be trained on a pedagogy of public health developed and mentored through a Standing Mentoring Group at National level incorporating best practices and implemented through active involvement of community health resource organizations.
- She will facilitate preparation and implementation of the Village Health Plan along with Anganwadi worker, ANM, functionaries of other Departments, and Self-Help Group members, under the leadership of the Village Health Committee of the Panchayat.

- She will be promoted all over the country, with special emphasis on the 18 high focus States. The government of India will bear the cost of training. Incentive and medical kits. The remaining components will be funded under Financial Envelope given to the States under the program.
- She will be given a drug kit containing generic AYUSH and allopathic formulations for common ailments. The drug kit would be replenished from time-to-time.
- Induction training of ASHA to be of 23 days in all, spread over 12 months. On the job training would continue throughout the year.
- Prototype training material to be developed at national level subject to state level modifications.
- Cascade model of training proposed through Training of Trainers including contract plus distance learning model.
- Training would require partnership with NGOs/ICDS Training Centers and State Health Institutes.

Component (B): Strengthening Sub-Centers

- Each sub-centers will have an united fund for local action @ Rs. 10,000 per annum. This fund will be deposited in a joint bank account of the ANM and Sarpanch and operated by the ANM, in consultation with the Village Health Committee.
- Supply of essential drugs, both allopathic and AYUSH, to the sub-centers.
- In case of additional outlays, multipurpose workers (Male) additional ANMs wherever needed, sanction of new sub-centers as per 2001 population norm, and upgrading existing sub-centes, including buildings for sub-centers functioning in rented premise will be considered.

Component (C): Strengthening Primary Health Centers

Mission aims at strengthening PHC for quality preventive, promotive curative, supervisory and outreach services.

- Adequate and regular supply of essential quality drug and equipment (including supply of Auto Disabled Syringes for immunization) to PHCs.
- Provision of 24 hours service in 50 percent PHCs by addressing shortage of doctors, especially in high focus states, through mainstreaming AYUSH manpower.
- Observance of standard treatment guidelines and protocols.
- In case of additional outlays, intensification of ongoing communicable disease control programs, new programs for control of noncommnuicable disease, upgaradation of 100 percent PHCs for 24 hours referral service, and provision of 2nd. Doctor at PHC level (1 male, 1 female) would be undertaken on the basis of felt need.

Component (D): Strengthening CHCs for First Referral Care

A key strategy of the Mission is:

- Operationalizing 3222 existing Community Health Center (30-50 beds) as 24 Hours First Referral Units, including of anesthetist.
- Codification of new Indian Public Health Standards, setting norms for infrastructure, staff, equipment, management, etc. for CHCs.
- Promotion of Stakeholder Committees (Rogi Kalyan Samitis) for hospital management.
- Developing standards of services and costs in hospital care.
- Developing, display and ensure compliance of Citizen's Charter at CHC/PHC level.
- In case of additional outlays, creation of new Community Health Centers (30-50 beds) to meet the population norm as per Census 2001, and bearing their recurring costs for Mission period could be considered.

Component (E): District Health Plan

- District Health Plan would be an amalgamation of field responses through Village Health Plans, State and Notional priorities for health, water supply, sanitation and nutrition.
- Health Plan would from the core unit of action proposed in areas like water supply, sanitation, hygiene and nutrition. Implementing departments would integrate into District Health Mission for monitoring.
- District becomes core unit of planning, budgeting and implementation.
- Centrally Sponsored Schemes could be rationalized/modified accordingly in consulation with States.
- Concept of "funneling" funds to district for effective integration of programs.
- All vertical Health and Family Welfare Programs at district and state level merge into one common—"District Health Mission (DHM)"at the district level and the "State Health Mission" at the state level.
- Provision of Project Management Unit for all district, through contractual engagement.

Component (F): Converging Sanitation and Hygiene under NRHM

- Total Sanitation Campaign (TSC) is presently implemented in 350 districts, and is proposed to cover all district, and proposed to cover all district in 10th Plan.
- Components of TSC include IEC activities, rural sanitary marts, individual household toilets, women sanitary complex, and School Sanitation Program.
- Similar to the DHM, the TSC is also implemented through Panchayat Raj Institutions (PRIs)

- The District Health Mission would, therefore, guide activities of sanitation at district level, and promote joint IEC for public health, sanitation and hygiene through Village Health and Sanitation Committee, and promote household toilets and School Sanitation Program. ASHA would be incentivized for promoting household toilets by the mission.

Component (G): Strengthening Disease Control Programs

- National Disease Control Programs for malaria, TB, kala azar, filaria, Blindness and Iodine Deficiency and Integrated Disease Surveillance Program shall be integrated under the Mission, for improved program delivery.
- New Initiative would be launched for control of Noncommunicable Diseases.
- Disease surveillance system at village level would be strengthened.
- Supply of generic drugs (both AYUSH and Allopathic) for common ailments at village, SC, PHC/CHC level.
- Provision of a mobile medical unit at District level for improved outreach services.

Component (H): Public-Private Partnership for Public Health Goals, including Regulation of Private Sector

- Since, almost 755 of health services are being currently provided by the private sector, there is a need to refine regulation
- Regulation to be transparent and accountable
- Reform to be regulatory bodies/creation where necessary
- District Institutional Mechanism for Mission must have representation of private sector
- Need to develop guidelines for public-private partnership (PPP) in health sector. Identifying areas of partnership, which are need based, thematic and geographic.
- Public sector to play the lead role in defining the framework and sustaining the partnership
- Management plan for PPP initiatives: At District, State and National levels.

Component (I): New Health Financing Mechanisms

A Task Group to examine new health financing mechanisms, including Risk Pooling for Hospital Care as follows:

- Progressively the District Health Mission to move towards paying hospitals of services by way of reimbursement on the principal of "money follows the patient."
- Standardization of services—outpatient, in-patient, laboratory, surgical interventions and costs will be done periodically by a committee of experts in each state.

- A National Expert Group to monitor theses standards and give suitable advices and guidance on protocols and cost comparisons.
- All existing CHCs to have wage component paid on monthly basis. Other recurrent costs may be reimbursed for services rendered from District Health Fund. Over the Mission period, the CHC may move towards all costs, including wages reimbursed for services rendered.
- A district health accounting system, and an ombudsman to be created to monitor the District Health Fund Management, and take corrective action.
- Adequate technical managerial and accounting support to be provided to DHM in managing risk pooling and health security.
- Where credible Community Based Health Insurance Schemes (CBHI) exits/launched, they will be encouraged as part of the Mission.
- The central government will provide subsidies to cover a part of the premiums for the poor, and monitor the schemes.
- The IRDA will be approached to promote such CBHIs, which will be periodically evaluated for effected delivery.

Component (J): Reorienting Health/Medical Education to support Rural Health Issues

- While district and tertiary hospitals are necessarily located in urban centers, they form an integral part of the referral care chain serving the needs of the rural people.
- Medical and paramedical education facilities need to be created in states, based on need assessment.
- Suggestion for Commission for Excellence in Health Care (Medical Grants Commission), National Institution for Public Health Management, etc.
- Task Group to improve guidelines/details.

INSTITUTIONAL MECHANISMS

- Village Health and Sanitation Samiti (at village level) consisting of Panchayat Representative/s, ANM/MPW, Anganwadi worker, teacher, ASHA, community health volunteers.
- Rogi Kalyan Samiti (or equivalent) for community management of public hospital.
- District Health Mission, under the leadership of Zila Parishad with District Health Head as Convener and all relevant departments, NGOs, private professionals, etc. represented on it.
- State Health Mission, chaired by Chief Minister and co-chaired by Health Minister and with the State Health Secretary as Convener—representation of related departments, NGOs, private professionals, etc.
- Integration of Departments of Health and Family Welfare, at National and State level.

- National Mission Steering Group chaired by Union Minister for Health and Family Welfare with Deputy Chairman, Planning Commission, Ministers of Panchayat Raj, Rural Development and Human Resource Development and public health professionals as members, to provide policy support and guidance to the Mission.
- Empowered Program Committee chaired by Secretary HFW, to be the Executive Body of the Mission
- Standing Mentoring Group shall guide and oversee the implementation of ASHA initiative
- Task Groups for Selected Tasks (time-bound).

TECHNICAL SUPPORT

- To be effective the Mission needs a strong component of technical support
- This would include reorientation into public health management
- Reposition existing health resource institutions, like Population Research Center (PRC), Regional Resource Center (RRC), State Institute of Health and Family Welfare (SIHFW)
- Involve NGOs as resource organizations
- Improved Health Information System
- Mission would require two distinct support mechanisms—Program Management Support Center and Health Trust of India.

Program Management Support Center

- For strengthening management system—basic program management, financial systems, infrastructure maintenance, procurement and logistics systems, Monitoring and Information System (MIS), non-lapsable health pool, etc.
- For developing manpower system—recruitment (induction of MBAs/ CAs/MCAs), training and curriculum development (revitalization of existing institutions and partnerships with NGO and private sector institutions), motivation and performance appraisal, etc.
- For improved governance—decentralization and empowerment of communities, indication of IT based systems like e-banking, social audit and right to information.

Health Trust of India

- Proposed as a knowledge institution, to be the repository of innovation —research and documentation, health information system, planning, monitoring and evaluation, etc.
- For establishing public accountability systems—external evaluations, community based feedback mechanisms, participation of PRIs/NGOs, etc.
- For developing a Framework for pro-poor innovations.
- For reviewing health legislations.
- A base for encouraging experimentation and action research.

- For inter- and intra-sector networking with National and International Organizations.

ROLE OF STATE GOVERNMENTS UNDER NRHM

- The Mission covers the entire country. The 18 high focus States are Uttar Pradesh, Bihar, Rajasthan, Madhya Pradesh, Orissa, Uttaranchal, Jharkhand, Chhattisgarh, Assam, Sikkim, Arunachal Pradesh, Manipur, Meghalaya, Tripura, Nagaland, Mizoram, Himachal Pradesh and Jammu and Kashmir. Government of India would provide funding for key components in these 18 high focus States. Other state would fund interventions like ASHA, Program Management Unit (PMU), and upgradation of SC/PHC/CHC through Integrated Financial Envelope.
- NRHM provides broad conceptual framework. States would project operational modalities in their State Action Plans, to be decided in consultation with the Mission Steering Group.
- NRHM would prioritize funding for addressing inter-state and intradistrict disparities in terms of health infrastructure disparities in terms of health infrastructure and indicators.
- State would sign Memorandum of Understanding with Government of India, indicating their commitment to increase contribution to Public Health Budget (Preferably by 10% each year), increased devolution to Panchyati Raj Institution as per 73rd Constitution (Amendment) Act, and performance for release of funds.

FOCUS ON THE NORTH EASTERN STATES

- All 8th North-East States, including Assam, Arunachal Pradesh, Manipur, Meghalaya, Mizoram, Nagaland, Sikkim and Tripura, are among the States selected under the Mission, for special focus.
- Empowerment to the Mission would mean greater flexibilities for the 10 percent Committed outaly of the Ministary of Health and Family Welfare, for North-East State.
- States shall be supported for creation/upgradation of Health infrastructure, increased mobility, contractual engagement, and technical support under the Mission.
- Regional Resource Center is being under supported under NRHM for the North Eastern States.
- Funding would be available to address local health issues in a comprehensive manner, through state specific schemes and initiatives.

ROLE OF PANCHAYATI RAJ INSTITUTIONS

The Mission envisages the following roles for PRIs:

- State to indicate in their Memorandum of Understandings (MoUs) the Commitment for devolution of funds, functionaries and programs for health, to PRIs.

- The District Health Mission to be led by the Zila Parishad. The DHM will control, guide and manage all public health institutions in the district, Sub-centers, PHCs and CHCs.
- ASHAs would be selected by and be accountable to the Village Panchayat.
- The Village Health Committee of the Panchayat would prepare the Village Health Plan, and promote integration.
- Each sub-center will have an United Fund for local action @ Rs. 10,000 per annum. This Fund will be deposited in a joint Bank Account of the ANM, in consultation with the Village Health Committee.
- PRI involvement in Rogi Kalyan Samitis for good hospital management.
- Provision of training to members of PRIs.
- Making available health related databases to all stakeholders, including Panchayats all levels.

ROLE OF NGOs IN THE MISSION

- Included in institutional arrangement at National, State and District levels, including Standing Mentoring Group for ASHA
- Member of Task Groups
- Provision of Training, Technical Support for ASHAs/DHM
- Health Resource Organizations
- Service delivery for identified population groups on selected themes
- For monitoring, evaluation and social audit

MAINSTREAMING AYUSH

- The Mission seeks to revitalize local health traditions and mainstream AYUSH infrastructure, including manpower, and drugs, to strengthen the public health system all level.
- AYUSH medications shall be included in the Drug Kit provided at village levels to ASHA.
- The additional supply of generic drugs for common ailments at Sub-center/PHC/CHC levels under the Mission shall also include AYUSH formulations.
- At the CHC level, two rooms shall be provided for AYUSh practitioner and pharmacist under the Indian Public Health System (IPHS) model.
- Single doctor PHCs shall be upgraded to two doctor PHCs by mainstreaming AYUSH practitioner at that level.

FUNDING ARRANGEMENTS

- The Mission is conceived as an umbrella program subsuming the existing programs of health and family welfare, including the RCHII,

National Disease Control Programs for Malaria, TB, Kala Azar, Filaria, Blindness and Iodine Deficiency and Integrated Disease Surveillance Program.
- The Budget Head For NRHM shall be created in 2006-07 at National and State levels. Initially, the vertical health and family welfare programs shall retain their Sub-Budget Head under the NRHM.
- The outlay of the NRHM for 05 to 06 is in the range of Rs 6700 crores.
- The Mission envisages an additionality of 30 percent over existing Annual Budgetary outlays, every year, to fulfill the mandate of the National Common Minimum Program to raise the outlays for Public Health from 0.9 percent of GDP to 2 to 3 percent of GDP.
- The outlay for NRHM shall accordingly be determined in the Annual Budgetary exercise.
- The States are expected to raise their contributions to Public Health Budget by minimum 10 percent p.a. to support the Mission activities.
- Funds shall be released to State through SCOVA, largely in the form of Financial Envelopes, with weightage to 18 high focus States.

TIMELINES (FOR MAJOR COMPONENTS)

Merger of Multiple Societies June 2005. Constitution of District/State Mission Provision of additional generic drugs at SC/PHC/CHC level December 2005, Operational Program Management Units 2005 to 2006 Preparation of Village Health Plans 2006, ASHA at village level (with drug kit) 2005-2008. Upgrading of Rural Hospitals 2005 to 2007, Mobile Medical Unit at district level 2005 to 2008.

OUTCOMES

National Level

- Infant mortality rate reduced to 30/1000 live births
- Maternal mortality ratio reduced to 100/100,000
- Total fertility reduction rate: 50 percent upto 2.1
- Malaria mortality reduction rate: 50 percent upto 2010 and sustaining elimination until 2012
- Kala azar mortality reduction rate: 100 percent by 2010 and sustaining elimination until 2012
- Filaria/Microfilaria reduction rate: 70 percent by 2010, 80 percent by 2012 and elimination by 2015
- Dengue mortality reduction rate: 50 percent by 2010 and sustaining at that level until 2012
- Japanese encephalitis mortality reduction rate: 50 percent by 2010 and sustaining at that level until 2012.
- Cataract operation: Increasing to 46 lakhs per year until 2012.

- Leprosy prevalence rate: Reduce from 1.8/10,000 in 2005 to less than 1/10,000 thereafter
- Tuberculosis DOTS services: Maintain 85 percent cure rate through entire Mission period.
- Upgrading Community Health Centers to Indian Public Health Standards
- Increase utilization of First Referral Units from less than 20 to 75 percent
- Engaging 250,000 female Accredited Social Health Activists (ASHAs) in 10 States.

Community Level

- Availability of trained community level worker at village level, with a drug kit for generic ailments
- Health Day at Anganwadi level on fixed day/month for provision of immunization, ante/postnetal checkups and services related to mother and child health care, including nutrition.
- Availability of generic drugs for common ailments at subcenter and hospital level
- Good hospital care through assured availability of doctors, drugs and quality services at PHC/CHC level
- Improved access to Universal Immunization through induction of Auto -Disabled Syringes, alternate vaccine delivery and improved mobilization services under the program
- Improved facilities for institutional delivery through provision of referral, transport, escort and improved hospital care subsidized under the Janani Suraksha Yojana (JSY) for the Below Poverty Line families.
- Availability of assured health care at reduced financial risk through pilots of Community Health Insurance under the Mission
- Provision of household toilets
- Improved outreach services through mobile medical unit at district level.

MONITORING AND EVALUATION

- Health MIS to be developed upto CHC level, and web-enabled for citizen scrutiny
- Subcenters to report on performance to Panchayats, Hospitals to Taluk, Panchayat Rogi Kalyan Samitis and District Health Mission to Zila Parishad
- The District Health Mission to monitor compliance to Citizen's Charter at CHC Level
- Annual District Reports on People's Health (to be prepared by Govt/ NGO collaboration)

- State and National Reports on people's Health to be tabled in assemblies, parliament
- External evaluation/social audit through professional bodies/NGOs.
- Mid course reviews and appropriate correction.

Is NRHM a New Program of the Government of India?

The NRHM is basically a strategy for integrating ongoing vertical programs of Health and Family Welfare, and addressing issues related to the determinants of Health, like sanitation, nutrition and safe drinking Water. The National Rural Health Mission seeks to adopt a sector wide approach and aims at systemic reforms to enable efficiency in health service delivery. NRHM subsumes key national programs, namely, the Reproductive and Child Health II project, (RCH II) the National Diseases Control Program (NDCP) and the Integrated Diseases surveillance Project (IDSP). NRHM will also enable the mainstreaming of Ayurvedic, Yoga, Unani, Siddha, and Homeopathy System of Health (AYUSH).

What is the Institutional Setup at National, State and District Levels?

The Mission Steering Group under the Chairmanship of the Union Minister for Health and Family Welfare will provide policy guidance and operational oversight at the National level. Ministrial/Secretary level representative of Planning Commission, Rural Development, Panchayati Raj, Human Resource Development and Health and Family Welfare.

NATIONAL URBAN HEALTH MISSION

As per Census 2001, 28.6 crores people live in urban area. The urban population is estimated to increase to 35.7 crores in 2011 and to 43.2 crores in 2021. Urban growth has led to rapid increase in number of urban poor population, many of whom live in slums and other squatter settlements.

The above situation is reflected in poor health indicators as per the reanalysis of the NFHS III data as follows:

	Urban poor	*Urban*
Under five mortality	72.7	51.9
Number of the children miss complete immunization	60%	42%
Piped water supply	18.5%	50%
Institutional deliveries	44%	67.5%

Therefore, there is need of the National Urban Health Mission to address the health economics of the urban poor by facilitating equitable access to available health facilities by rationalizing and strengthening of existing capacity of health care delivery for improving the health status of the urban poor.

Goal

To improve the health status of the urban poor particularly the slum dweller and other disadvantaged section.

Core Strategies

1. Improving the efficiency of public health system in the cities by strengthening, revamping and rationalizing urban primary health structure
2. Partnership with nongovernment provider for filling up of health delivery gaps
3. Promotion of access to improved health care at household level through community based groups; Mahila Arogya Samiti.
4. Strengthening the public health through preventing and promotive action
5. Increased access to health care through risk pooling and community health insurance model
6. IT enabled services (ITES) and e-governance and monitoring.
7. Capacity building of stakeholders
8. Prioritizing the most vulnerable among the poor.
9. Ensuring quality health care services.

Components of Urban Health Mission (UHM)

1. Planning and mapping
2. Program management
3. Outreach services
4. Primary urban health center
5. Referrals
6. Capacity building, training and orientation
7. Community risk pooling/insurance
8. Public private partnership
9. Monitoring and evaluation
10. Social program for vulnerable groups
11. Support for city level public health action
12. Additional support for National Health Programs

Targets

National Urban Health Mission is expected to achieve the following target in urban areas:

1. IMR reduced to 30/1000 live birth by 2012.
2. Maternal mortality reduced to 100/100,000 live birth by 2012.
3. TFR reduced to 2.1 by 2012
4. Malarial mortality reduction rate—50 percent by 2010 additional 10 percent by 2012
5. Kala-azar mortality reduction rate—100 percent by 2010 and sustaining elimination thereafter
6. Filarial reduction rate—70 percent by 2010, 80 percent by 2012 and elimination by 2015.
7. Dengue mortality reduction 50 percent by 2010 and sustaining it at that level till 2012.
8. Japanese encephalitis mortality reduction rate—50 percent by 2010 and sustaining at that level till 2012.
9. *Chikungunya:* Reduction in number of outbreaks and morbidity due to chikungunya by prevention and control strategy.
10. *Leprosy prevalence rate:* Reduced from 1.8 per 10,000 in 2005 to less than 1 per 10,000 thereafter.
11. *Tuberculosis DOTS Series:* Maintain 85 percent cure rate through the entire Mission period and also sustain planned case detection rate.
12. Reduce the prevalence of deafness by 25 percent (from existing level) by 2012.

Urban Health Delivery Model

a. At community level
b. Primary health center level
c. Referral units

At Community Level (Urban Social Health Activist, USHA)

The USHA would preferably be a women resident of the slummarried/widowed/divorced, preferably in the age group of 25 to 45 years.

She should also be a literate women with formal education upto class eight which may be relaxed only if no suitable person with this qualification is available.

Essential Service to be Rendered by the USHA

1. Active promoter of good health practices and enjoying community support.
2. Facilitate awareness on essential RCH services.

3. Facilitate access to health related services available at the Anganwadi/ Primary Urban Health Center and other services being provided by state/central government.
4. Formation and promotion of Mahila Arogya Samiti in her community.
5. Arrange/escort/accompany pregnant women and children requiring treatment to the nearest primary urban health center. Secondary/tertiary level health care facility.
6. Reinforcement of community action for immunization, prevention of water born and other communicable diseases like TB, malaria, chikungunya and Japanese encephalitis.
7. Carrying out preventive and promotive health activites with AWW/ Mahila Arogya Samiti
8. Maintenance of necessary information and records about birth and death, immunization, antinatal services in her assigned locality.

Performance Based Incentive Package for USHA

Activity	*Proposed incentive/month*
1. Organization of outreach services	Rs 200
2. Organization of monthly meeting of MAS	Rs 100
3. Attended monthly meeting at UHC	Rs 200
4. Organize Health and National Day in collaboration with AWW	Rs 100
5. Organize community meeting for strengthening preventive and promotive services	50 per meeting (200 upper limit)
6. Provide support to baseline survey and filling up of family health register	5 per house hold (once a year)
7. Maintain records as per the desired norms like household registers. meeting minutes, outreach camps register.	50 per month
8. Additional Immunization incentives for achiving complete immunization among the children in her area of responsibility.	5 per child

Primary Urban Health Center

- Generally one urban health center is for approximately 50,000 population.
- In slum area, one UHC for 20,000 to 30,000 population.
- In cities, UHC may be established for 75,000 population.
- In areas with very high density, isolated slum clusters or disadvantage group, one UHC can be established for 5000 to 10,000 population.

Services available under UHC: UHC can provide services for 4 hours in the morning and 2 hours in the evening. For provision of certain services evening OPD if required.

The services provided in UHC will include OPD, basic lab diagnosis, drug and contraceptive dispensing, distribution of health education material and counseling for all communicable and noncommunicable disease.

Staffing Pattern

- 1 Docter
- 1 Labtechnician
- 1 Pharmacist
- 2 Staff nurses
- 4 ANMs
- 1 Program manager/Community mobilization officer/Peon/ Sweeper.

Financial support: Annual financial support in the form of Rogi Kalyan Samiti/Hospital Management Committee fund of Rs. 50,000 per UHC per year.with the amount being proportional to the population covered @ Re 1.00 per head a PUHC covering 40,000 population will get Rs. 40,000.

Referral units: State government hospitals and medical colleges, apart from private hospitals will be empanelled/accredited to act as referral points for different types of health care services. The referral services will be cash-free for the beneficiary and will be financed by community health insurance or voucher scheme as per the PIP developed for the cities.

Chapter 19 Sanitation of Camps

CHAPTER OUTLINE

- CAMP SITE
- ACCOMMODATION AND EQUIPMENT
- FOOD AND COOKING ARRANGEMENTS
- DISPOSAL OF REFUSE AND EXCRETA
- DISPOSAL OF STABLE LITTER

INTRODUCTION

In view of the fact that camps and temporary lodgements have been freely set up all over the country, a description of the general sanitary control of camps demands special consideration. For all practical purposes, camps may be regarded as so many improvised townships where the different tents or temporary huts represent so many houses. Although the sanitation of camps is more or less based on the same principles as of ordinary houses or towns, in practice certain sanitary rules have to be followed because of their temporary nature and because very often they are located in places where sanitary conditions are not ideal. The following pointes require consideration with reference to camps:

1. Camp site.
2. Accommodation and equipment.
3. Water supply
4. Food and cooking arrangements.
5. Disposal of refuse, excretal matter and waste water.

CAMP SITE

The site should be on a high ground not subject to flooding or water logging and should have good approach from the main road. The soil should be porous and physical features suitable for easy and rapid surface drainage. Irrigated or marshy land or land with steep slope should be avoided; gentle slope however facilitates drainage. While the site should not be close to a bazaar, its accessibility, facility for transport and easy availability of supplies should be kept in mind.

The ground and its surroundings must be dry and free from dense vegetation. A high sub-soil water creates dampness and water-logging. All hollows and other excavations where water can collect should be filled up to prevent breeding of mosquitoes. For the same reason, digging or excavating the soil within the camp area is unwise.

Agricultural land, because of its propensity to breed flies, should be avoided. Wherever possible, there should be sufficient open land all around the camp area to sever as a protective boundary.

The most important consideration which should dominate selection of a camp site is the facility which exists for obtaining water. This is specially important in temporary camps. When camp sites are likely to be occupied for a longer period, the feasibility of bringing in filtered water by pipe from outside or sinking of deep tube wells locally may be considered.

ACCOMMODATION AND EQUIPMENT

The lay out of a camp should be properly planned after a survey of the site. In laying out a camp, the following particulars should be attended to:

i. The front of the camp should face the prevailing wind.
ii. The sleeping accommodation should be in front, with kitchens and messing accommodation nearby at one side.
iii. The bathing area and water point should be so at one side, well away from the conservancy area, and with drainage so arranged as to prevent the water logging of the camp.
iv. Camp roads should be so arranged that traffic for watering horses and the delivery of supplies do not cover the cooking and messing areas with manure-laden dust.
v. Surface drainage of the camp area should be provided.

Water

Supply of safe water is of primary importance and every effort should be made to see that the water is not only safe but the chances of accidental contamination are also nil. In camps where arrangements are made for supply of filtered water or deep tube well water, no inconvenience is experienced. The water is delivered from overhead reservoir and stand pipes. But attention should be paid to see that no contamination occurs due to defective storing or from other sources. The delivery taps should be near the kitchen.

FOOD AND COOKING ARRANGEMENTS

With regard to cook and cooking arrangement, attention should be paid to the following:

i. The kitchen should be located at a distance from latrines, urine pits and the receptacles for garbage and refuse, preferably at the opposite end but within easy access of the water cart. It should be well-lighted and ventilated preferably fly proofed and provided with a smoke outlet.

ii. There should be suitable provision for storage of food.
iii. All sullage water must be made to pass into pits from which it can drain into suitable dry trenches. In the alternative, it can be kept in special covered tubs or reservoirs and removed daily for sanitary disposal.
iv. Provisions should be made for washing cooking utensils, plates, dishes, etc. It is always convenient to have a special place allocated for this.
v. There should be provision of ample supply of hot water and a sufficiency of clean dish-cloths to secure a clean and wholesome food service.
vi. Everything used for food service namely, utensils, tables, knives and forks, plates and dishes, tables should be clean.

The practice of using earth. For cleansing cooking utensils, should be forbidden. Utensils should be cleaned by baked sand stored in a clean tin. Where ash is used, one should see that its preparation, collection and storing are sanitary.

DISPOSAL OF REFUSE AND EXCRETA

One of the important duties of the officer-in-charge of the camp is to ensure that disposal of refuse and excreta is carried out in such a way as these will be rendered innocuous.

These generally consist of:

a. Dry camp and kitchen refuse.
b. Liquid waste.
c. Feces.

Dry Camp and Kitchen Refuse

Dry camp and kitchen refuse generally consist of bits of papers and crockery.

These should be collected daily in sand bags or in specially provided receptacles by men detailed for the purpose.

Dry kitchen refuse consists of scraps of food, remnants of vegetables, fruits, etc. All these should be collected in covered metal receptacles and not allowed to scatter in and around the kitchen.

The solid refuse both from the camp and kitchen, should either be buried in deep pits at a safe distance or better still burnt in an incinerator. It may also be disposed of the special type of dustbins in which refuse can be burnt in the bin itself.

Liquid Waste

This consists of urine (human and animal), kitchen sullage and ablution water.

i. Kitchen sullage, consisting mainly of greasy water, soon becomes very foul if not properly disposed of. These should be collected in mental receptacles placed on a stand fitted with a cover. If allowed to run direct on to the soil, it makes a greasy quagmire covered with scum which attracts flies. When its disposal depends on the absorptive pits filed with hay, straw or coarse brushwood. Here the grease and other organic solids are entangled allowing the clear liquid to run away. The hay and straw loaded with greasy and other fatty matter should be buried or burnt and replaced by fresh material daily.
ii. Urine is disposed of in soakage pits. The pit may be combined with urinal. This consists of two parts, the urine receiving portion on top consisting of either a trough, funnel or tin; and the disposal portion consisting of the soakage pit below the ground consisting of the soakage pit below the ground.

Disposal of Feces

In permanent camps provided with piped water supply and where water-carriage system prevails, there is no trouble. But in places where such arrangement cannot be made, one should have recourse to trench system, earth-pet or service latrine.

The first principal in any form of trench system is to construct it in such a way as will not pollute the surrounding ground. Shallow trenches should be avoided. They should be regarded as an emergency measure and must not be used for more than two to three days.

Deep trenches cover less ground and are better suited for the purpose. These should be made fly-proof. Trenches should be source of water supply or kitchen. There should always be a superstructure for protection against inclement weather and partitions for privacy.

Where convenient, bored-hole, well or pit latrines may be provided. Boredhole latrines will be found suitable in places where the sub-soil water in not very high. Generally, one seat for every 12 persons will be found convenient.

If service latrines are used, the pans or pails should be daily emptied and the contents quickly removed for final disposal either by trenching or incineration, whichever will be available and convenient. After emptying, the pans should be thoroughly cleansed. Facilities for such cleansing should be available and convenient. After emptying, the pans should be thoroughly cleansed. Facilities for such cleansing should be provided with soakage pits for waster. The cleaned pans should be treated with crude oil before being replaced under the seats. There should be a small conservancy staff to look after the cleanliness of the latrines and urinals and also for removal of refuse. Washing facilities should be provided and there should be adequate supply of water for washing purposes. The approach to the latrines should always be kept clean and lighted at night.

DISPOSAL OF STABLE LITTER

Much nuisance is caused by stable litter which is generally horse manure or cow dung. Daily collection and complete removal of these ensure freedom from infestation by flies and biting insects to a large extent. Arrangements should be made for their sanitary removal and disposal either by incineration or by burying in deep pits.

Chapter 20

Indian Systems of Medicine

CHAPTER OUTLINE

- AYURVEDA SYSTEM OF MEDICINE
- UNANI SYSTEM OF MEDICINE
- YOGA
- ALLOPATHY
- SIDDHA SYSTEM OF MEDICINE
- HOMEOPATHY
- NATUROPATHY

INTRODUCTION

Indian systems of medicine covers both the systems of which originated in India and outside but got adopted in India in the course of time. These systems are Ayurveda, Siddha, Unani, Homeopathy, Yoga and Naturopathy. These systems have become a part of the culture and tradition of our country.

AYURVEDA SYSTEM OF MEDICINE

Ayurveda means the "science of life". Ayurveda or the Indian Science of Life oriented and developed around 1000 BC the knowledge of Ayurveda was documented by Charaka and Sushruta.

According to Ayurveda, health is considered a pre-requisite for achieving the goals of life. Ayurveda takes an integrated view of the physical and spiritual aspects of man.

The philosophy of Ayurveda is based on the theory of Panchmahabhutas of which all the objects and living bodies are composed of these five elements. The combination of these five elements are represented in the form of *tridosha*. For example, vata (Ether+Air), *pitta* (Fire) and *kapha* physiological entities in living beings. The mental-spiritual attributes are described as *satva*, *rajas* and *tamas*. The various permutations and combinations of satva, rajas and tamas constitute human temperament and personality. Ayurveda considers the human being as a combination of tridoshas, (Panchmahabhutas) (5 elements), seven body tissue (Saptadhatu), five senses (Panch-indriyas), mind (Manas), intellect (Budhi) and soul (Atman).The doctrine of Ayurveda aims to keep these structural and functional entities in a functional state of equilibrium which signifies good health. Any imbalance due to internal or external factors is a disease and restoring the equilibrium through various techniques, procedures, regimen, diet and medicine is the treatment.

In Ayurveda, diagnosis is done by questioning and examination, viz. pulse, urine, feces, tongue, eyes, visual/sensual examination and inference.

Treatment in Ayurveda has two complements:

a. Preventive measures
b. Curative measures.

Preventive aspects of Ayurveda is called Avasth Vritt and includes personal hygiene, appropriate social behavior and Rasayana Sevann, i.e. use of rejuvenate materials/drugs. The curative treatment consists of three major categories of procedures:

i. Aushdhi (drug)
ii. Anna (diets)
iii. Vihara (exercises and general mode of life).

SIDDHA SYSTEM OF MEDICINE

Introduction and Origin

Siddha system is one of the oldest systems of medicine in India. The term 'Siddha' means achievement and 'Siddhas' were saintly figures who achieved results in medicine through the practice of Yoga. Eighteen 'Siddha's are said to have contribute towards the development of this medical system Siddha literature is in Tamil and it is practiced in Tamil speaking parts of India. The system is also called Agasthyar system after its most famous exponent sage Agasthya. A number of medical works of this system are ascribed to him. The Siddha system is largely therapeutic in nature.

Basic Concepts

The principles and doctrines of this system, both fundamental and applied, have a close similarity to Ayurveda.

According to this system the human body is the replica of the universe and so are the food and drugs irrespective of their origin. Like Ayurveda, this system believes that all objects in the universe including human body are composed of five basic elements namely earth, water, fire, air, sky. The food which the human body takes and the drugs it uses all made of these five elements. The proportion of the elements in the drugs vary and their preponderance or otherwise is responsible for certain actions and therapeutic results.

Diagnosis and Treatment

The diagnosis of disease involved identifying its cases identification of causative factors is through the examination of pulse, urine, eyes, study of voice, color of body, tongue and status of the digestive system of

also believed that the external influences such as bacteria, viruses could not cause sickness unless the vital resistance of an individual is reduced beyond a certain level.

In treatment, primary emphasis is given to increasing the defensive mechanism of the individual through holistic approach of individualization. Here the treatment is directed in correcting the imbalance in the immune mechanism and restoring health to the sick. Here two sick individuals are never considered identical for selection of medicine, though they may be suffering from the same disease. Individualization through a detailed and exhaustive case taking is the most important aspect in homeopathy.

Homeopathy has definite and effective treatment for individuals with chronic diseases such as diabetes; arthritis; bronchial asthma; skin, allergic and immunological disorders and for several other diseases, for which there is less or no treatment in other system.

YOGA

Yoga is a way of life propounded by Patanjali in a systematic form. It consists of eight components namely restraint, observance of austerity. Physical postures, breathing exercises, restraining of sense organs, contemplation, meditation and samadhi. These steps in the practice of Yoga have potential for improvement of social and personal behavior, improvement of physical health by encouraging better circulation of oxygenated blood in the body, restraining the sense organs and thereby the mind and inducing tranquility and serenity of mind. The practice of Yoga prevents psychosomatic disorders/diseases and improves individuals resistance and ability to endure stressful situations. Meditation, one of the eight components, if regularly pracused, has the capacity to reduce unwholesome bodily responses to a bare minimum so that the mind can be directed to perform more fruitful functions.

A number of physical postures are described in Yogic works to improve bodily health, to prevent diseases and to cure illness. The physical postures are required to be chosen judiciously and have to be practiced in the right way to drive the benefits of prevention of diseases, promotion of health and for therapeutic purposes.

Studies have revealed that the Yogic practices improved intelligence and memory and help in developing resistance to endure situations of strain and stress and also to develop an integrated psychosomatic personality. Meditation is an exercise which can stabilize emotional changes and prevent abnormal functions of vital organs of the body. Studies have shown that meditation not only restrain the sense organs but also controls the autonomic nervous system.

NATUROPATHY

Naturopathy is not only a system of treatment but also a way of life. It is often referred to as a drugless treatment of diseases. It is based mainly on the ancient practice of the application of the simple laws of Nature. The system is closely allied to Ayurveda as far as it fundamental principals are concerned. There are two schools of thought regarding the approach to Naturopathy. One group believes in the Indian methods while the other mainly adopts Western methods, which are more akin to modern physiotherapy.

The advocates of naturopathy pay particular attention to eating and living habits, adoption of purificatory measures, use of hydrotherapy, cold packs, mud packs, baths, massage uses a variety of methods, measures, based on various innovations.

This system believes that properly boundless organized way of life and deliver energy, health and happiness. For prevention of disease, promotion health and to get therapeutic advantages, it is required to adopt natural means to avoid distortion of nature.

ALLOPATHY

Allopathy is a method of treating disease with remedies that produce effects different from those caused by the disease itself.

The term "allopathy" was *invented by German Physician Samuel Hahnemann* he referred it to harsh practices of his time which included bleeding, purging, vomiting and administration of highly toxic drugs.

Four humorous theory—attributed diseases to an imbalance of four humors (i.e. blood, phlegm and black, yellow bile) and four bodily conditions (i.e. hot, cold, wet and dry) that corresponded to four elements (earth, air, fire and water). Physicians follow the Hippocratic tradition attempted to balance the humors by treating symptoms with 'opposites' during 18th century, it started to loose ground to several new and conflicting systems that attempted to several one or two basic causes for all diseases.

It was well known to the physician that their drugs were damaging, thus by mid century scientific medicine took a back seat.

Methods

Methods are used for:

1. Bleeding
2. Blistering
3. Plastering
4. Leaching
5. Blood letting
6. Cupping
7. Poulticing
8. Puking
9. Swatting
10. Fumigation
11. Purging
12. Ointments
13. Dehydrations.

Chapter 21 Adolescent Health

CHAPTER OUTLINE

- PHYSICAL CHANGES DURING ADOLESCENT
- PUBERTY CHANGES IN ADOLESCENT
- EMOTIONAL PROBLEMS
- EDUCATIONAL PROBLEMS
- BENEFICIARIES

INTRODUCTION

The term adolescence is derived from the Latin word "adolescere" meaning to grow, to mature. It is considered as a period of transition from childhood to adulthood. They are no longer children yet not adults. It is characterized by rapid physical growth, significant physical, emotional, psychological and spiritual changes. Adolescents constitute 22.8 percent of population of India as on 1st march 2000. They are not only in large numbers but are the citizens and workers of tomorrow. The problems of adolescents are multi- dimensional in nature and require holistic approach.

Adolescent has been defined by WHO as the period of life spanning between 10 to 19 years and the youth as between 15 to 24 years. Young people, when referred to as such, are those between 10 to 24 years of age. They are no longer children, but not yet adults.

Population Profile: Ages 10 to 24 Years in India

Population age: 10 to 24 (yrs)	284.2 millions
10 to 24 years as percent of total population	30
Percentage of males enrolld in secondary school	59
Percentage of females enrolled in secondary school	38
Average age at first marrige	20
Total fertility rate	3.4
Percentage of adolescent TFR contributed by 15 to 19 years	9
Percentage of adolescent using contraceptives	7

Characteristics

- A—Aggressive, anemic, abortion
- D—Dynamic, developing, depressed
- O—Overconfident, overindulging, obese

- L—Loud but lonely and lacking information
- E—Enthusiastic, explorative, and experimenting
- S—Social, sexual and spiritual
- C—Courageous, cheerful, and concern
- E—Emotional, eager, emulating
- N—Nervous, never say no to peers
- T—Temperamental, teenage pregnancy.

Early Adolescence (10 to 13 years)

In early adolescent period spurt of growth of development of secondary sex will take place.

Middle Adolescence (14 to 16 Years)

In middle adolescent period they will have separate identity from parents, new relationship to peer groups, with opposite sex and desire for experimentation.

Late Adolescence (17 to 19 Years)

In late adolescent period they will have distinct identity, well formed opinion and ideas.

The following changes are taking place during adolescent period:

a. Biological changes—onset of puberty
b. Cognitive changes—emergence of more advanced cognitive abilities
c. Emotional changes—self-image, intimacy, relation with adults and peers group
d. Social changes—transition into new roles in the society.

PHYSICAL CHANGES DURING ADOLESCENT

	Age group
In girls, physical changes may begin at around	10 years
Reaches their maximum growth by around	14 years
Thereafter, growth continues at slower rate till the age of	18 years

Puberty in boys usually appears later than in girls.

During adolescence there is considerable gain in the weight and height, it accounts for nearly 20 to 25 percent of adult height and 50 percent of weight. Puberty height spurt begins at an average age of 12 years for girls and 14 years for boys.

During puberty girls gain 25 cm height and boys 38 cm height. At the cessation of growth boys are taller than girls by 13 cm.

PUBERTY CHANGES IN ADOLESCENT

Puberty in Girls

During this period, in female, subjects the secondary sexual characteristics appear such as appearance of hair in pubic area, and breast begin to grow. Other changes include accelerated growth and development of genital organs.

Ovaries begin to ovulate at around 11 to 14 years once every 28 days. Menarche is the onset of first menstruation which occurs in a young girl at around 12 years.

Psychological and Behavioral Changes

1. During this transition phase from childhood to adulthood due to rapid physical and sexual changes in the body, the adolescent develops anxiety and apprehension.
2. In case they are not given appropriate information and education on these normal physical, sexual and psychological changes they are prone to health risk behavior such as sex experiments and drug abuse leading to teenage pregnancy, contracting RTI/STI, HIV/AIDS, injuries, accidents, violence, rape, homicides, suicides, etc.

Impact of Adolescence

1. Lack of formal or informal education
2. School dropout and childhood labor
3. Malnutrition and anemia
4. Early marriage, teenage pregnancies
5. Habits and behaviors picked up during adolescence period have lifelong impact
6. Lot of unmet needs regarding nutrition, reproductive health and mental health
7. They require safe and supportive environment
8. Desire for experimentation
9. Sexual maturity and onset of sexual activity
10. Transition from dependence to relative independence
    - Ignorance about sex and sexuality
    - Lack of understanding
    - Suboptimal support at family level
    - Social frustration
    - Inadequate school syllabus about adolescent health
    - Misdirected peer pressure in absence of adequate knowledge
    - Lack of recreational, creative, and working opportunity.

Adolescent Health Problems

1. Anorexia nervosa
2. Obesity and overweight
3. Adolescent pregnancy
4. Micronutrient deficiency
5. Emotional problems
6. Behavioral problems
7. Substance abuse and injuries
8. Sexually transmitted infection
9. Thinking and studying problems
10. Identity problems
11. Respiratory infection, asthma
12. Goiter
13. Bed wetting
14. Dandruff
15. Alopecia
16. Skin patches
17. Pimples
18. Nutritional problem
19. Menstrual problem.

EMOTIONAL PROBLEMS

1. *Lack of freedom:* Worry about future and career, loneliness. Worries regarding love marriage and child birth, struggle for identity and inferiority complex.
2. *Lack of confidence:* Failed love affairs, stranger anxiety, difficulty in adjusting with others, parental expectation, problems dealing with elders.
3. *Lack of emotional stability:* Depression, suicide, homicidal tendencies.

EDUCATIONAL PROBLEMS

1. Lack of proper counseling and guidance.
2. Inferiority complex due to poor performance in studies.
3. Constant nagging of teachers.
4. Lack of opportunities for preferred profession.
5. Difficulty in adjusting with fellow students.
6. Lack of peer acceptance.
7. Difficulty in talking with teachers.
8. Examination fear.
9. Not achieving academic goals like entrance examination.
10. Stage fear.

Reasons for Adolescent Reluctant to seek Help

- Fear
- Uncomfortable with of opposite sex health worker
- Poor quality perception
- Lack of privacy
- Confidentiality
- Cumbersome procedure
- Long waiting time
- Parental consent
- Operational barrier
- Lack of information
- Feeling of discomfort.

Prevention

- Health education
- Skill based health education
- Life skill education
- Family life education
- Counseling for emotional stress
- Nutritional counseling
- Early diagnosis and management of medical and behavioral problem.

Syllabus for Adolescent Health Education

- Development of secondary sexual characters and menarche
- Problems associated with menstrual cycle and menstrual hygiene
- Body image
- Nutritional needs (micronutrients)
- Managing emotional stress
- Early marriage
- RTI/HIV/AIDS
- Safe sex
- Family life including pregnancy
- Child rearing and responsible parenthood
- Stress management
- Substance abuse.

Inclusion of life skill training in school and college to empower adolescent in making informed choice to face the complex life situation.

Life Skills

Decision making: Assessing option and what effects different decisions may have.

Problem solving: Unresolved problems may cause tension.
Creative thinking: Consequences of both action and non-action, looking beyond direct experience.
Critical thinking: Factors that influence attitudes and behavior.
Effective communication: To express not only opinions and desires but also needs and fears.
Interpersonal skill: To develop and nurture supportive networks, to be able to end relationships constructively.
Self-awareness: Recognition of our self-positives and negatives .
Coping with emotions and stress.

Adolescent Friendly Health Center Services

- Reproductive health services
- Sexual and reproductive health education
- Contraception
- Pregnancy testing and option
- MTP
- STD/HIV screening counseling and treatment
- Prenatal and postpartum care
- Well baby care
- Nutritional services
- Growth and development monitoring
- Anticipatory guidance about substance abuse and other risk taking behavior
- Counseling for life skill development
- Screening for various disorders.

Criteria for Adolescent Friendly Health Worker

- Welcoming and friendly nature
- Knowledgeable
- Presentable
- Have good communication skill
- Maintain confidentiality
- Punctuality
- Flexibility
- Understanding
- Good listener
- Nonjudgemental.

Criteria for Adolescent Friendly Health Center

- Good reception
- All facilities

- Accessibility
- Quality care service
- Well trained people
- Security
- Easy communication to the outside
- Privacy
- Conducive environment.

Adolescent Girls Scheme

There are two schemes:
- Scheme I: Girl-to-girl approach
- Scheme II: Balika Mandal.

BENEFICIARIES

Scheme I: Girl-to-Girl Approach

This has been designed for adolescent girl (AG) in the age group 11 to 15 years belonging to families with income level below Rs. 6400/- per annum and school dropouts in urban and in the rural areas.

These girls are selected per Anganwadi and attached to the local Anganwadi center for six months duration for learning and training. These girls act as resource person for other girls in their neighborhood.

Intervention focal point of services is an Anganwadi. These girls are provided supplementary nutrition equivalent to the entitlement of pregnant/lactating women for six days in a week.

Simple and practical messages are provided on preventive health, hygiene, nutrition, working of Anganwadi centers and family life education. This is provided through initial three days training program, followed by six continuing education sessions of one day each, every month. This exercise is aimed at building confidence and encouraging adolescent girls to become active participants in the development process. Anganwadi workers act as role models for these girls.

Scheme II: Balika Mandal

All eligible in the age bracket 11 to 18 years irrespective of income levels of the family are eligible to receive assistance in this scheme; preference is given to 11 to 15 years age group. In each community development block and urban ICDS areas 10 percent of total Anganwadi centers are selected to serve as Balika Mandals 20 girls in the age bracket 11 to 18 are identified. These girls are enrolled for a period of 6 months in Balika Mandal. Thus, in a year each Balika Mandal will reach out to 40 adolescent girls.

Interventions

- These girls are provided supplementary nutrition for six days in a week to provide 500 calories and 20 g of protein.
- Activities cover the areas of personal hygiene, environmental sanitation, nutrition, home nursing, first aids, communicable diseases, vaccine preventable diseases, family life, child care and development and the impact of constitutional rights on the quality of life.
- Participate in creative activities and recreation. Learning through sharing of experiences and discussions on issues that affect their lives.
- Training in vocational skills/agro-based skills/household related appropriate technology.

The Anganwadi worker is regular honorary instructor for the Balika Mandal and provides general education and literacy to adolescent girls. She is also responsible for overseeing the work related to skills improvement/upgradation.

Kishori Shakti Yojna (KSY) has much wider scope than the earlier AG scheme and involves the entire network of Government of state/union Territory and district as supportive skills of local self-Government.

Training

Under the AG scheme, a nine days training program has been designed for selected girls, three days training period is spent at circle headquarter and remaining six days are devoted for continuing education, spread over to six months. The training is conducted by supervisors. There are 10 themes for training-environmental sanitation, nutrition, home nursing, first aid, family life education, child development, legal rights of women, home economics, positive attitudes and motivation.

The National Population Policy 2000, National Health Policy 2002 identifies the adolescent girls as under-served group for priority intervention. Similarly, National Nutrition Policy focuses on adolescent girls to improve their nutritional status, to remove the intergenerational gap.

Chapter 22 Integrated Disease Surveillance Project (2004-2009)

CHAPTER OUTLINE

PROJECT OBJECTIVES

- To establish a decentralized state based system of surveillance for communicable and noncommunicable disease, so that timely and effective public health action can be initiated in response to health challenges in the country at the state and national level.
- To improve the efficiency of the existing surveillance activities of disease control programs and facilitate sharing of relevance information with the health administration, community and other stakeholders so as to detect disease trends over time and evaluate control strategies.

SPECIFIC OBJECTIVES

- To integrate, coordinate and decentralize surveillance activities
- To surveil a limited number of health conditions and risk factors
- To establish system for quality data collection, reporting, analysis and feedback using information technology
- To improve laboratory support for disease surveillance
- To develop human resources for disease surveillance
- To involve all stakeholders including private sector and communities in surveillance.

PHASING OF IDSP COVERING THE STATES OF INDIA

Phase I (commencing from financial year 2004-2005): Andhara Pradesh, Himachal Pradesh, Karnataka, Madhya Pradesh, Maharashtra, Uttaranchal, Tamil Nadu, Mizoram and Kerala.

Phase II (commencing from finacial year 2005-2006): Chhattisgarh, Goa, Gujarat, Rajasthan, West Bengal, Manipur, Meghalaya, Orissa, Tripura, Chandigarh, Pondicherry, Delhi

Phase III (commencing from financial year 2006-2007): Uttar Pradesh, Bihar, Jammu and Kashmir, Jharkhand, Punjab, Arunachal Pradesh, Assam, Nagaland, Sikkim. Andaman and Nicobar, Dadra and Nagar Haveli, Daman and Diu, Lakshadweep.

Project Activities

1. Upgradation of laboratories
   - Renovation and furnishing laboratories
   - Supply of laboratory equipments
   - Laboratory material and supplies
2. Information technology and communication
   - Computer hardware and office equipment
   - Software for surveillance
   - Leasing of wide area networking
3. Human resources and development
   - Consultant/Contract staff
   - Training
   - Information education and communication
4. Operational activities and response
5. Monitoring and evaluation.

Diseases and Conditions Covered under IDSP (Table 22.1)

Table 22.1: Diseases and conditions covered under IDSP

Category	*Disease and condition*
Regular surveillance	
Vector borne diseases	1. Malaria
Water borne diseases	2. Acute diarrheal disease (Cholera)
	3. Typhoid
Respiratory diseases	4. Tuberculosis
Vaccine preventable diseases	5. Measles
Disease under eradication	6. Polio
Other conditions	7. Road traffic accidents
Other international commitments	8. Plague

SENTINAL SURVEILLANCE UNDER IDSP

A. STDs/Blood borne diseases: HIV, HBV, HCV
B. Other conditions: Water quality, air quality.

REGULAR PERIODIC SURVEY

Noncommunicable risk factors:
Antropometry, BP, pulse, tobacco, blindness, BMI, etc.

NATIONAL SURVEILLANCE UNIT

1. Execution of approved annual plan of action.
2. Monitor progress of implementation of project.
3. Obtain reports and expenditure statements from state.
4. Seek reimbursement from world bank.
5. Production of prototype guide lines, manuals, modules.
6. Analysis of data from states and provide feedback on trends observed.
7. Coordinating with other national organizations.
8. Conduct periodic meetings with state surveillance officers.
9. Organize independent evaluation of various activities.

STATE SURVEILLANCE UNIT

- Chair person: State Secretary for Health
- Analysis of data received by districts and sending it to Central Surveillance Unit (CSU).
- Formation of rapid response teams and deputing them
- Coordinating with state public health lab, medical colleges, state level institutes
- Sending regular feedback to districts unit
- Coordinating training activity and meetings of state surveillance units.

DISTRICT LEVEL UNIT

1. Chair person: DC or district magistrate
2. Data analysis and transmitting it to State Surveillance Unit (SSU)
3. Constituting rapid response teams
4. Coordinating with other organizations
5. Organizing surveys on infections/noncommunicable diseases and risk factors
6. Periodic review meetings with State Surveillance Officers.

DISTRICT SURVEILLANCE UNIT (FLOW CHARTS 22.1 TO 22.4)

Functions of the District Surveillance unit

Flow chart 22.1: Chief medical and health officer

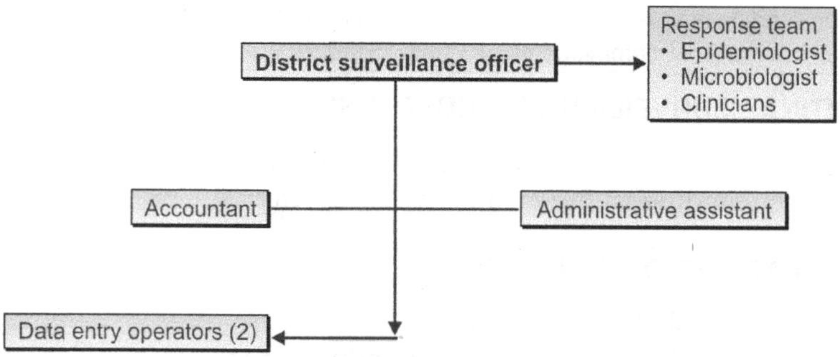

Flow chart 22.2: The role of the district within the surveillance system

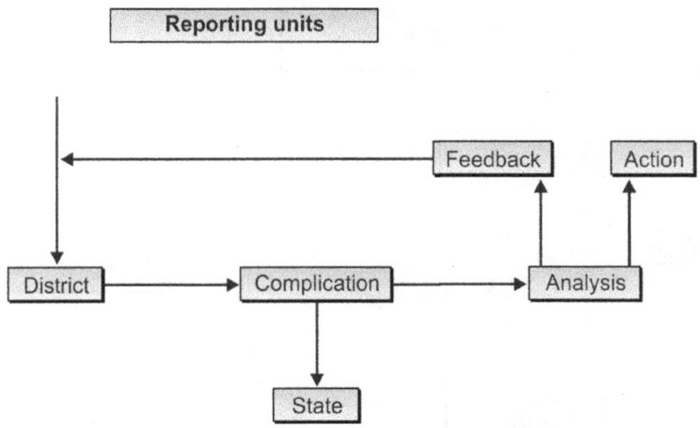

Flow chart 22.3: District surveillance committee

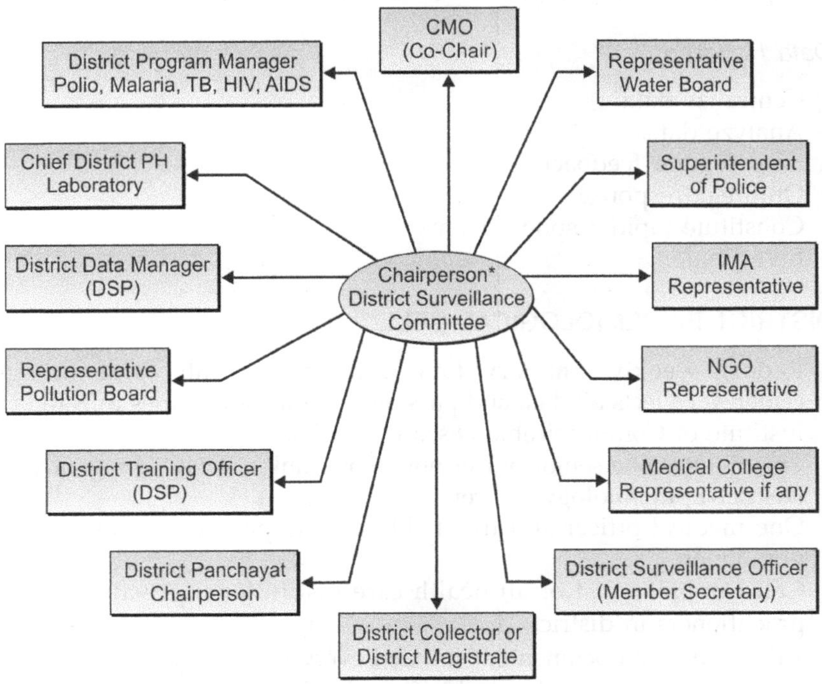

Flow chart 22.4: District epidemic investigating team (DEIT)

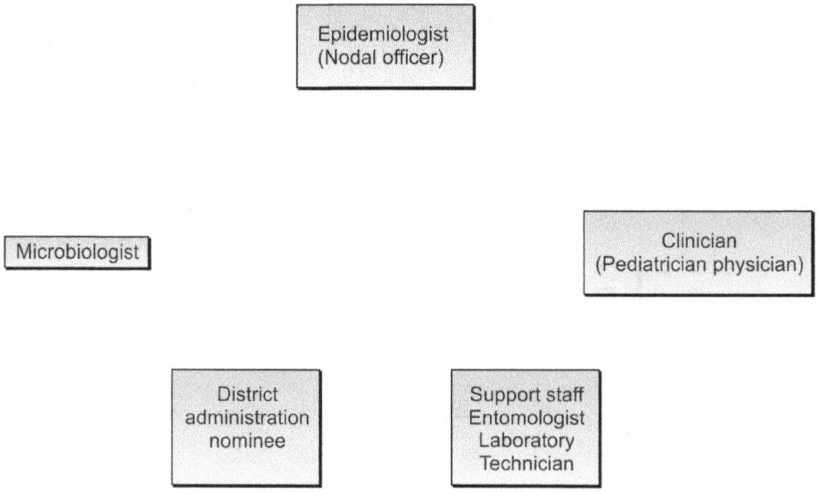

Managerial

- Implement and monitor all project activities
- Coordinate with laboratories, medical colleges, nongovernmental organizations and private sector
- Organize training and communication activities
- Organize district surveillance committee meetings.

Data Handling

- Centralize data
- Analyze data
- Send regular feedback
- Outbreak response
- Constitute rapid response teams
- Investigate.

DISTRICT EPIDEMIOLOGICAL CELL

- Reports weekly summary data on disease to state epidemiology center. It collects all data and pass on monthly summaries to National Institute of Communicable Disease (NICD).
- This cell has one senior officer not below rank of DHO, designated as District Epidemiology Officer
- One medical officer and five field workers per two million or less population
- Cell completes list of all health care institutions, private medical practitioners in district
- All reports are documented, scanned every day to rule out clustering of cases, analyzed weekly and is forwarded to state epidemiology unit

- District cell is responsible for defining and designing interventions
- Implements and monitors all project activity in coordination with labs, private sector and medical colleges
- Conducts training and communication activity
- Organize district surveillance unit meetings
  Triggers in the context of the Indian Integrated Disease Surveillance Program (IDSP) (Flow chart 22.5)
- Threshold for diseases under surveillance that trigger predetermined actions at various levels
- Based upon the number of cases in weekly report
- Trigger levels depend on:
  - Type of disease
  - Case fatality (Death/case ratio)
  - Number of evolving cases
  - Usual trend in the region.

Flow chart 22.5: Structural framework of IDSP

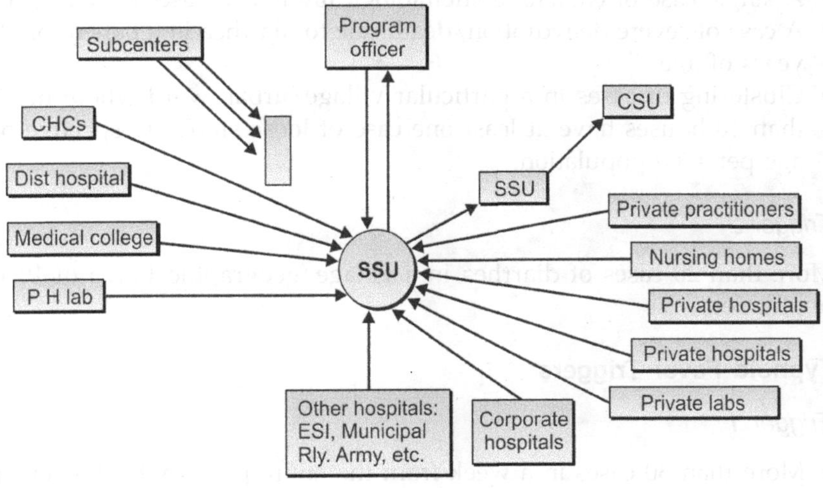

LEVELS OF RESPONSE TO DIFFERENT TRIGGERS (TABLE 22.2)

Table 22.2: Levels of response to different triggers

Trigger significance	*Levels of response*
1. Suspected/limited outbreak	• Local response by health worker and medical officer
2. Outbreak	• Local and district response by district surveillance officer and rapid response team
3. Confirmed outbreak	• Local, district and state
4. Wide spread epidemic	• State level response
5. Disaster response	• Local, district, state and center

Malaria Triggers

Trigger 1

- Single case of smear positive in an area where malaria was not present for a minimum of three months
- Slide positivity rate doubling over last three months
- Single death from clinically/microscopically proven malaria
- Single *falciparum* case of indigenous origin in a free region.

Trigger 2

- Two fold rise in malaria in the region over last three months
- More than five cases of *falciparum* of indigenous origin.

Cholera Triggers

Trigger 1

- A single case of cholera/epidemiologically linked cases of diarrhea
- A case of severe dehydration/death due to diarrhea in a patient of >5 years of age
- Clustering of cases in a particular village/urban ward where more than 10 houses have at least one case of loose stools irrespective of age per 1000 population.

Trigger 2

More than 20 cases of diarrhea in a village/geographical area of 1000 population.

Typhoid Fever Triggers

Trigger 1

- More than 30 cases in a week from the entire primary health center area
- Five or more cases per week from one sub-center of 5,000 population
- More than two cases from a single village/urban ward/1000 population
- Clustering of cases of fever.

Trigger 2

More than 60 cases from a primary health centre or more than 10 cases from a subcenter.

Polio Trigger

One single case.

Plague Triggers

- Trigger 1
  - Rat fall
- Trigger 2
  - At least one probable case of plague in community.

Japanese Encephalitis Triggers

- Trigger 1
  - Clustering of two or more similar case from a locality in one week
- Trigger 2
  - More than four cases from a PHC (30,000 population) in one week.

Dengue Triggers

Trigger 1

- Clustering of two similar cases of probable dengue fever in a village
- Single case of dengue hemorrhagic fever.

Trigger 2

More than four cases of dengue fever in a village with population of about 1000.

Triggers for Syndromic Surveillance

- Fever
  - More than two similar case in the village (1000 population)
- Diarrhea
  - See cholera
- Acute flaccid paralysis
  - 1 case
- Jaundice
  - More than two cases of jaundice in different houses irrespective of age in a village or 1000 population.

When to Sample?

- Isolation of agent, PCR or antigen:
  - At the earliest
  - Before antimicrobial administration
- For antibody estimation:
  - Ideally two paired specimens
    - i. At earliest
    - ii. After 7 to 10 days
  - Alternately, one specimen 4 to 5 weeks after onset

Whom to Sample During a Classical Outbreak?

- Typical cases
  - Should represent the majority of the specimens
- Untreated patients
  - Without antibiotics
- Cases likely to carry the pathogen
  - Children
- Atypical cases
  - Few specimens
- Healthy contacts
  - Few specimens.

Rule of Thumb Regarding the Number of Specimens to take during a Cholera Outbreak

- 10 specimens to confirm the outbreak
- Five specimens per week during the outbreak

Specimens at the end to confirm that the outbreak is over.

How many Specimens to take?

- Ensure sufficient number of specimens (At least 20)
  - Avoid sampling error
  - Obtain reliable results
- Avoid overwhelming the laboratory with excessive specimens
- Repeat sampling in some case-patients
  - Acute and convalescent sera
  - Exploration of chronic carriage
  - Intermittent shedding (e.g. Stool microscopy for parasites)
  - Unknown etiology.

Transport Medium

- Allows organisms to survive under adverse conditions
- Does not allow organisms to proliferate
- Available for bacteria, e.g. Cary Blair
- Available for viruses
- Virus transport media (VTM).

What is a Viral Transport Medium?

- Sterile buffered solution (Pink colored) containing antibiotics for preservation of viruses
- Used in the collection of specimens for viral isolation and testing

- Save the viruses from drying
  - Nutrient, glycerol
- Prevents specimen from drying out
- Prevents bacterial and fungus growth
- Prepared in the lab or commercially obtained
- Storage for short periods at 4 to 8°C.

Vacutainers

- Vacuum tube with rubber stopper mounted on a needle system
- Tubes may be changed for collection of different tubes for different purposes
- Smooth blood flow, lower risk of hemolysis
- Reduces risk of spillage.

Collecting Blood for Cultures

- Collect within 10 to 30 minutes of fever
- Aseptic technique
- Quantity
- Venous blood for infants—0.5 to 2 ml
- Venous blood for children—2 to 5 ml
- Venous blood for adults—5 to 10 ml
- Take three sets of blood culture when suspecting bacterial endocarditis.

To Avoiding Hemolysis for Blood Specimens

- Fine needles
- Forced suction of blood with syringe
- Unclean tube (residual detergents)
- Shaking tube vigorously
- Forced expulsion of the blood through needle
- Freezing/thawing of blood
- High speed centrifugation before complete clotting.

Handling and Transporting Blood for Cultures

- Collect in blood culture bottles with infusion broth
  - Change the needle to inoculate the broth
- Travel at ambient temperature.

Handling and Transporting Serum

- Transport at 4 to 8°C if transport lasts less than 10 days
- Freeze at –20°C if storage for weeks or months before processing and shipment to reference laboratory
  - Ship frozen

- Avoid repeated freeze-thaw cycles
  - Destroy IgM (e.g. Measles diagnosis)

Collecting and Handling Cerebrospinal Fluid

- Collection
  - Lumbar puncture
    - i. Aseptic conditions
    - ii. Trained person
  - Sterile tubes
- Handling and transportation
  - For bacteria, transport at ambient temperature or preferably in trans-isolate medium (pre-warmed to 25-37°C before inoculation)
  - For viruses, transport at 4 to 8°C for up to 48 hours or at –70°C for longer duration.

Collecting a Sputum

- Instruct patient to take a deep breath and cough up sputum directly into a wide-mouth sterile container
- Avoid saliva or postnasal discharge
- Minimum volume should be about 1 ml.

Handling and Transportation of Respiratory Specimens

- All respiratory specimens except sputum are transported in appropriate media
  - Amie's or Stuart's transport medium for bacteria
  - Viral transport medium for viruses
- Transport as quickly as possible to the laboratory to reduce overgrowth by oral flora
- For transit periods up to 24 hours
  - Ambient temperature for bacteria
  - For viruses 4 to 8°C

Collecting Stool Specimens for Parasites

- Timing
  - As soon as possible after onset
- Specimen amount and size
  - At least 3 × 5 to 10 ml fresh stool from patients (and controls)
- Method
  - Mixed with 10 percent formalin or polyvinyl chloride, 3 parts of stool to 1 part preservative
  - Unpreserved specimens for antigen detection and PCR
- Storage
  - Refrigerate at 4°C
  - Store at –15°C for antigen detection and PCR

Transport
- 4°C (Do not freeze)
- Dry ice for antigen detection and PCR.

Collecting stool Specimens for Bacteria

- Timing
  - During active phase
- Specimen amount and size
  - Fresh specimens and two swabs from patients, controls and carriers (if indicated)
- Method
  - In Cary-Blair medium (+ specimen without transport medium for antigen detection/PCR)
- Storage
  - Refrigerate at 4°C if testing within 48 hours, –70°C if longer.

Collecting Stool Specimens for Viruses

- Timing
  - Within 48 hours of onset
- Specimen amount and size
  - At least 5 to 10 ml fresh stool from patients (and controls)
- Method
  - Fresh stool unmixed with urines in clean, dry and sterile container
- Storage
  - Refrigerate at 4°C. Do not freeze
  - Store at –15°C for antigen detection and protein chain reaction (PCR)
- Transport
  - 4°C Do not freeze at 4°C
  - Dry ice for antigen detection and PCR.

Rectal Swabs

- Advantage
  - Convenient
  - Adapted to small children, debilitated patients and other situation where voided stool specimen collection is not feasible
- Drawbacks
  - No macroscopic assessment possible
  - Less materials available

    i. Not recommended for viruses.

Collecting and Handling Stool Specimens

- Take freshly passed stool specimen
  - Avoid collecting specimen from a bed pan
- Collect specimen in sterile container (if available) or clean container (not cleaned with a disinfectant)

Collecting Serum

- Collect venous blood in a sterile test tube
- Let specimen clot for 30 minutes at ambient temperature
- Place at 4 to 8°C for clot retraction for at least 1 to 2 hours
- Centrifuge at 1500 RPM for 5 to 10 min
- Separate the serum from the clot with pipette/micro-pipette.

Triple-packaging of Specimens: Two Goals

- Protect the environment and the carrier
- Protect the specimen.

Early Warning Signals for an Outbreak (Flow chart 22.6)

- Clustering of cases of deaths
- Increase in cases or deaths
- Single case of disease of epidemic potential
- Acute febrile illness of an unknown etiology
- Two or more linked cases of disease with outbreak potential
  - (e.g. measles, cholera, dengue, Japanese encephalitis or plague)
- Unusual isolate (Cholera O 139)
- Shifting in age distribution of cases (Cholera O 139)
- High vector density
- Natural disasters.

Flow chart 22.6: Components of early warning surveillance

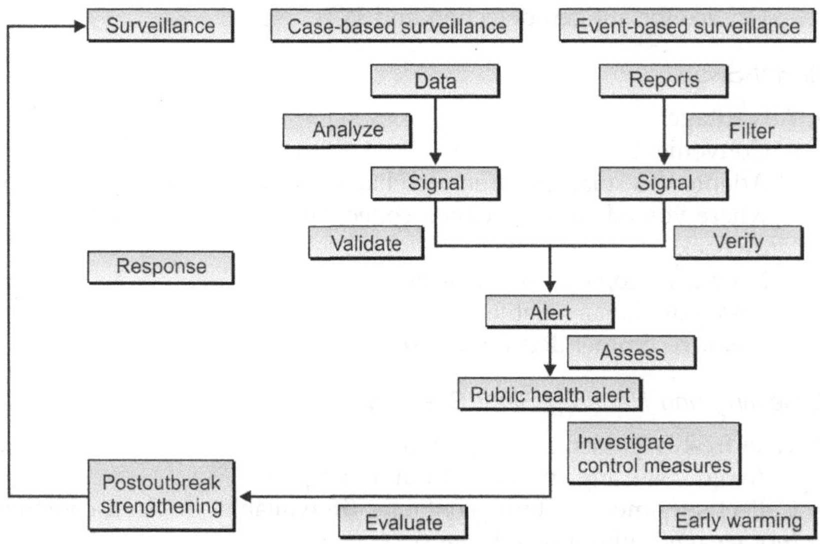

Steps in Outbreak Response (Flow chart 22.7)

1. Verifying the outbreak
2. Sending the rapid response team
3. Monitoring the situation
4. Declaring the outbreak over
5. Reviewing the final report.

Step 1: Verifying the Outbreak

- Validate the source of information
  - Change in the reporting system
  - Change in the population size
  - Acute reporting of old, chronic cases
- Check with the concerned medical officer
  - Abnormal increase in the number of cases
  - Clustering the cases
  - Epidemiological link between cases
  - Triggering event
  - Deaths

Step 2: Sending the Rapid Response Team

- Review if the source and mode of transmission are known
- If not, constitute team with:

Flow chart 22.7: Investigation of an epidemic

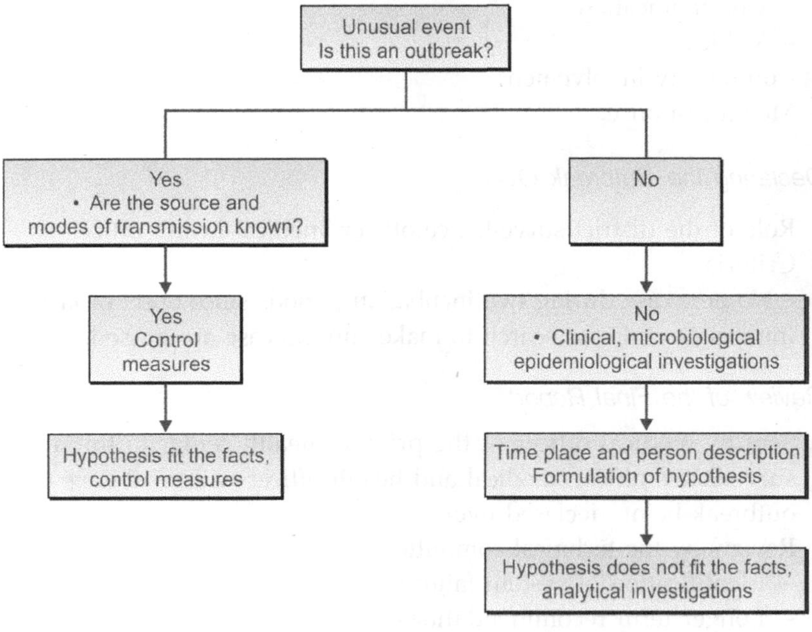

- Medical officer
- Epidemiologist
- Laboratory specialist
- Formulation of hypothesis on basis of the description by time, place and person (Descriptive epidemiology)
  - Does the hypothesis fits the fact
    Yes: Propose control measures
    No: Conduct analytical studies.

The rapid response team:

- Composition
  - Epidemiologist, clinician and microbiologist
    i. Entomologist when vector-borne disease
  - Gathered on ad hoc basis when needed
- Role
  - Confirm and investigate outbreaks
- Responsibility
  - Assist in the investigation and response
  - Primary responsibility rests with local health staff

Monitoring the situation:

- Trends in cases and deaths
- Implementation of containment measures
- Stocks of vaccines and drugs
- Logistics
  - Communication
  - Vehicles
- Community involvement
- Media response.

Declaring the Outbreak Over

- Role of the district surveillance officer/medical health officer
- Criteria
  - No new case during two incubation periods since onset of last case
- Implies careful case search to make sure no case are missed.

Review of the Final Report

- Sent by medical officer of the primary health center to the district surveillance officer/medical and health officer within 10 days of the outbreak being declared over
- Review by the technical committee
  - Identification of system failures
  - Longer term recommendations

Control Measures for an Outbreak

- General measures
  - Till source and route of transmission identified
- Specific measures, based upon the results of the investigation
  - Agent
    i. Removing the source
  - Environment
    i. Interrupting transmission
  - Host
    i. Protection (e.g. immunization)
    ii. Case management.

Sources of Information to detect Outbreaks

- Event-based surveillance
  - Rumor register
    i. To be kept in standardized format in each institution
    ii. Rumours need to be investigated
  - Community informants
    i. Private and public sector
  - Media
    i. Important source of information, not to neglect
- Case-based surveillance
    i. Review of routine surveillance data and triggers

Outbreaks versus Epidemics

- Occurrence of cases of an illness in excess of expected numbers
- Scale
  - Outbreak
    i. Limited to a small area, within one district or few blocks
  - Epidemic
    i. Covers larger geographic areas
    ii. Linked to control measures in district/state
  - No exact precise threshold: Use a word or the other according to whether you want to generate or deflect attention
    i. Be aware of legal implications of the use of the term "Epidemic" in India (Epidemic Disease Act, being revised)
- Endemic versus epidemic
  - Endemicity
    i. Disease occurring in a population regularly at a usual level
      - Tuberculosis, Malaria
- Epidemics
  - Unusual occurrence of the disease in excess of its normal expectation
    i. In a geographical location
    ii. At a given point of time
    For example, hepatitis E, measles, cholera

SURVEILLANCE OF NONCOMMUNICABLE DISEASES

Aims

1. To monitor trends of important risk factors of NCD's in community over a period of time.
2. Evolve strategies for intervention of these risk factors so as to reduce the burden of diseases due to NCD's.
3. Strengthen NCD surveillance and integrate risk factors surveillance.

NCD Risk Factors

1. Behavioral: Tobacco, alcohol, diet habits
2. Physical: Levels of inactivity
3. Biochemical: Blood sugar, cholesterol
4. Measurements: Height, weight, pulse, BP, wiast circumference

Program for Control and Treatment of Occupational Diseases

Major occupational illness are listed based on three criterias:
1. Frequency
2. Severity
3. Potential for prevention.

List

- Occupational injuries
- Occupational lung disorders
- Occupational cancer
- Occupational dermatoses
- Occupational toxicology
- Occupational mental illness.

Etiological Classification of Occupational Disorders

1. Chemical: Dust, gases, acids, alkali, metals.
2. Biological factors
3. Behavioral factors
4. Social occupational factors.
5. Physical: Noise, heat, radiation.

Proposed Projects for Occupational Diseases under National Program for Control and Treatment of Occupational Diseases

1. Prevention, control, treatment of silicotuberculosis
2. Occupational health problems of tobacco harvestors

3. Hazardous process and chemicals database generation, documentation and information dissemination.
4. Capacity building to promote research, education, training at National Institute.

Global Strategy of Occupational Health (Fig. 22.1)

- Developing healthy work environment and healthy work practices to promote health at work.
- Strengthening occupational health services
- Support services for occupational health
- Developing health standards on scientific risk assessment.
- Developing human resources for occupational health
- Strengthening research and developing collaboration in occupational health services and organizations.
- Strengthening international and national policies.

Monitoring and Evaluation

Monitoring

1. Number and percent of districts providing monthly surveillance reports on time by state and overall.
2. Number and percent response to disease specific triggers on time by state and overall.

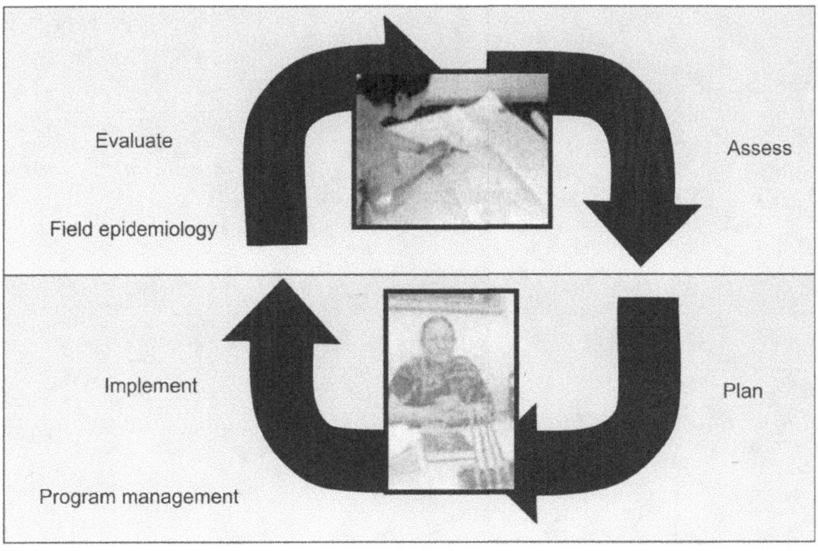

Fig. 22.1: Recommendations link field epidemiology and program management

3. Number and percent of labs providing adequate quality of information by state and center.
4. Number of districts in which private providers are contributing to disease information
5. Publication by CSU of consolidated annual surveillance report.

Evaluation

1. *Baseline study:* Existing quality of lab services and waste management practice.
2. *Sample surveys:* Surveys of risk factors of NCDs.
3. *Mid-term evaluation:* Evaluation of training activities at various levels.
4. Trends on lab quality assurance and waste management practices.
5. *End line evaluation:* Evaluation of training activities at various levels.
6. Effectiveness information technology in surveillance, cost-benefit analysis of a project.

Chapter 23 Integrated Management of Neonatal and Childhood Illnesses

CHAPTER OUTLINE

- COMPONENTS OF IMNCI IN INDIA
- IMNCI STRATEGY IN INDIA

INTRODUCTION

Most illness contributing to under five deaths are preventable. Only a few, mostly developing countries, account for a large proportion of child deaths worldwide. Internationally, there has been a call to reduced burdens contributing to infant, neonate, child morbidity and mortality such as the world summit for children (1990) and the Millennium Development Goals (2001). From this, the Integrated Management of Childhood Illness (IMCI) strategy was developed by WHO, UNICEF and other agencies, institution and individuals to address issues related to morbidity among children under five years of age.

Problem Statement

- In India 2.1 million children die before reaching the age of 5 years
- India accounts for one-fifth of the global child morbidity burden
- IMR—60 to 7 per 1000 live births of which two-third are neonates.
- NMR—40 to 45 per 1000 live births.
- National Goals of India by 2015
  - IMR—27 and NMR—20.

COMPONENTS OF IMNCI IN INDIA

1. Care of newborns and young infants (<2 months)
2. Care of infants and children (2 months to 5 years)
3. Home visits
4. Skill based training
5. Strengthening the Health Systems and Referral
6. Improvements of family and community practices
7. Collaboration with other departments, PRIs, SHGs, MSS.

IMNCI STRATEGY IN INDIA

Implementation of Integrated Management of Neonatal and Childhood Illness, in the district is a component of the Child Health Strategy under the National Rural Health Mission/Reproductive and Child Health Program Phase II. The IMNCI strategy has been developed by child health researchers, academicians, the Indian Academics of Pediatrics (IAP) and National Neonatology Forums (NNFs). According to operational guidelines developed by the Indian Ministry of Health and Family Welfare, Governments of India, the IMNCI package includes the following components:

I. Care of newborns and young infants (under-two months):
   - Keeping the baby warm
   - Initiation of breastfeeding immediately after birth and counseling for exclusive breastfeeding and non-use of prelacteal feeds
   - Cord, skin and eye care
   - Recognition of illness in newborn and management and/or referral
   - Immunization
   - Home visits in postnatal period.

II. Care of *infants* (*2 months and 5 years*):
   - Management of diarrhea, acute respiratory infections (pneumonia), malaria, measles, acute ear infection, malnutrition and anemia
   - Recognition of illness, risk conditions and their management and referral
   - Prevention and management of iron and vitamin A deficiency
   - Counseling on feeding for malnourished children between two to five years
   - Immunization.

III. *Home visits:* Home visits made by ANMs, ASHAs and link volunteers are integral part of this intervention which help mothers and families to understand and provide essential newborn care at home.

IV. *Training:* IMNCI involves two categories of skill based training. One for medical officers and a second for front Line functionaries including ANMs and AWWs. For ASHA and link volunteers if any a separate package focusing on home care of newborn and children is being prepared.

V. *Improvements to health systems:* Essential elements include:
   - Ensuring availability of essential drugs
   - Improves referral to identified referral health facility
   - Referral mechanism to ensure that an identified sick infant or child can be swiftly transferred to a higher level of care
   - Functioning referral centers, especially where health care systems are weak, referral institutions need to be reinforced or private/public need to be established
   - Ensuring availability of health workers/providers at all levels.

- Ensuring supervision and monitoring follow-up visits by trained supervisors.

VI. Improvements of family and community practices: Counseling of families and creating awareness among community on healthy behaviors through IEC campaigns and counseling of caregivers and families as part of management of the sick child.

VII. Collaboration/Community Medicine coordination with other departments, PRIs, Self-Help Groups, MSS, etc.

Globally

Integrated Management of Childhood Illness (IMCI)

India

Integrated Management of Neonatal and Childhood Illness (IMNCI) (Table 23.1)

Table 23.1: Integrated management of neonatal and childhood illness

Feature	*Generic IMCI*	*Indian IMNCI*
Coverage of 0-6 days (early new born period)	No	Yes
Basic health worker module	No	Yes
Home visit module by provider for care of new born and young infants	No	Yes
Home based training	No	Yes
Duration of training on newborn/ young infant	2 of 11 days	4 of 8 days
Sequence of training	*Child first then young infant*	*Newborn/young infant then children*

Timeline of IMNCI

1. Instrument Development (July-Sep, 2006)
2. Program Managers Meeting (August, 2006)
3. International Advisory Board meeting (September, 2006)
4. National Orientation and Protocol Finalization Workshop (September, 2006)
5. Second International Advisory Board meeting (November, 2006)
6. Regional Training Workshops (February-March, 2007)
7. Data Collection (March-May, 2007)
8. Data Analysis (ongoing)
9. Draft Report Writing (ongoing)
10. Dissemination of Results (July, 2009)
11. Final Report (August, 2009).

The IMNCI-PLUS

- The objective of IMNCI-PLUS strategy in RCH II are to implement by 2010, a comprehensive newborn and child health package at the level of all subcenters (through ANMs). Primary health centers (through medical officers, nurse and LHVs) and first referral units (through medical officers and nurses).
- Implement by 2010 a comprehensive newborn and child health package at household level in 250 districts (through AWWs).

Chapter 24 Community-based Rehabilitation

CHAPTER OUTLINE

INTRODUCTION

Community-based Rehabilitation (CBR) strategy was developed by the WHO after 1978. Alma Ata declaration, which stated that comprehensive primary health care, should include promotive, preventive, curative and rehabilitative care. The major objective of CBR is to ensure that people with disabilities (PWD) are able to maximize their physical and mental abilities, have access to regular services and opportunities and achieve full social integration within their communities. CBR is a comprehensive approach, which encompasses disability prevention and rehabilitation in primary health care activities and integration of disabled children in ordinary school and provision of opportunities for the gainful economic activities for disabled adults.

Community-based Rehabilitation (CBR) may be defined, according to three United Nation Agencies, ILO, UNESCO, and the WHO, as a strategy within community development for the rehabilitation, equalization of opportunities, and social integration of all people with disabilities. CBR is implemented through the combined efforts of disabled people themselves, their families and communities, and the appropriate health, education, vocational and social services.

HARD FACTS

- One billion population distributed over 27 states and 7 union territories that are further divided into 557 administrative units called districts.
- About five percent persons with disabilities.
- Seventy eight percent population lives in rural areas.
- Fifteen percent people who live in urban areas have access to some kind of rehabilitation service whereas in rural areas it is only one percent.
- On average 5 to 10 percent person with disabilities has access to basic rehabilitation services.

NEED OF REHABILITATION SERVICE

Only 15 percent people living in urban areas and three percent people living in rural areas can avail rehabilitation service in India, total coverage according Ministry of Social Justice and Empowerment is only 5.7 percent

Seven National Levels Institutes

- National Institute for the Visually Handicapped, Dehradun
- National Institute for the Hearing Handicapped, Mumbai
- National Institute for the Mentally Handicapped, Secunderabad
- National Institute for the Orthopedically Handicapped, Kolkata
- National Institute of Rehabilitation Training and Research, Cuttack
- Institute for the Physically Handicapped, New Delhi
- National Institute for the Empowerment with Persons with Multiple Disabilities, Chennai

Government Rehabilitation Services

The Ministry of Social Justice and Empowerment is the nodal agency of the Central Government that promotes services for the people with disabilities through its various schemes.

Objectives

The primary object is to promote services for people with disabilities through government and non government organizations, so that they are encouraged to become functionally independent and productive members of the nation through opportunities of education, vocational training, medical rehabilitation, and socioeconomic rehabilitation.

Emphasis is also placed on coordination of services particularly those related to health, nutrition, education, science and technology, employment, sports, cultural, art and craft and welfare programs of various government and nongovernment organizations.

- District Rehabilitation Center (DRC) Project
- Regional Rehabilitation Training Center (RRTC)
- National Information Center on Disability and Rehabilitation (NICDR)
- National Council for Handicapped Welfare
- National Handicapped Finance and Development Corporation
- Assistance through Overseas Development Administration, UK
- Training in the UK under the Colombo Plan
- UNICEF Assistance in collaboration with the Government of India National Awards.

District Rehabilitation Center (DRC) Project

The District Rehabilitation Center scheme was launched in early 1985 to provide comprehensive rehabilitation services to the rural disabled.

This was done in collaboration with the National Institute of Disability and Rehabilitation Research (NIDRR), Washington, USA. A Central Administrative and Coordinaiton Unit (CACU) for coordinating and administering the activities of DRC was setup.

The aims and objectives of the DRCs include surveys of disabled population, prevention, early detection and medical intervention and surgical correction, fitting of artificial aids and appliances, therapeutic services—physiotherapy, occupational therapy and speech therapy, provision of educational services in special and integrated schools, provision of vocational training, job placement in local industries and trades, self-employment opportunities, awareness generation for the involvement of community and family to create a cadre of multidisciplinary professionals to take care of major categories of disabled in the district. At present, 11 DRCs function in 10 states in India.

Regional Rehabilitation Training Center (RRTC)

Four Regional Rehabilitation Centers have been functioning under the DRCs scheme at Mumbai, Chennai, Cuttack and Lucknow since 1985 for the training of village level functionaries, training of DRCs professionals, orientation and training of State Government officials, research in service delivery and low cost aids, etc. Apart from developing training material and manuals for actual field use, RRTCs also produce material for creating community awareness through the medium of folders, posters, audiovisuals, films and traditional forms.

National Information Center on Disability and Rehabilitation (NICDR)

A National Information Center on Disability and Rehabilitation was set up under CACU in 1987 to provide a database for comprehensive information on all facilities and welfare services for the disabled within the country. It also acts as a nodal agency for awareness creation, preparation/collection and dissemination of materials/information on disability relief and rehabilitation. The computerized data so far collected relates to institutions/professionals working for the disabled, aids and appliances, scholarships, national awards and physical/financial performance of DRCs/RRTCs. It publishes the Indian Journal of Disability and Rehabilitation.

The Media Cell is responsible for the publication of awareness-generation material/journals, hold seminars/workshops, organization of film festival/exhibitions, production of films, etc. UNICEF assistance is obtained for different activities on awareness creation.

Proposed Program for Rehabilitation of the Disabled in the Ninth Five-year Plan

- At the Gram Panchayat level the local panchayat committee will manage the CBR program. Preferably, two CBR workers—one male and one female, for about 5,000 population, may be employed and suitably trained at the Gram Panchayat level.

- At the PHC level 2 multirehabilitation workers (MRWs) for about 30,000 population will be responsible to provide services to the persons with disabilities. They will provide information to community leaders, to the persons with disabilities and their families about disability. They will also provide services and opportunities using already available resources. The MRW will cooperate with PHC, education, labor, NGOs and other persons, which will make services available and open opportunities for PWDs. They will also make appropriate referral of cases to the District Rehabilitation Center (DRC).
- At the district level DRC will be headed by District Rehabilitation Officer who will monitor and guide the work carried out at peripheral levels. Functionaries of the department of rural development, social welfare, labor and employment and women and child development will also provide specialist services at the district level.
- At the state level, an apex level institution will be set up to serve as resource center in the field of disability prevention and rehabilitation. This institute will train the functionaries of DRCs, PHCs and CHCs. The institute will also undertake long and short term training program to develop the manpower required in the state for the delivery of rehabilitation services. It will also establish linkages with the existing medical professionals, training and employment infrastructure and also promote and conduct research in the area of disability prevention and rehabilitation.
- At the national level, it is proposed that there should be a national center for disability rehabilitation under the national program of rehabilitation.

Role of Primary Health Centers for Disability Rehabilitation

Various services for persons with disabilities in India are very short in supply and do not cover more than even one percent of the entire disabled population. In order to face the challenges of increased population and the lack of proper services to match the needs and expectations of the persons with disability, their family members and the society as a whole, a suitable framework having wide coverage has to be developed in the country for effective management of the disabled. It is in view of these primary and basic needs, the primary health center (PHC) network in India assumes great importance. A PHC is the only existing minimum necessary infrastructure to provide various disability prevention and rehabilitation services. By sensitizing the medical officers and health teams in PHCs on some of the important aspects of disability prevention, early identification, referral and rehabilitation, valuable services could be rendered to people with disabilities in the rural areas.

Primary health care in India is provided by a network of primary health centers and its subcenters in rural areas and health posts in urban areas. Health workers at subcenters get help from village health guides (VHGs), traditional birth attendants (TBAs) and Anganwadi workers in their functioning. This huge manpower can help in identification of disabled along with CBR workers and community level functionaries of DRC with the help of training packages developed by WHO.

Multi-rehabilitation workers (MRWs) at PHC with the help of Medical Officer will attend to referred disabled and help in training of personnel engaged at subcenter and village level. Vocational rehabilitation centers will provide support in relation to generating various occupational opportunities for disabled along with NGOs and other concerned personnel at district level.

Model Method of Implementation of CBR Using Primary Health Centers

Community level functionaries (CLF) at village and subcenter level for a population of 5000. The village rehabilitation committee (VRC) of the Panchayat members will manage the activities.

Manpower

- Person with disabilities
- Family trainee
- Community rehabilitation worker
- MPHW male and female
- VHG, TBA and Anganwadi worker
- NGOs, teachers and volunteers.

Functions

- Micromanagement
- Community preparation
- Resources
- Monitoring.

Tasks

- Locate and identify PWD
- Referral
- Assess functions and activities
- Select training material and trainees
- Teach and motivate family training
- Increased acceptance by family
- Facilitate school admission
- Refer to social and vocational organization

- Assess record and report results to VRC
- Stimulate awareness of community about disability.
- Continuing education for CLF and teach them about health care needs of disabled persons.

At PHC and CHC level for a population of 30,000 to 1 lakh. The Medical Officer-in-charge of PHC and CHC will manage the activities.

Manpower

- Multirehabilitation worker (MRW)
- Health assistant male and female.

Functions

- Provide technical training, supervision and support of CBR program
- Report on effectiveness of CBR center
- Provide first level referral advice and refer to higher level if required
- Interact with middle level personnel in other sectors like social, education and labor and coordinate supports to community.

Orientation of Medical Officers Working in Primary Health Centers to Disability Management

Rehabilitation Council of India has launched the National Program on Orientation of Medical Officers working in Primary Health Centers to Disability Management on 15th July 1999, with a view that the Medical Officers of PHCs could be trained in various disability issues, PHC is the only health infrastructure, which is spread over the country. Training the Medical Officers in Disability Prevention and Rehabilitation can bring significant benefits to the persons with disabilities. Most of the disable people live in the rural areas with very poor infrastructure for providing rehabilitation services. In view of such gross neglect of rural areas, this program has been designed for rural disabled.

The program is being implemented in two stages. In the first stage, a master training program is imparted in each state to a team of medical practitioners/rehabilitation professionals working in the institutions selected to conduct the master training program. In the second stage, the trained Master Trainer's Services are utilized for taking up the training of the Medical Officers working in the PHCs. The ingenuity of program is the utilization of the rehabilitation professionals taken from all the disability areas for the training of Medical Officers. This has been consciously done with a view to add thrust to program by way of transferring the rich knowledge and experience of these professionals to the Medical Officers regarding various intricate disability issues. Another notable feature of the program is the selection of institutions, which have rich experience and possess laboratories in one or more areas of disability. This not only gives an opportunity to the doctors to observe themselves the various facets of disability and also allow them to gain practical insight into managing the problems in the locality covered under their PHCs.

Expected Benefits of the Program

1. The program is expected to generate in the country, the following benefits in the short as well as in the long run.
2. Large scale direct benefit of various services like prevention, early identification, referral and rehabilitation to the rural population.
3. Wide and improved service network for the persons with disabilities even in the remotest corners of the country.
4. Decrease in the severity and extent of disability in millions of cases.
5. Increase in the GDP, as the impact of disability prevalence will be less.
6. Awareness generation among the Health Workers through the PHC Medical Officers which will percolate to the lowest level as the lower level health workers function within the community.
7. Social and economic empowerment of the persons with disability.
8. Leadership building in the PHC Medical Officers to help create better sensitization at the grass root level which will ultimately ensure better implementation of the Persons with Disabilities Act, 1995.

BIBLIOGRAPHY

1. Disability Prevention and Rehabilitation in primary health care—a guide for district health and rehabilitation managers. Rehabilitation, WHO, 1995.
2. National programme on orientation of medical officers working in primary health centres to disability management-status of implementation 2001, Rehabilitation Council of India.
3. Proceedings of workshop on Community-based Rehabilitation WHO sponsored—department of Physical Medicine and Rehabilitation, Safdarjang Hospital, New Delhi, 1997.
4. The Persons with Disabilities (equal opportunities, protection of rights and full participation) Act 1995—Ministry of Law, Justice and Company affairs.

Chapter 25 Social Security

CHAPTER OUTLINE

- WORKFORCE IN INDIA
- FUNCTIONS OF SOCIAL SECURITY DIVISION

INTRODUCTION

Social security protects not just the subscriber but also his/her entire family by giving benefit packages in financial security and health care. Social security schemes are designed to guarantee at least long-term sustenance to families when the earning member retires, dies or suffers a disability. Thus, the main strength of the social security system is that it acts as a facilitator—it helps people to plan their own future through insurance and assistance. The success of social security schemes, however, requires the active support and involvement of employees and employers.

In the Indian context, social security is a comprehensive approach designed to prevent deprivation, assure the individual of a basic minimum income for himself and his dependents and to protect the individual from any uncertainties. The state bears the primary responsibility for developing appropriate system for providing protection and assistance to its workforce. Social security is increasingly viewed as an integral part of the development process. It helps to create a more positive attitude to the challenge of globalization and the consequent structural and technological changes.

WORKFORCE IN INDIA

The dimensions and complexities of the problem in India can be better appreciated by taking into consideration the extent of the labor force in the organized and unorganized sectors.

Organized and Unorganized Sectors

The organized sector includes primarily those establishments which are covered by the Factories Act, 1948, the Shops and Commercial Establishments Acts of State Governments, the Industrial Employment Standing Orders Act, 1946, etc. This sector already has a structure through which social security benefits are extended to workers covered under these legislations.

The unorganized sector on the other hand, is characterized by the lack of labor law coverage, seasonal and temporary nature of occupations, high labor mobility, dispersed functioning of operations, casualization of labor, lack of organizational support, low bargaining power, etc. all of which make it vulnerable to socioeconomic hardships. The nature of work in the unorganized sector varies between regions and also between the rural areas and the urban areas, which may include the remote rural areas as well as sometimes the most inhospitable urban concentrations. In the rural areas it comprises of landless agricultural laborers, small and marginal farmers, share croppers, persons engaged in animal husbandry, fishing, horticulture, bee-keeping, toddy tapping, forest workers, rural artisans, etc. where as in the urban areas, it comprises mainly of manual laborers in construction, carpentry, trade, transport, communication, etc. and also includes street vendors, hawkers, head load workers, cobblers, tin smiths, garment makers, etc.

FUNCTIONS OF SOCIAL SECURITY DIVISION

List of Subjects

- Matters concerning framing of social security policy especially for the organized sector of workers.
- Administration of Employees' State Insurance Act, 1948.
- Administration of the Employees' Provident Funds and Miscellaneous Provisions Act, 1952 and three schemes framed there under, namely:
  - The Employees' Provident Fund Scheme, 1952
  - The Employees' Pension scheme, 1995
  - The Employees' Deposit linked Insurance Scheme, 1976.
- Workmen's Compensation Act, 1923.
- Maternity Benefits Act, 1961.
- Payment of Gratuity, Act, 1972.
- Establishment matters relating to the Employees' State Insurance Corporation—Constitution of ESI Corporation, Standing Committee and Medical Benefit Council of ESIC as also Regional Board.
- Administrative matters of ESI Corporation including implementation of ESI Scheme in New Geographical Areas, opening of Sub-Regional Offices of ESIC and up-gradation of medical facilities.
- Annual report, budget and accounts, and matters connected with auditing of accounts of the ESIC and EPFO
- Issues relating to International Social Security Association (ISSA); and other International Social Security Organizations. Processing of ILO Conventions relating to social security.
- All parliamentary matters and MP/VIP References in relation to the above as also legislative matters/amendment in respect of the aforesaid Acts.

- Vigilance matters/Disciplinary proceedings relating to officers of EPFO and ESIC.
- Representations from employees of ESIC and EPFO, and general public grievances on ESIC/EPFO/Social Security measures in India.
- All matters relating to setting up of EPF Appellate Tribunal-establishment matters and appointment of staff.
- Constitution of the Central Board of Trustees and Regional Committees, EPFO.
- All matters relating to:
  - Pattern of investment of provident fund money.
  - Declaration of rate of interest on the provident fund.
  - Enhancement of the rate of provident fund contributions.
  - Budget of the EDLI Scheme and EPS;
  - Payment of central government contribution and administrative charges for Family Pension Scheme, Deposit Linked Insurance under the EPF Act as well as the Assam Tea Plantation Provident Fund Act.
  - References relating to recovery of EPF/ESI dues/exemptions and Exclusions from the EPF and MP Act and also the ESI Act.

EPFO Programs at a Glance (Table 25.1)

Table 25.1: EPFO programs at a glance

Program name	*Program type*	*Financing*	*Coverage*
Employees provident fund	Mandatory	• Employer: 1.67–3.67% • Employee: 10–12% • Government: None	Firms with + 20 employees
Employees pension scheme (EPS)	Mandatory	• Employer: 8.33% • Employee: None • Government: 1.16%	Firms with + 20 employees
Employees deposit linked insurance Scheme (EDLI)	Mandatory	• Employer: 0.5% • Employeees: None • Government: None	Firms with+20 employees

ESI contribution rates
- Employees: 1.75 percent of wages
- Employers: 4.75 percent of wages
- State Govts.: 1/8th share of expenditure.

A few examples of other retirement programs giving social security (Table 25.2).

(Information on extent of coverage of the labor force under these programs is not available).

Table 25.2: Retirement programms in social security

Program name	*Program type*	*Financing*	*Coverage*
Civil service pension scheme	Mandatory	State or central Government	Civil servants at state and central government level
Government provident fund	Mandatory	Employee contribution	Civil servants at state and central government level
Special provident particular funds	Mandatory	Employer and employee contributions	Applies to worker in sectors: Coal, mines, tea plantation, Jammu and Kashmir seamen, etc.
Public provident fund	Voluntary	Contributions	All individuals are eligible to apply
Personal pension	Voluntary	Contributions	Employees as decided by respective establishments
Personal pension	Voluntary	Purchase of annuity type products	All individuals
State level social assistance	Government sponsored social assistance	State Government	Varies by state and type of scheme
National old age pension scheme	Government sponsored social assistance	Central Government	Poor persons above age 65

New Initiative in Social Security

Varishtha Pension Bima Yojana (VPBY): This scheme proposed in the 2003-04 budget by the Ministry of Finance is to be administered by the Life Insurance Corporation of India (LIC). Its main features are summarized below:

- Under VPBY, any citizen above 55 years of age could apy a lump-sum and get a monthly pensions are pegged at Rs. 250 and Rs. 2000 per month respectively. These amounts are not indexed to inflation.
- There is a guaranteed return of nine percent per annum for this scheme.
- The difference between the actual yield by the LIC under this scheme and the 9 percent will be made up by the central government.
- The EPF and MP Act is proposed to be amended suitably to allow EPF subscribes to invest in the VBPY.

Chapter 26 Swine Flu

CHAPTER OUTLINE

- Transmission
- Signs and Symptoms

INTRODUCTION

Swine influenza was first proposed to be a disease related to human influenza during the 1918 flu pandemic. When pig became sick at the same time as human. The first identification of an influenza virus as a cause of disease in pigs occurred about ten years later, in 1930. For the following 60 years, swine influenza strain were almost exclusively H1N1. Then, between 1997 and 2002, new strain of three different subtype and five different genotype emerged as cause of influenza among pigs in North America. In 1997 to 1998, H_3N_2 strain emerged. These strain, which include genes derived by reassortment from human, swine and avian virus, have become a major cause of swine influenza in North America.

Outbreak in Human, 2009

The H1N1 viral strain implicated in 2009 flu pandemic among human often is called "swine flu" because initial testing showed many of genes in the virus were similar to influenza viruses normally occurring in North American swine.

TRANSMISSION

The main route of transmission is through direct contact between infected and uninfected animals. These close contacts are particularly common during transport. Intensive farming may also increase the risk of transmission, as the pigs are raised in very close proximity to each other. The direct transfer of the virus probably occurs either by pigs touching noses or through dried mucus. Airborn transmission through the aerosols produced by pigs coughing or sneezing are also an important means of infection. The virus usually spread quickly through a herd, infect all the pigs within a few days. Transmission may also occur through wild animals, such as:

Transmission to Human

People who work with poultry and swine, especially people with intense exposures, are at increased risk of zoonotic infection with influenza virus endemic in these animal and constitute a population of human host in which zoonosis and reassortment can co-occur.

SIGNS AND SYMPTOMS

The symptoms of swine flu H1N1 virus are similar to those of influenza and of influenza like illness in general. Symptoms include fever, cough, sore throat, body aches, headache, chills, and fatigue. The 2009 outbreak has shown an increased percentage of patient reporting diarrhea and vomiting.

Cause of Death

Common cause of death is respiratory failure. Other cause of death are pneumonia (leading to sepsis) high fever (leading to neurological problem), dehydration (excessive diarrhea and vomiting) and electrolyte imbalance. Fatality are more likely in young children and the elderly.

Prevention

i. Prevention in swine
ii. Prevention of transmission to human
iii. Prevention of its spread among humans.

Prevention in Swine

i. Facility management
ii. Herd management
iii. Vaccination.

Facility Management

Facility management includes using disinfectant and ambient temperature to control virus in environment.

Herd Management

Herd management includes not adding pigs carrying influenza to herds that have not been exposed to the virus. The virus survives in healthy carrier pigs for upto three months.

Prevention of human-to-human transmission: Frequent washing of hands with soap and water or with alcohol-based hand sanitizers, especially after being out in public.

Social distancing is another tactic. It means staying away from other people who might be infected and can include avoiding large gatherings, spreading out a little at work or perhaps staying home and lying low if an infection is spreading in a community.

Treatment in human being: If the person become sick with swine flu, antiviral drugs can make illness milder and make the patient feel better faster. They may also prevent serious flu complications. For treatment antiviral drugs work best if started soon after getting sick (within 2 days of symptoms). Beside antivirals, supportive care at home or in hospital, focuses on controling fevers, relieving pain and maintaining fluid balance, as well as indentifying and treating any secondary infections or other medical problems. The US Centers for Disease Control and Prevention recommends the use of Tamiflu (oseltamivir) or Relenza (zanamivir) for the treatment and prevention of infection with swine influenza viruses; however, the majority of people infected with the virus make a full recovery without requiring medical attention or antiviral drugs. The virus isolates in the 2009 outbreak have been found resistant to amantadine and rimantadine.

Chapter 27 Hospital Statistics

CHAPTER OUTLINE

- DAILY ANALYSIS
- CENSUS
- MONTHLY REPORTS
- DEATH RATE

DAILY ANALYSIS

- Daily census of admissions, births, transfer in, transfers out and death complied by ward and by specialty.
- Daily discharge analysis.

MONTHLY REPORTS

- Summary of outpatient visits (first and repeat).
- Summary of inpatient activity speciality wise: number of admissions, discharges, death, hospital days, mean length of stay, bed turnover ratio, occupancy rate, mortality rate, operations, infections, specialized procedures.

CENSUS

- Inpatient bed occupancy ratio:
  Total inpatient service days for a period × 100
  Total inpatient bed count × number of days for a period
- Average daily newborn inpatient service days for a period. Total number of days in the period.

DEATH RATE

- Hospital death rate (Gross death rate):

$$= \frac{\text{No. of inpatient deaths in a period}}{\text{No. of discharges (including deaths) in the same period}} \times 100$$

- Postoperative death rate:

$$= \frac{\text{Total no. of deaths within 10 days postoperative for a period}}{\text{Total no.of patients operated upon for the period}} \times 100$$

- Anesthesia death rate:

$$= \frac{\text{Total number of deaths due to anesthetic agents for a period}}{\text{Total no. of patients administered anesthesia for the period}} \times 100$$

- Maternal death rate (Maternal mortality rate):

$$= \frac{\text{Total no.of direct maternal deaths for a period}}{\text{No. of obstetric discharges (incl. deaths) for the period}} \times 100$$

- Neonatal death rate

$$= \frac{\text{Total number of newborn deaths for a period}}{\text{No of newborn infant discharges (incl. deaths) for the period}} \times 100$$

- Perinatal mortality rate:
  Intermediate (20-28 weeks gestation or 500-1000 gm weight) and late fetal (after 28 weeks) deaths + neonatal

$$= \frac{\text{Deaths (less than 28 days)}}{\text{Births and fetal deaths for the period}} \times 100$$

- Hospital admission rate
  Hospital admission rate denotes the number of hospital admissions per 1000 population per year. Hospital admission rate

$$= \frac{\text{Total admissions during the year}}{\text{Midyear population}} \times 100$$

- Per capita hospitalization rate
  Per capita hospitalization rate is the per capita days of hospital care given per 1000 population for a particular geographical area. During a particular period. It expresses the volume of hospitalizations in terms of number of hospitalization days per person per year.

$$= \frac{\text{Total number of days inpatient care}}{\text{Midyear population}} \times 100$$

  The rang varies from 0.3 to 1.5 in India, it is approximately 0.3.
- Bed turnover rate (BTR)
  Bed turnover rate gives the number of discharges per hospital bed over a given period, i.e. how many times a bed was "turned over" during the period, say a year. It is directly related to the average length of stay (ALS) and bed turnover interval (BTI).

$$\text{Bed turnover rate: } \frac{\text{No. of discharges for a given period of time}}{\text{Average bed count for that period of time}}$$

$$\text{Average length of stay} = \frac{\text{Total patient days during a given period}}{\text{Total discharges (including deaths) during the same period}}$$

- Average length of stay (ALS)
  Average length of stay (ALS) is the average period in hospital (in days) per patient admitted, i.e. the average number of days of service rendered to each inpatient
  Number of inpatient days care (excluding) healthy newborn during the year
  ALS = Total number of discharges and deaths.

Other Statistics

- Autopsy rate
  This relates to autopsies carried out on patients who died in hospital Therefore, it excludes stillbirths. Dead on arrival/brought in dead. and medicolegal cases.

$$\text{Autopsy rate} = \frac{\text{No of autopsies}}{\text{No of deaths in hospital}} \times 100$$

- Consultation (written only) rate

$$\frac{\text{No. of patients receiving consultations}}{\text{No. of patients discharged (and dead)}} \times 100$$

Cesarean Section Rate

$$= \frac{\text{Total no. of cesarean sections in a period}}{\text{No. of deliveries (incl. cesarean sections) in the period}} \times 100$$

Infection Rates

Hospital infection rate:

$$= \frac{\text{Total no. of nosocomial infections in the hospital (or specific clinical unit) for a period}}{\text{Total no. of discharges (incl. deaths) in the hospital (or specific clinical unit) for the period}} \times 100$$

- Postoperative infection rate:

$$= \frac{\text{No. of infections in clean surgical cases for a period}}{\text{Number of clean surgical operations for the period}} \times 100$$

Chapter 28 Biostatistics

CHAPTER OUTLINE

- COLLECTION AND PRESENTATION OF DATA
- GRAPHICAL REPRESENTATION OF DATA
- CENTERING CONSTANTS (MEASURES OF CENTRAL TENDENCY)
- MEASURES OF VARIATION
- INTERNATIONAL DEATH CERTIFICATE—CAUSE OF DEATH

INTRODUCTION

Definitions of Statistics

The word "statistics" used in plural means 'figures' but while used in singular it implies "science of figures" such as collection, presentation, analysis and interpretation of data.

Quantitative Medicine

Since, every thing in medicine be it research, diagnosis, or treatment depends on measurement and counting the medical biostatistics is defined as quantitative medicine.

Science of Variation

For defining normal health and prescribing the normal limits for health, the variations in the characteristics like pulse rate, blood pressure, height, weight, etc. are noted and studied. In this sense it is defined as science of variation.

Science of Averages

Many types of averages are computed in course of the analysis of a statistical data to arrive at an inference or interpretation. In this connection it is also defined as the science of averages.

Biostatistics in the real sense means "Science of figures about any life".

The three important branches of biostatistics are: (a) Health statistics, (b) Medical statistics, and (c) Vital statistics.

a. The Health Statistics are collected in connection with the assessment of health and for prescribing the normal limits of health.

b. The medical statistics deal with the study of injury defect and disease. The efficiency of various drug. Seraline of treatment are also tested statistically in this branch.
c. Vital statistics deal with the figures of births deaths and marriages in populations.

Use of Biostatistics

1. Interpretation of observation
2. Assessment of patient/situation/problem
3. Management of patient/situation/problem
4. Evaluation of patient/situation/problem.

COLLECTION AND PRESENTATION OF DATA

The data collected in respect of any characteristics will be full of figures and lies in a haphazard manner. It conveys no meaning unless the figures are sorted out properly and presented systematically.

The following are the principles of presentation:

1. To arrange the data in such a way that it should create interest in the reader's mind at the first sight.
2. To present the information in a compact and concise form without losing important details.
3. To present the data in a simple form so as to draw the conclusion directly by viewing at the data.
4. To help in the further statistical analysis.

Presentation of Data (Flow chart 28.1)

Flow chart 28.1: Presentation of data

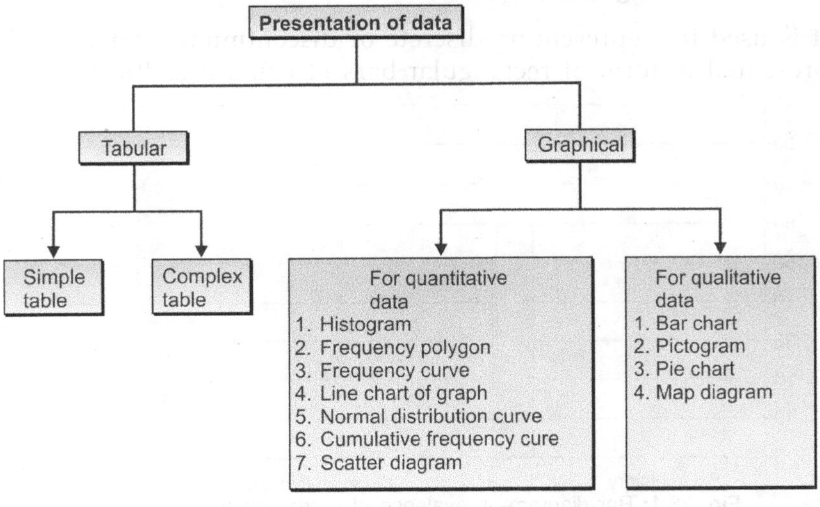

Frequency Table

It is a table showing the frequency with which the values are distributed in different groups or classes with some defined characteristic.

Construction of a Frequency Table

Rules: Rules to be followed in the construction of a frequency table.

a. The class interval should not be too large or too small.
b. The number of classes to be framed more than 8 and less than 15.
c. Class interval should be equal and uniform throughout the classification.
d. After the construction of the table, proper and clear heading should be given to it.
e. The base or source of a data should be mentioned with the pattern of analysis in a footnote at the end of the table.
f. If some observations are omitted or missing the details of exclusion of such observations should be mentioned.

GRAPHICAL REPRESENTATION OF DATA

Graphs

1. The data is presented diagramatically.
2. It gives better grasp than the table.
3. Interpretation is done by rough translation of the points into the actual figures as a change in the scale will give different patterns.
4. Graphs should never be substituted for statistical table because the graphs cannot have the mathematical treatment whereas table can be treated mathematically.
5. Whenever comparing graphs note the difference in the scale if any.

Bar Diagram (Fig. 28.1)

It is used for representing discrete or discontinuous data. Data is presented in form of rectangular bars of equal breadth. Each bar

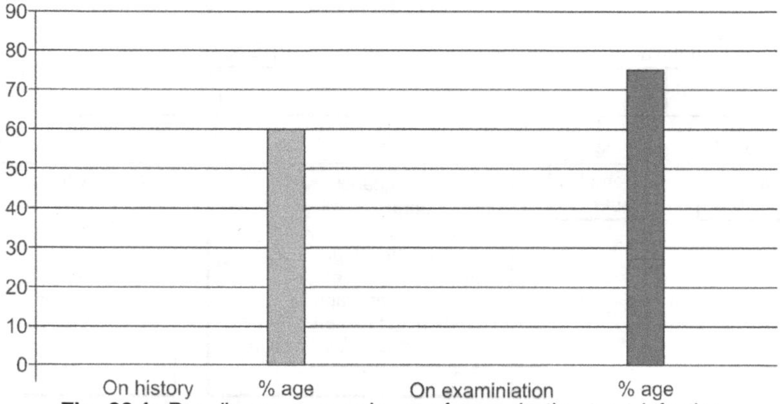

Fig. 28.1: Bar diagram—prevalence of reproductive tract infection

represents one attribute/variate. The width of the bar and the gaps between the bars should be the same throughout. Scale must from zero if not it may be indicated by broken bar.

1. Breadth of all bars is equal.
2. Length of each bar is proportional to the frequency of the characteristic it is representing.
3. Distance between the bars is smaller than the breadth of each bar.
4. Scale has been indicated.
5. Scale starts from zero.
6. Available space is used.

Proportional Bar Diagram (Fig. 28.2)

The bar is colored differently to show various proportions.

Gynecological morbidity

Age group years	Vaginitis		Cervicitis		Cervical erosion		Genital prolapse		Pelvic inflamma-tory disease		Firm bulley uterul	
	No%	No%	No%	No%	No%	No%	No%	No%	No%	No%	No%	No%
15-25	12	18.2	34	31.7	21	20.6	4	10	11	31.4	02	14.3
26-35	37	56.1	57	53.3	61	59.8	10	25	18	51.4	08	57.1
36-45	16	24.2	11	10.3	18	17.6	20	50	5	14.3	02	14.3
46+	01	1.5	05	4.7	02	2.0	6	15	01	2.9	02	14.3
Total	66	100	107	100	102	100	40	100	35	100	14	100

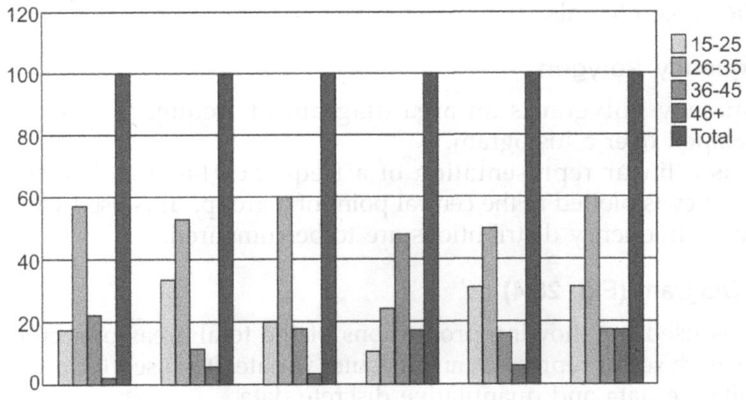

Fig. 28.2: Proportional bar diagram—age-wise distribution of gynecological morbidity on clinical examination

Histogram (Fig. 28.3)

1. This method is useful for presenting frequency of quantitative continuous variate.
2. It is an area diagram composed of a series of adjacent rectangles. The area of each rectangle is proportional to the frequency of that group or class.

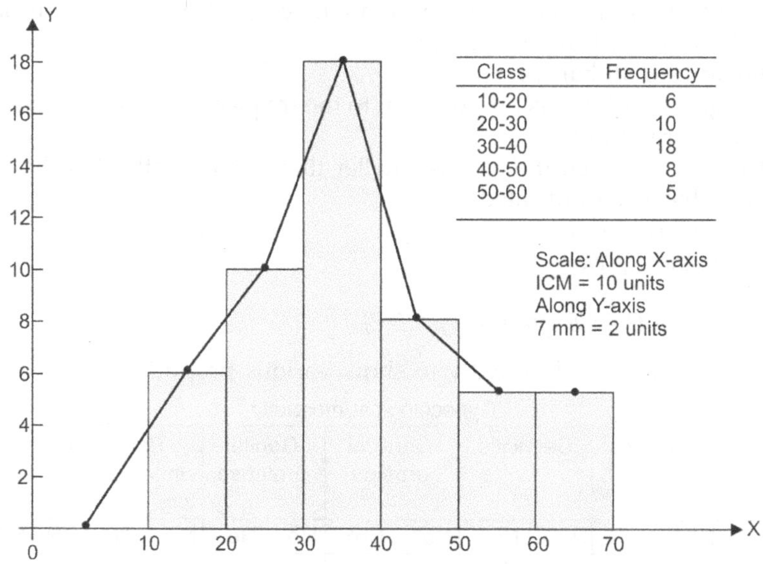

Fig. 28.3: Histogram with frequency polygon

3. The width of the rectangles is equal.
4. Histogram is useful to represent the mode graphically.
5. The only disadvantage of this graph is that it varies accordingly to the class intervals.

Frequency Polygon

Frequency polygon is an area diagram of frequency distribution developed over a histogram.

It is a linear representation of a frequency table and histogram. Frequency is plotted at the central point of a group. It is used when two or more frequency distributions are to be compared.

Pie Diagram (Fig. 28.4)

This is used for showing proportions of the total areas of sectors of a circle each sector represents an attribute/variate. It is used for presenting qualitative data and quantitative discrete data.

The Ogive

The ogive is graph of the cumulative relative frequency distribution.

This is curve plotted on X- and Y-axis with the corresponding cumulative frequency of each class or group. This curve is useful to find the median and the quartiles graphically.

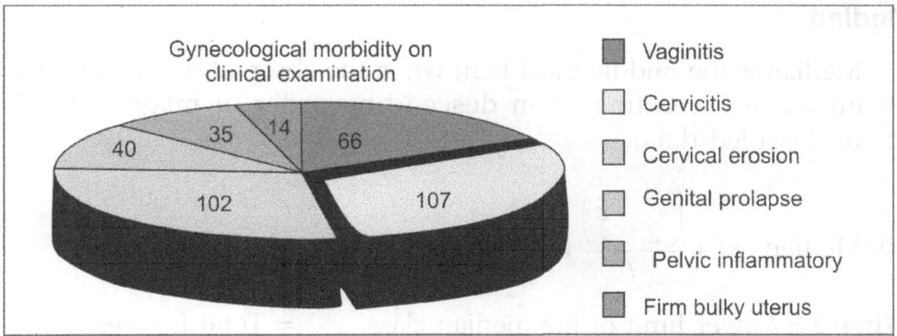

Gynecological morbidity	Number of women	Percentage
Vagintis	66	22.75
Cervicitis	107	36.89
Cervical erosion	102	35.17
Genital prolapse	40	13.79
Pelvic inflammatory disease	35	12.06
Firm bulky uterus	14	4.82

Fig. 28.4: Pie diagram—gynecological morbidity on clinical examination

CENTERING CONSTANTS (MEASURES OF CENTRAL TENDENCY)

Measures of central tendency is measurement of variate which represents a group of individual measurement in a simple and precise manner.

After collecting and presenting the data in frequency distribution, it is essential to calculate certain values which may be used as descriptive characteristic of that distribution. With the help of these values it is possible to make the comparisons between two series of observations as they represent the entire data. A majority of the observations are very close to this value.

There are three measures of central tendency.

There are helpful in measuring closeness of each observation to the central value and to understand the homogenicity of the information collected.

a. Mean b. Median c. Mode

Arithmetic Mean

It is the sum of observations divided by the total number of observations and is noted by $\overline{x}$.

By Definition

i. $\overline{x} = \frac{\Sigma x}{n}$ (for unclassified data) ii. $\overline{x} = \frac{\Sigma fx}{N}$ (for classified data)

The arithmetic mean is used usually when the data is quantitative.

Median

i. Median is the middle most item when the observations are arranged either in ascending or in descending order of magnitude (for unclassified data).

ii. Median $= l + \dfrac{\left(\dfrac{N}{2} - c\right)}{f} \times i$ (for classified data)

Where l = Lower limit of the median class N= Total frequency
f = Frequency of the median class i = Class interval
c = Cumulative frequency of the class preceeding to the median class. Median is usually preferred in case if the data is quantitative type.

Mode

Mode is that value of variate for which the frequency is maximum.

It is calculated if median and mean are known by using the relation.

$$\text{Mode} = 3\ (\text{Median}) - 2\ (\text{Mean})$$

In case of normal distribution, Mean = Median = Mode

Mode is generally used in the field of industrial statistics to control the quality of the products produced.

MEASURES OF VARIATION

Measures of variation are computed to know the degree of scatteredness of each value from the central value. The important measures of variation are larger scatteredness indicate not normal condition while less or no scatteredness suggest to the normal conditions.

- Range
- Mean deviation
- Standard deviation
- Coefficient of variation
- Quartile deviation
- Inter-quartile range
- Percentile.

Range

It is the difference between the maximum and minimum value of the observation. It quantities the variation in one number. The nature of variation between the observations is not taken into account.

$$\text{Range} = X_{max} - X_{min}$$

Mean Deviation (MD)

It is arithmetic average of each observations from the mean neglecting the sign of the deviation. It measures the absolute distance of each observation from the central value as an average.

$$\text{Mean deviation (MD)} = \frac{\Sigma|(X - \overline{x})|}{n} \quad \text{(for unclassified data)}$$

Or

$$= \frac{\Sigma f\,|(X - \overline{x})|}{N} \quad \text{(for classified data)}$$

Standard Deviation (SD)

It is defined as 'Root-Means—Square-Deviation'.

$$SD = \sqrt{\frac{\Sigma(x - \overline{x})^2}{n - 1}} \quad \text{for } n < 30$$

If the number of observation is less than 30, then the sum of squares of deviation is divided by (n – 1) instead of n. It is the most sensitive measures of variation lesser SD reveals smaller variation and a bigger SD suggests the deviation from normal condition.

$$SD = \sqrt{\frac{\Sigma(x - \overline{x})^2}{n}} \quad \text{for large size}$$

Coefficient of Variation (CV)

It is a relative measure of dispersion defined as the ratio of SD to the mean and expressed in percentage.

$$CV = \frac{SD}{\text{Mean}} \times 100\%$$

If the CV is small then observations are considered to be more consistent as it reveals little variation from the normal value higher value of CV. Suggests uncomfortable situation.

Quartile Deviation (QD)

It is obtained by dividing the range between the lower and upper Quartiles by 2.

$$QD = \frac{Q_3 - Q_1}{2},$$

where Q_1 = lower Quartile and Q_3 = upper Quartile

$$\text{Coefficient of QD} = \frac{Q_3 - Q_1}{Q_3 + Q_1}$$

Percentile

In inter-quartile range, we divide the set of observations into four parts. If the series is divided into 10 equal parts then each part is called as 'decile' if it is divided into 100 equal parts, each part is called "percentile".

Tests of Statistical Comparison of Two Groups

Tests of statistical comparison of two groups where the cause effect relationship is to be established for a certain factor under consideration.

Tests of Statistical Significance (Flow chart 28.2)

Flow chart 28.2: Tests of statistical significance

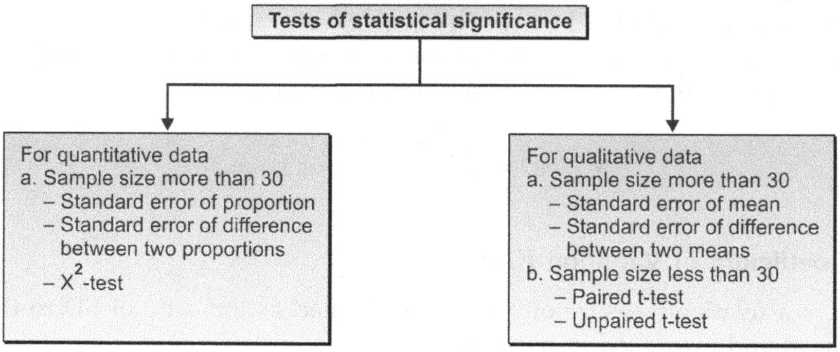

- **Chance:** Something unexpected
- **Probability:** May be defined as possible chances of occurrence. With which an event is expected to occur on an average, such as of giving birth to a boy in the first pregnancy.
- **Null hypothesis:** Assumption is made that external factor plays no role in the condition under study. Such an assumption is called Null Hypothesis (Ho). This hypothesis nullifies the claim that the experimental result is different from or better than the one observed already.

Test of Significance (for Large Size)

Standard Error of Mean

Definition: Standard error (SE) of any statistical value is a measure of variability that would occur merely by chance in the repeated samples of the same size drawn from the same population. The standard error of mean is given by $SE_{\bar{x}} = \frac{SD}{\sqrt{n}}$, i.e. the SE varies directly with SD and inversely as square root of the size the sample.

Uses of SE of Mean

1. To find the confidence limits of population mean if the standard deviation of the sample is known.
2. To tell whether a sample is drawn. From the same population or not.
3. To test the significant difference between two sample means.
4. To calculate the approximate size of a sample in order to have the desired confidence limits.
5. It measures variation due to chance (or biological factors).

Standard Error of difference between Two Means

Definition: If repeatedly independent random samples are drawn in pairs from the same population and each time the difference between two means of each pair is calculated. There will be a series of difference between means. It is shown mathematically that these differences are also normally distributed around the population mean. The standard deviation of difference is called as standard error of difference between two means.

Whenever we want to test the significance of the observed difference between two given means the standard error is applied directly by making use of the individual standard deviation. In case the observed difference is more than 1.96 times the standard error, then it is said to be statistically significant at 95 percent confidence limits.

Formulae

Let $\bar{X}_1$ and $\bar{X}_2$ be the means of the first and the second samples respectively.

Next the steps involved in the calculation of standard error of difference between two means are:

i. $|\bar{X}_1 - \bar{X}_2|$

ii. $$\text{SED} = \sqrt{\frac{SD_1^2}{n_1} + \frac{SD_2^2}{n_2}} = \sqrt{SD^2\left(\frac{1}{n_1} + \frac{1}{n_2}\right)} = \text{SD}\sqrt{\left(\frac{1}{n_1} + \frac{1}{n_2}\right)}$$

iii. $$\frac{|\bar{X}_1 - \bar{X}_2|}{SED}$$

Note: > 1.96 the difference is significant.
The Ho is rejected (Variation is due to external factors)
< 1.96 the difference is not significant.

The Ho is accepted (Variation is due to chance).

Where Ho is null hypothesis Ho is a tentative statement related to the population and always stated negatively, e.g. there is no difference in the birth weight of babies born in two different hospitals.

Or

There is no difference in growth rate of babies belonging to two different socioeconomic groups.

Test of Significance (for Small Sample Size)

t-Distribution

If we have to test the difference between two sample means of small size (usually less then 30) the sample standard deviation will not be the accurate estimate of the population SD. Secondary it has been shown mathematically that the ratio of difference between two means to their SD will not be following the normal distribution. But it will follow a slightly different distribution known as "Students t-distribution". The tests based on this distribution are known as t-tests. There are two t-tests.

i. t-tests for unpaired data
ii. t-tests for paired data.

Criteria for Applying t-test

1. Random samples
2. Quantitative data
3. Variable normally distributed
4. Sample size less than 30.

t-tests for Unpaired Data

This test is used when two types of observation one on controlled group and the other on experimental group are available to test the significance of difference between means of the two groups.

Steps involved in the test: Suppose X and Y are two series of observations.

1. Make the null hypothesis that there is no difference between the two sample means.
2. Calculate the difference between the two sample means.
3. Calculate combined standard deviation.

$$CSD = \sqrt{\frac{\Sigma(X - \bar{X}) + \Sigma\,(Y - \bar{Y})^2}{n_1 + n_2 - 2}}$$

Standard Error of Difference

Standard error of difference is then calculated as

$$SED = CSD\sqrt{\frac{1}{n_1}+\frac{1}{n_2}}$$

$$tc = \frac{(\bar{X}-\bar{Y})}{SED}$$

Note: $> t$ 0.05 for df $(n_1 + n_2 - 2)$ the difference is significant
Ho is rejected (Variation is due to external factors)
$< t$ 0.05 for df $(n_1 + n_2 - 2)$ the difference is not significant
Ho is accepted (Variation is due to chance for biological variation)

t-tests for Paired Data

The paired t-test is used when paired observations are available. This is when:

i. Observation are made on the same individual before and after exposure to some factor (or treatment) under study.
ii. The same sample is tested by two methods.

Before proceeding with the test we first frame the null hypothesis that there is no real difference between the two sets of observations.

Steps for Paired t-test

1. Calculate the difference in each set of observations ($x - y = z$). This will form the new set of observation (z series).
2. Find out the mean of this series (Z).
3. Compute the *SEz* by the formula.

i. $SDz = \sqrt{\frac{\Sigma Z^2 - \left(\frac{\Sigma Z}{n}\right)^2}{n-1}}$ ii. $SE_2 = \frac{SD_2}{\sqrt{n}}$ iii. $t = \frac{\bar{Z}}{SE_2}$

$t = \frac{\bar{Z}}{SE_2}$ $> t$ 0.05 for df (n – 1) the difference is significant.

$< t$ 0.05 for df (n – 1) the difference is not significant. Ho is accepted.

Standard Error of Proportion (Large Sample Size)

Whenever the statistical value is of qualitative type it is the customary to express it in proportion of percentages.

The SE of proportions is computed to know the variation in proportions of different samples drawn from the same population due to chance it is given by:

$$SE_P = \sqrt{\frac{P \times q}{n}}$$

p = Sample proportion (expressed in percentage)
$q = 1 - p$ (expressed in percentage)

When p is the percentage of individuals belonging to one category and q is the percentage of the individuals belonging to the other category and n is the number of individuals in the sample. Since, all sample proportions p and q follow the normal distribution the confidence limits can be calculated to find the range for p the population percentage.

As a convention we take 1.96 times. SE as a criteria. If the difference exceeds 1.96 (SE) the difference is said to be significant statistically. This rule applies for a large sample size (>30) taken from the same population. For small sample this does not hold good. Since, the distribution of proportion follows the normal distribution the CL can also be computed.

P ± 1. SEp Contains 68.27 percent of sample proportions
P ± 2. SEp Contains 95.45 percent of sample proportions
P ± 3. SEp Contains 99.73 percent of sample proportions

Standard Error of Difference between Two Proportions (Large Sample)

As we have tested the standard error of difference between two means in case of quantitative data, we can similarly test the difference between two proportion in case of qualitative data by using SE of proportions.

The difference between proportions in a pair samples will vary from pair to pair and from even sample to sample though they are drawn from the same population or universe.

The object of the test is to determine the size of difference that is likely to occur by chance in samples of given size and how far it can deviated by chance. In reasonably large sample the SE of difference may be taken as the sum of square root of the two individual standard errors of values in two samples.

Steps for Calculation

1. Compute the difference between proportion $|(P_1 - P_2)|$

2. $SE_{(p_1 - p_2)} = \sqrt{\frac{p_1 q_1}{n_1} + \frac{p_2 q_2}{n_2}}$

3. $Z = \frac{|P_1 - P_2|}{SE_{(p_1 - p_2)}}$

Probability of a Larger Value of 't' (Table 28.1)

Table 28.1: Probability (P)

df	*0.10*	*005*	*001*	*0.001*
1	6.31	12.71	63.66	636.62
2	2.92	4.30	9.39	31.60
3	2.35	3.18	5.84	12.94
4	2.13	2.78	4.60	8.61
5	2.02	2.57	4.03	6.89
6	1.94	2.47	3.71	5.96
7	1.90	2.37	3.50	5.41
8	1.86	2.31	3.36	5.04
9	1.83	2.26	3.25	4.78
10	1.81	2.23	3.17	4.59
11	1.80	2.20	3.11	4.44
12	1.78	2.18	3.06	4.32
13	1.77	2.16	3.01	4.22
14	1.76	2.15	2.98	4.14
15	1.75	2.13	2.95	4.07
16	1.75	2.12	2.92	4.02
17	1.74	2.11	2.90	3.97
18	1.73	2.10	2.88	3.92
19	1.73	2.09	2.86	3.88
20	1.73	2.09	2.85	3.85
21	1.72	2.08	2.83	3.82
22	1.72	2.07	2.82	3.79
23	1.71	2.07	2.81	3.77
24	1.71	2.06	2.80	3.75
25	1.71	2.06	2.79	3.73
26	1.71	2.06	2.78	3.71
27	1.70	2.05	2.77	3.69
28	1.70	2.05	2.76	3.67
29	1.70	2.05	2.76	3.66
30	1.70	2.04	2.75	3.65
35	1.69	2.03	2.72	—
40	1.68	2.02	2.71	3.55
45	1.68	2.02	2.69	—
50	1.68	2.01	2.68	—
100	1.66	1.98	2.63	3.37
—	1.64	1.96	2.58	3.29

P = Probability of getting a larger value of 't' than indicated in the column by mere chance

df = Degrees of freedom

Note: > 1.96 the difference is significant
Ho is rejected
< 1.96 the difference is not significant
Ho is accepted

If the sample is small, then it follows *t*-test with prescribed degrees of freedom.

Normal Distribution

If we take large number of observations of a characteristic and if the observations are arranged in a frequency distribution with small class interval, the frequencies will be very small in the beginning and at the end, while the largest frequency is found to have concentrated somewhere in the middle class. The frequency curve drawn of such data will give us a smooth symmetric curve. This curve is normal curve. This is a curve of great importance in statistics theory as it is the basis of all statistical tests of significance. It is useful:

1. To estimate the population value based on a small sample.
2. To study whether two samples are drawn from the same population.
3. To know whether two samples values differ significantly or not.

Normal Curve

The normal curve is as shown in Figure 28.5.

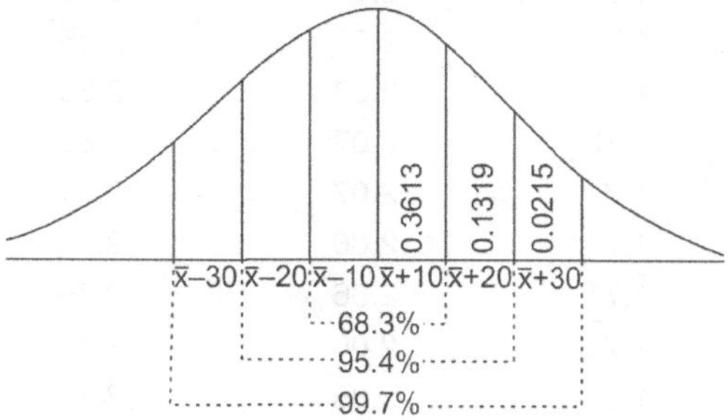

Fig. 28.5: Normal curve

Characteristics of the Normal Curve

The normal curve has the following characteristics—it is bell shaped curve.

1. The mean, median and the mode all coincide.
2. It is smooth symmetrical curve. The smoothness is due to small and equal class intervals. Symmetry means that the curve has one peak and its skewness is zero.
3. The whole area under the curve is unity.
4. By knowing the sample mean and standard deviation we can calculate

Table of the Unit Normal Distribution (Table 28.2)

Table 28.2: The normal distribution with mean zero and standard deviation unity

The normal variate with and standard deviation unity	*Proportion of individuals who do not exceed the value (Z)*	*Normal variate with mean = 0*	*Proportion of individuals who do not exceed the value (Z)*
	1	2	3 4
0.0	0.50000	2.3	0.98928
0.1	0.53983	2.4	0.99180
0.2	0.57926	2.5	0.99379
0.3	0.61791	2.6	0.99534
0.4	0.65542	2.7	0.99653
0.5	0.69146	2.8	0.99744
0.6	0.72575	2.9	0.99813
0.7	0.75804	....	....
0.8	0.78814	3.0	0.99865
0.9	0.81594	3.1	0.99903
....	....	3.2	0.99931
1.0	0.81434	3.3	0.99952
1.1	0.86433	3.4	0.99966
1.2	0.88493	3.5	0.99977
1.3	0.90320	3.6	0.99984
1.4	0.91924	3.7	0.99989
1.5	0.93319	3.8	0.99993
1.6	0.64520	3.9	0.99995
1.7	0.95543	....	....
1.8	0.96407	4.0	0.99997
1.9	0.97128	4.1	0.99998
....	....	4.2	0.99999
2.0	0.97725	4.3	0.99999
2.1	0.99214	4.4	0.99999
2.2	0.98610	....	....

the number of observations falling on both sides of mean at any multiple of SD by the help of this curve.

a. $\bar{X} \pm 1\ \sigma$ contains 68.27 (68.3) percent of observations

b. $\bar{X} \pm 2\ \sigma$ contains 95.45 (95.4) percent of observations

c. $\bar{X} \pm 3\ \sigma$ contains 99.73 (99.7) percent of observations

We thus find that the values that differ from the mean by more than twice the SD(s) are fairly large (5%) and that differ more than three times the SD(s) are very few (0.27) in normal distribution.

If mean height $\bar{X}$ is 160 cms, SD (σ) = 4 cms and height X is 166 cms. Z will be $\frac{X - \bar{X}}{\sigma} = \frac{166 - 160}{4} = 1.5$ corresponding $Z_{1.5}$ we find 0.93 out of one 93 percent height do not exceed 160 cms only seven percent of the subjects will be taller. To find proportion for negative values of Z subtract the corresponding proportion from one.

Chi-square Test (χ^2-Test)

Chi-square (χ^2): Test offers an alternate method of testing the significance of difference between two proportions. It can also be used when more than two groups are to compared.

It was developed by Karl Pearson and has got the following three common but very important application in medical statistics as test of:

1. Proportion
2. Association
3. Goodness of fit.

The test is usefull to know whether the observed frequencies in the distribution differ significantly from the expected frequencies calculated according to same assumed hypothesis like the other tests of significance it only shows the probability of chance operation.

a. Chi-square-test (χ^2-test) is done with the actual observations.

Table of Chi-square (Table 28.3)

Table 28.3: Probability (P)

d.f.	*.50*	*.10*	*.05*	*.02*	*.01*	*005*	*.001*
1	0.45	2.71	3.84	5.41	66.3	7.88	10.83
2	1.39	4.61	5.99	7.82	9.21	10.60	13.82
3	2.37	6.25	7.82	9.84	11.34	12.84	16.27
4	3.35	7.78	9.46	11.67	13.38	14.86	18.47
5	4.35	9.24	11.07	13.39	16.09	16.75	20.52
6	4.35	10.64	12.59	5.03	16.81	18.55	22.46
7	6.35	12.02	14.07	16.62	18.48	20.28	24.32
8	7.31	13.36	15.51	18.17	20.09	21.96	26.13
9	8.34	14.68	16.92	19.68	21.67	23.59	27.88
10	9.34	15.99	18.31	21.16	23.21	25.19	29.59
11	10.34	17.28	19.68	22.62	24.72	26.70	31.26
12	11.34	18.55	21.03	21.05	26.22	28.30	31.91

chi-square

P = Probability of getting a larger value of χ^2 by chance alone

df = Degrees of freedom

b. Degrees of freedom (df) are not related to the actual number of observations but on the number of columns and rows in the table, i.e.

d.f = $(c - 1)(r - 1)$, c for columns, and r for rows

c. Yate's correction is to be applied to the 2 × 2 contingency tables if any of the frequency in the cells is less than 5.

d. If the expected frequency in any group is less than five, it is to be clubed with the frequency of the previous group so that the total frequency is greater than five.

Formula

1. $x^2 = \sum \frac{(O - E)^2}{E}$

where O = observed frequency and E = expected frequency

2. $x^2 = \frac{(ab - bc)^2 N}{(a + b)(c + d)(a + c)(b + d)}$,

where $N = a + b + c + d$ and r = row c = columns

Yates correction – $x^2 = \frac{\left(|ab - bc| - \frac{N}{2} \right)^2 \times N}{(a + b)(c + d)(a + c)(b + d)}$

$$x^2 = \sum \frac{(|O - E| - 0.5)^2}{E}$$

Reject Ho if $x_c^2 > x^2$ 0.05 for df = $(c - 1)(r - 1)$

Accept Ho if $x_c^2 < x^2$ 0.05 for df = $(c - 1)(r - 1)$

Fallacies in Biostatistics

1. Comparison of dissimilar groups.
2. Use of different standard for classification.
3. Generalization from not representative sample.
4. Conclusions based on biased sample.
5. Conclusions from the relative values or proportion rates without considering absolute values or population.
6. Mixture of noncomparable records.
7. Consideration of association direct or indirect as the cause and effect.
8. Conclusion based on statistical significance alone without other important practical consideration.

Causes

1. Personal error
   - Interviewee
   - Interviewer
2. Institutional errors
   - Records

– Selection of the facts for reporting
3. Spurious correlation
4. Correlation of unusual situations.

Vital Statistics

Definition

Data which gives quantitative information on vital events occurring in life, i.e. births, deaths, marriages, etc.

Measures of Population

Mid-year population
Arithmetical progression method
$P_t = P_0 + rt$
where t is the period in years after the last census.
P_t = Population at the required time, i.e. t years after the last census.
P_o = Population of last census
r = Annual increase rate.

Geometrical Progression Method

$P_t = P_0 (1 + r)^t$ where P_o = Population of any census years and r = Annual increase per person in intercensal years. P_t = Population after t years

Measures of Vital Statistics

Measures of Fertility

1. Crude birth rate (CBR)

$$= \frac{\text{Number of live births which occurred among the population of a given geographical area during a given year}}{\text{Mid-year population of the same geographical area during same year}} \times 1000$$

2. General fertility rate (GFR)

$$= \frac{\text{Number of live births in one year}}{\text{Number of women aged 15-49 years}} \times 1000$$

3. Age specific fertility rate (ASFR)

$$= \frac{\text{Number of live births to mothers of a specified age group}}{\text{Mid-year female population of the same age group}} \times 1000$$

4. Gross reproduction rate (GRR)

$$= \frac{\text{Total number of female children born to women in the cohort sample}}{\text{Total number of women in the same cohort sample}}$$

5. Net reproduction rate (NRR)

$$= \frac{\text{Number of girls survived after the mortality experience}}{\text{Number of cohort women survived at the end of reproductive period as per their mortality experience}}$$

6. Sex ratio at birth

$$= \frac{\text{Number of female live births}}{\text{Number of male live birth}} \times 1000$$

Measures of Mortality

1. Crude death rate (CDR)

$$= \frac{\text{Number of death which occurred among the population of a given geographical area during a given year}}{\text{Mid-year population of the same geographical area during same year}} \times 1000$$

$$\text{CDR} = \frac{\text{D}}{\text{P}} \times 1000,\ \text{where D = Total death and P = Total population}$$

2. Age specific death rate (ASDR)

$$= \frac{\text{Number of deaths in the specified age group}}{\text{Mid-year population of the same age group}} \times 1000$$

3. Infant mortality rate (IMR)

$$= \frac{\text{Number of deaths under one year of age}}{\text{Number of live births}} \times 1000$$

4. Still or late fetal death rate

$$= \frac{\text{Fetal deaths of after 28 weeks of gestation}}{\text{Live births + still births}} \times 1000$$

5. Perinatal mortality rate (PMR)

$$= \frac{\text{Late fetal deaths (after 28 weeks or more)} + \text{deaths under 1 week}}{\text{Live births} + \text{still births}} \times 1000$$

6. Neonatal mortality rate (NMR)

$$= \frac{\text{Number of deaths up to 28 days of life}}{\text{Number of live births}} \times 1000$$

7. Post-neonatal mortality or late infant mortality rate

$$= \frac{\text{Deaths after 28 days of life up to one year}}{\text{Live births}} \times 1000$$

8. Cause specific mortality rate (CSMR)

$$= \frac{\text{Number of deaths in a year due to some cause}}{\text{Mid-year population}} \times 100000$$

9. Case fatality rate (CFR)

$$= \frac{\text{Number of deaths due to a particular disease}}{\text{Number of cases of the same disease}} \times 100$$

10. Proportional mortality rate (PMR)

$$= \frac{\text{Number of deaths from the specific disease in a year}}{\text{Total deaths from all causes in that year}} \times 100$$

Morbidity Statistics

1. Incidence rate (IR)

$$= \frac{\text{Number of persons becoming sick in a specified period of time}}{\text{Number of exposed to risk at the same period}} \times 1000$$

2. Period prevalence rate (PPR)

$$= \frac{\text{Number of person sick (Old + New) within a specific of time}}{\text{Number exposed to risk at the same period}} \times 1000$$

3. Point prevalence rate (PPR)

$$= \frac{\text{Number of person sick (Old + New) at a specified point of time}}{\text{Number of exposed to risk at the point of time}} \times 1000$$

4. Average duration of sickness

$$= \frac{\text{Point prevalence rate}}{\text{Incidence rate}}$$

INTERNATIONAL DEATH CERTIFICATE—CAUSE OF DEATH (TABLE 28.4)

Table 28.4: International death certificate—cause of death

Name of patients:	Approximate interval between onset and death
Address:	
Part 1	
Disease or condition directly leading to death (a) ________________	
Antecedent cause: Morbid condition if any:	
Giving rise to the above (b)	
Cause stating the underlying condition last (c)	
Part 2	
Other significant condition contributing to the death but not related to the death or condition causing it.________________	
	Signature

BIBLIOGRAPHY

1. Kulkarni AP, Baride JP. Textbook of community medicine, 2nd edn, 2002.
2. Mahajan BK. Methods in Biostatics, 6th edn, 1997.
3. Park's Textbook of PSM, 16th edn, 2000.

Chapter 29 Problems

CHAPTER OUTLINE

- ENVIRONMENTAL PROBLEMS
- CORRELATION AND REGRESSION
- EPIDEMIOLOGICAL AND NUTRITIONAL EXERCISES
- BIOSTATISTICS
- DEMOGRAPHY

ENVIRONMENTAL PROBLEMS

1. 1 cubic feet = 6.25 gallons of water
2. 1 cubic meter = 1000 liters of water
3. 1 gallon of water = 4.55 liters.
4. If blue color appears in I, II, and III up of Horrock's apparatus the required amount of bleaching powder to disinfect the well is 2,4, 6 gm for 100 gallons of water.
5. Standard bleaching powder contains 33 percent of available chlorine.
6. If available chlorine is 25 percent, i.e. ¼ for 1 gm, it is taken as inverse proportion and while calculating, multiply 1000 liter of water 5×4. This will give you required amount of bleaching powder to disinfect 1000 liters of water. If available chlorine in given sample of water is 20 percent in $\frac{1}{5}$ of 1 gram multiply by 2.
7. If the well is circular and measurement is in feet, calculate the total amount of water by using the formula $5D^2h$.
   Where D = diameter of well , h = depth of water
8. If the measurements are in meters, then:

   $$\pi r^2 h \text{ or } \frac{22}{7} r^2 h \text{ or } 3.14\, r^2 h$$

   where r = radius of well, h = depth of water
9. If the well is rectangular well then:
   $L \times b \times h \times 6.25$ which gives, gallons of water.
10. If measurements are in meters, then:
    $L \times b \times h \times 1000$ gives liters of water.

Problems

1. *Calculate the amount of bleaching powder required to disinfect a circular well having a diameter of 6 m and depth of water is 12 m. The Horrock's test shows blue color in 4th cup.*

Sol. Given $D = 6$ m, $R = 3$ m, $H = 12$ m

– The given data for circular well is in meters, so

$= 3.14\ r^2 h$

$= 3.14 \times 3^2 \times 12$

$= 3.14 \times 9 \times 12$

$= 3.14 \times 108$

$= 339.12$ m

– 1 cubic meter = 1000 liters of water

– 339.12 meter = ?

339.12 × 1000 = 339120 liters of water

– 4.55 liters = 1 gallon of water

– 339.120 liter = ?

– 339120/4.55 = 74531.868 gallons

– 100 gallons = 8 gm of bleaching powder

– 74531.868 = ?

– 74531.868 × 8/ 100 = 5962.5 gm

2. *Calculate the amount of bleaching powder required to disinfect a circular well where D = 5 feet and depth of water is 10 feet. Available chlorine is 33 percent in bleaching powder.*

Sol. Given D = 5 feet and h = 10 feet

– The given data for circular well is in feet, so

$5\ D^2 h = 5 \times 5^2 \times 10$

$= 5 \times 25 \times 10 = 1250$ feet

– 1 cubic feet = 6.25 gallons of water

1250 feet = ?

1250 × 6.25 = 7812.5 gallons of water.

– 1 gallon of water = 4.55 liters

7812.5 gallons of water = ?

7812.5 × 4.55 = 35546.87 liters

– 1000 liters – 2.5 gm of bleaching powder

35546.85 liters = ?

35546.85 × 2.5/1000 = 88867.18/1000

= 88.867 gm of bleaching powder.

3. *A well measuring 10 m in diameter having depth of water 20 m. Available chlorine is 25 percent in bleaching powder. Calculate the amount of bleaching powder required.*

Sol. Given D = 10 m, H = 20 m, R = 5 m

The given data for circular well is in meters, so

$= 3.14\ r^2 h$

$= 3.14 \times 5^2 \times 20$

$= 3.14 \times 25 \times 20$

= 3.14 × 500

= 1570 m

Available chlorine is 25 percent, i.e. ¼ of gm = 0.25 gm

Hence,

= 1570 × 0.25 × 4

= 1570 × 1 = 1570 gm

= 1.57 kg.

4. *Calculate the amount of bleaching powder required if L = 6 feet, B= 8 feet, D = 25 feet Horrock's apparatus shows blue color in 12th cup.*

Sol. The given data for rectangular well is in feet, so

= $L \times b \times h \times 6.25$

= 6 × 8 × 25 × 6.25

= 48 × 156.25

= 7500 gallons of water

– 100 gallons = 24 gm of bleaching powder, then:

7500 gallons = ?

7500 × 24 = 1800 gm

= 1.8 kg

5. *An annual fair has been organized in summer season in a village on the bank of river. What arrangements you shall make for the safe drinking water for the fair?*

Sol.
- The survey should be done by Medical Officer (MO). The fair consists of a large number of people.
- Gathered at one place it is the site for the spread of many diseases.

Arrangements:
- The site should be surveyed by Medical Officer.
- As the fair is to be conducted on the bank of rivers, all the precautions should be taken to prevent contamination of water.
- Fencing of river should be done, to prevent people going in for wash.
- Safe drinking water should be provided by constructing reserviours tanks separately away from the gathering place, which should be provided with taps to prevent contamination.
- The surrounding should be kept clean or platform should be constructed so that there is no stagnation of water.
- Water should be changed regularly *one* for two days.
- Health education to the people regarding water-borne disease.

6. *There is an NCC camp of 100 students in the outskirts of the city. What type of sanitary measures you suggest?*

Sol. *Arrangements:*
- The site should be surveyed by Medical Officer.
- It should be selected in such a way that it should be clean, free from endemic diseases.

- It should be free from mosquito and fly-breeding sites.
- Trench latrine should be provided for some days, shallow latrines, for weeks and for months deep trench latrine.
- Disposal of refuse should be done by controlled tipping.
- Safe water should be provided by boiling and cooling the water and chlorine tablets.
- All the students should be advised to have separate beds, towels, to prevent communicable diseases.

BIOSTATISTICS

1. *Following are the respiratory rates of 10 infants suspected to be suffering from acute respiratory infection.*
   53, 52, 55, 48, 54, 59, 46, 58, 49 and 60.
   Find the measures of central tendency.

Sol.

i. Mean $= \dfrac{\sum_{i=1}^{n} x_i}{n} = \dfrac{534}{10} = 53.4$

ii. Median $= \left(\dfrac{n+1}{2}\right)^{th}$ value in the arranged series.

Arranging the data in ascending order:

46, 48, 49, 52, 53, 54, 55, 58, 59, 60

$= \left(\dfrac{10+1}{2}\right)^{th}$ value

$= \left(\dfrac{11}{2}\right)^{th}$ value = 5.5th

i.e. Average of 5th and 6th value

$= \dfrac{53+54}{2} = 53.5.$

iii. Mode: Mode does not exist.
Mode is most repeated value or the value which possesses the highest frequency. Here, in this problem not any value repeats, i.e. it indicates mode does not exist in this distribution.

2. *During the MCH clinic at Devarayasamudra RHTC, the Hb% of 10 ANC and 10 PNC women were recorded as follows:*
   ANC (gm%) : 12, 11, 10, 12, 12, 11, 08, 06, 09, 08
   PNC (gm%) : 11, 09, 10, 11, 10, 11, 07, 08, 05, 07
   Calculate the measures of dispersion and compare the coefficient of variation.

Sol. i. Take ANC group. Write the data in ascending order:
6, 08, 08, 09, 10, 11, 11, 12, 12, 12

Range = H – L
= 12 – 6
= 6

$$\text{Mean deviation (from Mean)} = \frac{\sum_{i=1}^{n} |(x_i - \overline{x})|}{n}$$

$$= \frac{17.2}{10} = 1.72$$

X	$\overline{x}$	$\lvert(x_i - \overline{x})\rvert$	$(x_i - \overline{x})^2$
12		2.1	4.41
11		1.1	1.21
10		0.1	0.01
12		2.1	4.41
12	9.9	2.1	4.41
11		1.1	1.21
08		1.9	3.61
06		3.9	15.21
09		0.9	0.81
08		1.9	3.61
		17.20	38.90

(for $n < 30$)

$$\text{Standard deviation} = \sqrt{\frac{\sum_{i=1}^{n}(x_i - \overline{x})^2}{n-1}}$$

$$= \sqrt{\frac{38.9}{9}}$$

$$= \sqrt{4.3222}$$

$$\text{SD} = 2.0790 = \sigma$$

$$\text{Coefficient of variation} = \frac{\sigma}{\overline{x}} \times 100$$

$$\left[\text{where mean } (\overline{x}) = \frac{\sum_{i=1}^{n} x_i}{n} = \frac{99}{10} = 9.9 \right]$$

$$\text{CV} = \frac{2.0790}{9.9} \times 100 = 0.2100 \times 100$$

CV for ANC group = 21

ii. Take PNC group:
Write the data in ascending order:
05, 07, 07, 08, 09, 10, 10, 11, 11,11
Range = 11 – 05 = 6
Range = 6

$$\text{Mean deviation} = \frac{\sum_{i=1}^{n} |x_i - \bar{x}|}{n}$$

x_1	$\bar{x}$	$\lvert(x_{i1} - \bar{x})\rvert$	$(x_{i1} - \bar{x})^2$
11		2.1	4.41
09		0.1	0.01
10		1.1	1.21
11		2.1	4.41
10	8.9	1.1	1.21
11		2.1	4.41
07		1.9	3.61
08		0.9	0.81
05		3.9	15.21
07		1.9	3.69
		17.2	38.9

$$\left(Mean = \frac{\sum_{i=1}^{n} x_i}{n} = \frac{89}{10} = 8.9 \right)$$

$$\text{Mean deviation} = \frac{\sum_{i=1}^{n} |(x_i - \bar{x})|}{n}$$

$$= \frac{17.2}{10} = 1.72$$

$$\text{Standard deviation} = \sqrt{\frac{\sum_{i=1}^{n} (x_i - \bar{x})^2}{n-1}}$$

$$= \sqrt{\frac{38.9}{9}}$$

$$= \sqrt{4.3222}$$

$$SD = 2.0790$$

$$\therefore CV = \frac{\sigma}{\bar{x}} \times 100 = \frac{2.0790}{8.9} \times 100$$

$$= 0.2336 \times 100$$

$$= 23.36$$

CV of ANC group is less than CV of PNC group

3. *The following data represents the total weight gain in kg of 15 women at the end of 9th month of pregnancy:*
   06, 08, 07, 10, 06, 07, 07, 08, 09, 11, 10, 10, 12, 14, 12.
   Calculate the measures of central tendency and discuss the limitations of the mean.

Sol. i. Mean $= \bar{x} = \frac{\sum_{i=1}^{n} x_i}{n} = \frac{137}{15} = 9.1333$

ii. Median is the middle most value in the arranged series:
06, 06, 07, 07, 07, 08, 08, 09, 10, 10, 10, 11, 12, 12, 14.

$$\text{Median} = \left(\frac{n+1}{2}\right)^{th} \text{ value}$$

$$= \left(\frac{15+1}{2}\right)^{th} \text{ value}$$

$$= \left(\frac{16}{2}\right)^{th} \text{ value} = 8\text{th value}$$

Median = 9

iii. Mode = Most repeated value
In this problem 07 and 10 repeat three times. Therefore, this is a
"Bimodel"distribution. Both 7 and 10 are the modes.

Limitations of the Mean

- It is unduly influenced by an abnormal value in the distribution.
- It cannot be easily calculated in the case of distributions containing open-end class-interval.
- If one of value of the items is missing, the arithmetic mean cannot be calculated.
- Sometimes it gives fallacious conclusions.
- It has an upward bias. It gives less importance to smaller items and more importance to larger items in the data, i.e. a large item in the series can push-up the value of arithmetic mean considerably, but a small item cannot pull down the value of it to the same extent.

4. *In a series of boys during admission to a college the mean height was 160 cm and the standard deviation was 10 cm. In the same series, the mean weight was 55 kg and the standard deviation was 5 kg. Find which of the above two characters show greater variation.*

Sol. CV of 1st character $= \frac{\sigma}{\bar{x}} \times 100$

$$\therefore \quad CV = \frac{10}{160} \times 100$$

and $$CV = 6.25\%$$

CV of IInd character $= \frac{\sigma}{\bar{x}} \times 100$

$$\therefore \quad CV = \frac{5}{55} \times 100$$

$$CV = 9.09\%$$

Thus, we find that the 2nd character shows greater variation.

5. *The systolic BP of male and female interns posted to UHC, Gulpet, is as follows:*

Males : 130, 120, 126, 128, 122, 142, 116 and 160
Females : 110, 120, 100, 114, 108, 102, 110 and 110

Calculate arithmetic mean and standard deviation.
Comment on the above data.

Sol. For males:

X_1	$\bar{x}$	$\lvert(x_i - \bar{x})\rvert$	$(x_i - \bar{x})^2$
130		0.5	0.25
120		10.5	110.25
126		4.5	20.25
128		2.5	6.25
122	130.5	8.5	72.25
142		11.5	132.25
116		14.5	210.25
160		29.5	870.25
1044			1422

Arithmetic mean for males $= \bar{x}$

$$\bar{x} = \frac{1044}{8} = 13.05.$$

$$\text{Standard deviation} = \sqrt{\frac{\sum_{i=1}^{n}(x_i - \bar{x})^2}{n-1}}$$

$$= \sqrt{\frac{1422}{8-1}} = \sqrt{\frac{1422}{7}}$$

$$\therefore \text{SD} = \sqrt{203.1428}$$

$$\text{SD} = 14.25$$

For females:

x_1	$\bar{x}$	$\lvert(x_i - \bar{x})\rvert$	$(x_i - \bar{x})^2$
110		0.75	0.56
120		10.75	115.56
100		9.25	85.56
114		4.75	22.56
108	109.25	1.25	1.56
102		7.25	52.56
110		0.75	0.56
110		0.75	0.56
874			279.48

$$\text{Arithmetic mean for females} = \frac{\sum_{i=1}^{n} x_i}{n} = \frac{874}{8} = 109.25$$

$$\text{Standard deviation} = \sqrt{\frac{\sum_{i=1}^{n}(x_i - \bar{x})^2}{n-1}}$$

$$= \sqrt{\frac{279.48}{8-1}} = \sqrt{\frac{279.48}{7}}$$

$$\therefore \text{SD} = \sqrt{39.9257}$$

$$\text{SD} = 6.3186$$

Comments: On comparing the SD values for males and females, it is concluded that:

(SD value for male = 14.25 and
SD value for female = 6.31)

The deviation of values from mean in the male is greater than the female values.

6. *The respiratory rate in 10 persons was as follows:*
   20, 21, 22, 16, 19, 18, 19, 17, 20 and 18.
   Calculate the range, mean deviation, standard deviation and coefficient of variation.

Sol. Range = H – L = 22 – 16
Range = 4

x_i	$\bar{x}$	$(x_i - \bar{x})$	$(x_i - \bar{x})^2$
20		1	1
21		2	4
22		3	9
16		3	9
19		0	0
18	19	1	1
19		0	0
17		2	4
20		1	1
18		1	1
190		14	30

$$\text{Mean deviation} = \frac{\sum_{i=1}^{n}|(x_i - \bar{x})|}{n} = \frac{14}{10} = 1.4$$

$$\text{Standard deviation} = \sqrt{\frac{\sum_{i=1}^{n}(x_i - \bar{x})^2}{n-1}}$$

$$= \sqrt{\frac{30}{9}}$$

$$\therefore \text{SD} = \sqrt{3.3333}$$

$$\text{SD} = 1.8257$$

$$\text{CV} = \frac{\sigma}{\bar{x}} \times 100$$

$$= \frac{1.82}{19} \times 100$$

$$= 0.0957 \times 100$$

$$\text{CV} = 9.57$$

CORRELATION AND REGRESSION

1. Here the variables are non-correlated. Because the points spread all over the graph.

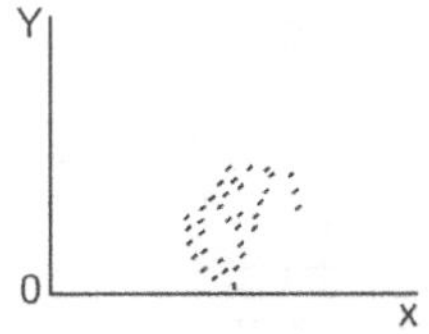

2. The variables are positively correlated. Because the points cluster around a line with positive slope. (It is also called partially positive correlation)
(Moderately + ve correlation)

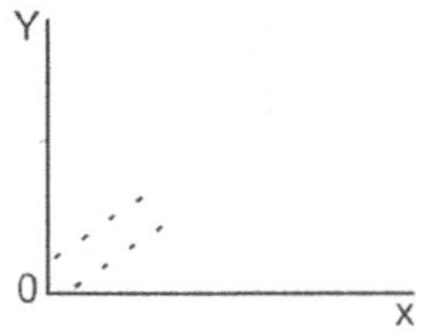

3. The variables are positively and perfectly correlated. Because the points form a line with positive slope.

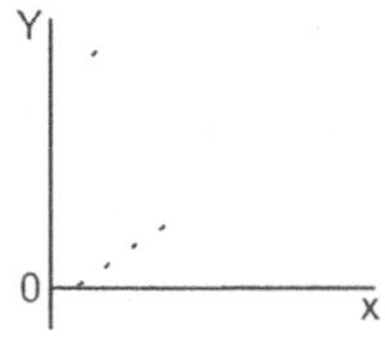

4. There is a curvilinear relation between the variables.

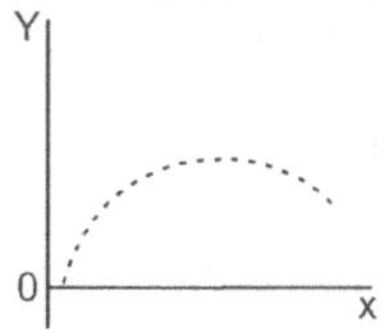

5. The variables are negatively very correlated. Because the points cluster around a line with negative slope (It is also called partially negative correlation)
(Moderately –ve correlation)

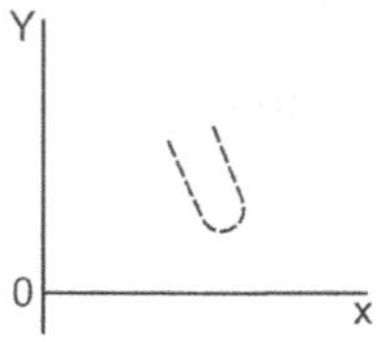

6. This diagram indicates curvilinear relation between the variables.

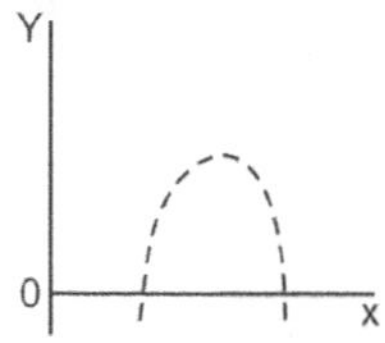

7. The variables are perfect –ve correlation. Because the points form a line with –ve slope

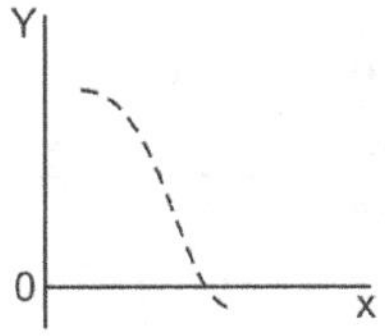

8. The variables are perfectly –vely correlated.

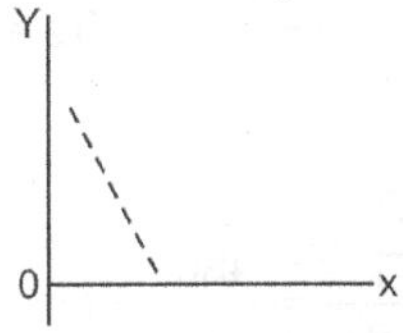

Problems

1. *Find the value 'r' for the following data:*
   X—48, 52, 60, 45, 65, 72, 80, 50
   Y—50, 55, 72, 50, 60, 60, 78, 55.

Sol. Karl Pearson's coefficient of correlation between two variables X and Y is:

$$r_{xy} = \frac{\text{Covariance } (x, y)}{\sqrt{\text{var } (x) \times \text{var } (y)}} = \frac{\text{Cov } (x, y)}{\sigma_x \, \sigma_y}$$

$$r_{xy} = \frac{\Sigma(x-\bar{x})(y-\bar{y})}{\sqrt{\Sigma(x-\bar{x})^2 \, \Sigma(y-\bar{y})^2}}$$

X	Y	$(x-\bar{x})$	$(y-\bar{y})$	$(x-\bar{x})(y-\bar{y})$	$(x_i-\bar{x})^2$	$(y-\bar{y})^2$
48	50	–11	–10	110	121	100
52	55	–7	–5	35	49	25
60	72	1	12	12	1	44
45	50	–14	–10	140	196	100
65	60	6	0	0	36	0
72	60	13	0	0	169	0
80	78	21	18	378	441	324
50	55	–9	–5	45	81	25
				720	1094	718

$$\therefore \qquad r_{xy} = \frac{\Sigma(x-\bar{x})(y-\bar{y})}{\sqrt{\Sigma(x-\bar{x})^2(y-\bar{y})^2}}$$

[When means are not known, we can use:

$$r = \frac{n\Sigma\, xy - (\Sigma x)(\Sigma y)}{\sqrt{\left[n\Sigma x^2 - (\Sigma x)^2 \times \sqrt{\left[n\Sigma y^2 - (\Sigma y)^2\right]}\right.}}$$]

$$\bar{x} = \frac{\sum_{i=1}^{n} x_i}{n} = \frac{472}{8} = 59 \text{ and}$$

$$\bar{y} = \frac{\sum_{j=1}^{n} y_i}{8} = \frac{480}{8} = 60.$$

From the table,

$$= \frac{720}{\sqrt{1094 \times 718}} = \frac{720}{\sqrt{785492}}$$

$$= \frac{720}{886.2815} = 0.8123 = 0.8 = r_{xy} = 0.8$$

i.e. the variables are +vely correlated.

2. *Find the regression coefficients for:*

X : 10, 15, 16, 20, 21, 17, 12, 13, 18 and 8

Y : 7, 16, 20, 18, 19, 21, 10, 14, 19, 6

Sol. The regression coefficients are:

$$b_{xy} = \frac{\Sigma(x-\bar{x})(y-\bar{y})}{\Sigma(x-\bar{x})^2}$$

$$\text{and } b_{yx} = \frac{\Sigma(x-\bar{x})(y-\bar{y})}{\Sigma(y-\bar{y})^2} \text{ if means are known.}$$

[If the means are not known, then we can use

$$b_{xy} = \frac{r \cdot \sigma_x}{\sigma_y} = \frac{n\Sigma\, xy - (\Sigma x)(\Sigma y)}{n\Sigma\, y^2 - (\Sigma y^2)}$$

$$\text{and } b_{yx} = \frac{r \cdot \sigma_y}{\sigma_x} = \frac{n\Sigma\, xy - (\Sigma x)(\Sigma y)}{n\Sigma\, x^2 - (\Sigma x^2)}$$]

Applying the first formulae for b_{xy} and b_{yx}

x	y	$(x-\bar{x})$	$(y-\bar{y})$	$(x-\bar{x})(y-\bar{y})$	$(x_i-\bar{x})^2$	$(y-\bar{y})^2$
10	7	–5	–8	40	25	64
15	16	0	1	0	0	1
16	20	1	5	5	1	25
20	18	5	3	15	25	09
21	19	6	4	24	36	16
17	21	2	6	12	4	36
12	10	–3	–5	15	9	25
13	14	–2	–1	2	4	1
18	19	3	4	12	9	16
8	6	–7	–9	63	49	81
Total=150	150			188	162	274

$$\bar{x} = \frac{\Sigma x}{n} = \frac{150}{10} = 15$$

$$\bar{y} = \frac{\Sigma y}{n} = \frac{150}{10} = 15$$

$$b_{xy} = \frac{(x-\bar{x})(y-\bar{y})}{(x-\bar{x})^2} = \frac{188}{162}$$

$$\therefore \quad b_{xy} = 1.16$$

$$\therefore \quad b_{yx} = \frac{(x-\bar{x})(y-\bar{y})}{(y-\bar{y})^2} = \frac{188}{274}$$

$$\therefore \quad b_{yx} = 0.6861$$

3. *For the following data calculate correlation coefficient to determine association if any between fluoride content of drinking water and community fluorosis index:*

Drinking water fluoride level mg/L	*Community fluorosis index*
0.8	0.1
1.3	0.4
1.5	0.9
1.9	0.6
2.3	0.7
2.4	1.1
2.6	0.8
3.5	1.1

Sol. Karl Pearson's correlation coefficient '*r*'

$$r_{xy} = \frac{Cov\,(x, y)}{\sqrt{\text{var}\,(x) \times \text{var}\,(y)}} = \frac{Cov\,(x, y)}{\sigma_x \sigma_y}$$

$$r_{xy} = \frac{\Sigma(x-\bar{x})\,(y-\bar{y})}{\sqrt{\Sigma(x-\bar{x})^2\,\Sigma(y-\bar{y})^2}}$$

X	y	$(x-\bar{x})$	$(y-\bar{y})$	$(x-\bar{x})\,(y-\bar{y})$	$(x-\bar{x})^2$	$(y-\bar{y})^2$
1.8	0.1	– 0.36	– 0.6	0.216	0.1296	0.36
1.3	0.4	– 0.86	– 0.3	0.258	0.7396	0.09
1.5	0.8	– 0.66	0.1	– 0.066	0.4356	0.01
1.9	0.6	– 0.26	– 0.1	+ 0.026	0.0676	0.01
2.3	0.7	0.14	0	0.000	0.0196	0
2.4	1.1	0.24	0.4	0.096	0.0576	0.16
2.6	0.8	0.44	0.1	0.044	0.1936	0.01
3.5	1.1	1.34	0.4	0.536	1.7956	0.16
Total: 17.3	5.6			1.11	3.4388	0.8

$$\bar{x} = \frac{\Sigma x_i}{n} = \frac{17.3}{8} = 2.16$$

$$\bar{y} = \frac{\Sigma y_i}{n} = \frac{5.6}{8} = 0.7$$

$$r_{xy} = \frac{\Sigma(x-\bar{x})\,(y-\bar{y})}{\sqrt{\Sigma(x-\bar{x})^2\,\Sigma(y-\bar{y})^2}}$$

$$= \frac{1.11}{\sqrt{3.4388 \times 0.8}} = \frac{1.11}{\sqrt{2.7510}} = \frac{1.11}{1.65}$$

$$r_{xy} = \frac{1.11}{1.6586} = 0.6692 \qquad r_{xy} = \quad 0.7.$$

This indicates there is +ve correlation between these two variables.

DEMOGRAPHY

1. *The census population of Kolar town.*

1981	: 75,000
1982	: 87,000
No. of live births in 1988	: 1250
Total no. of deaths in 1988	: 750
No. of infant deaths	: 70
Deaths of infants within 1 month of births	: 30

   a. *Calculate all vital statistics rates for 1988*

   b. *Compare with current national rates and comment.*

Sol. a. For the calculation of 1988 vital rates,

CBR = (Total births/Mid year population of 1988) × 1000

Mid year population (MYP) of 1988

Pt = P + rt

MYP of 1988 = 75000 + rt

Increase in 10 years

= 87000 – 75000

= 12000

Average increase per year = 12000/10 = 1200

MYP of 1988 = 75000 + (1200 × 7) + (1200 × 1/3)

= 75000 + 8400 + 400

= 83800

b. i. CBR = (Total births/Mid year population of 1988) × 1000

= (1250/83800) × 1000

= 0.0149 × 1000

CBR = 14.9

ii. CDR = (No. of deaths registered during a year in an area/Mid year population of 1988) × 1000

= (750/83800) × 1000

= 8.9498

iii. IMR = (Number of deaths under one year of age or infants/ No. of live births) × 1000

= (70/1250) × 1000

IMR = 7000/125 = 56

iv. NMR = Neonatal mortality rate

= (No. of deaths up to 28 days of life/ No. of live births) × 1000

NMR = (30/1250) × 1000 = 3000/125 = 24

2. *The following vital events are recorded in Kolar district for 1991:*

MYP of 1991	:	22,00000
Total no. of deaths in 1991	:	20,000
Total no. of live birth in 1991	:	40,000
Newly diagnosed TB cases	:	220
Old cases of TB	:	880
No. of deaths due to TB	:	140

Calculate all vital indices for 1991 [comment on the growth rate of the district with reference to the current year].

Sol. CBR = (No. of live births/Mid year population of 1991) × 1000

= (40000/2200000) × 1000

= 18.1818

CDR = (No. of deaths/MYP of 1991) × 1000

= (20000/2200000) × 1000

CDR = 200/22 = 9.0909

3. *The following is the data of DSRM. PHC area for 1997:*

Midyear popn	:	70000
Total deaths	:	1050
Total birth	:	2500
Total infant deaths	:	300
No. of maternal deaths	:	15
No. of death with in 28 days	:	120

Calculate all vital rates of the PHC area for 1997. *Compare with the goal for* 2000 AD.

Sol. i. CBR = (No. of live births/Mid year population of 1997) × 1000
= (2500/70000) × 1000
CBR = 250/7 = 35.742

ii. CDR = (Total no. of deaths/MYP of 1997) × 1000
= (1050/70000) × 1000
CDR = 105/7 = 15

iii. Infant mortality rate
= (Total infant deaths/No of live births) × 1000
IMR = (300/2500) × 1000
= 3000/25
∴ IMR = 120

iv. Maternal mortality rate
MMR = (No. of maternal deaths/Total of live births) × 1000
= (15/2500) × 1000
= 150/25 = 6
MMR = 6

v. Neonatal mortality rate
= (No. of deaths with 28 days of life
No. of live births) × 1000
NMR = (120/2500) × 1000
= 1200/25
= 48

4. *The MYP of Kolar town in 1998 was 90,000 and the following vital indices were reported:*

CBR = 24/1000 MYP
CDR = 10/1000 MYP
IMR = 80/1000 LB
MMR = 3/1000 LB

Calculate :

i. No. of births
ii. No. of deaths
iii. Infant deaths
iv. Maternal deaths
v. Growth rate for 1998.

Sol. i. CBR = (No. of births/MYP of Kolar) × 1000

∴ No. of births = (CBR × MYP)/1000

= (24 × 90,000)/1000 = 2160

∴ No. of births = 2160

Similarly

ii. No. of deaths = (CDR × MYP)/1000

= (10 × 90,000)/1000

∴ No. of deaths = 900

iii. IMR = (No. of infant deaths/Total no. of live births) × 1000

∴ No. of infant deaths = (80 × 2160)/1000

= 1728/10 =172.8

∴ Infant deaths = 172.8

iv. MMR = (No. of maternal deaths/No. of live births) × 1000

Maternal deaths = (3 × 2160)/1000

= 6480/1000 = 6.48

∴ Maternal deaths = 6.48

v. Growth rate for 1998 = Birth rate – Death rate

= 24 –10

∴ GR = 14/1000 MYP

5. *The MYP of PHU is 35,000. The age wise population of women and live births is given below :*

Age group	*No. of women*	*No. of live births*
15-25	3500	300
25-35	5500	600
35-45	3000	200
Total	12000	1100

Calculate

i. CBR

ii. Age specific fertility rate

iii. Total fertility rate

iv. Comment on the results.

Sol. i. CBR = (Total births/Mid year population) × 1000

= (1100/35000) × 1000

∴ CBR = 31.4285

ii. Age specific fertility rate

In the first group, i.e. for 15 to 25 age group

ASFR = (No. of live births reported at 15-25 age group/ No. of mothers at the same age group) × 1000

ASFR = (300/3500) × 1000

= 3000/35

= 85.71

ASFR for the age-group 25 to 35 i.e.

ASFR = (600/5500) × 1000
= 6000/55 =109.0909
= 109.1

and ASFR for the age group 35 to 45

ASFR = (200/3000) × 1000

ASFR = 2000/30 = 66.66

iii. Total

Fertility rate = Addition of the ASFR gives us TFR

TFR = 85.71 + 109.1 + 66.66
= 261.47

6. *The following is the data related to Mulbagal town for 1996:*

MYP	:	64000
No. of live births	:	1856
No. of deaths	:	704
No. of fetal deaths > 1000 gms	:	40
No. of deaths age < 1 week	:	20
No. of deaths aged < 4 weeks	:	120
No. of infant deaths	:	160
No. of maternal deaths between 28 weeks of pregnancy and 42nd day of delivery	:	8

Calculate CDR, CBR, MMR, perinatal mortality rate, NMR, IMR, GR.

Sol. i. CDR = (No. of deaths registered during a year in an area/Mid year population) × 1000
= (704/64000) × 1000

CDR = 11

ii. CBR = (No. of live births/Mid year population) × 1000

$$= \frac{1856}{64000} \times 1000 = 0.029 \times 1000 = 29$$

iii. MMR = (No. of female deaths registered during a year due to pregnancy and its complication/No. of live births during that year) × 1000

∴ MMR = (8/1856) × 1000

∴ MMR = 4.3103

iv. Perinatal mortality rate

= PMR = [Late fetal deaths (after 28 weeks or more) + deaths under one week/Total births (live + still)] × 1000
= [(40 + 20)/1856] × 1000
= (60/1856) × 1000
= 60000/1856

∴ PMR = 32.32

v. NMR = Neonatal mortality rate
= (Number of deaths upto 28 days of life/ Number of live births) × 1000
= (120/1856) × 1000
= 0.0646 × 1000 = 64.6

vi. IMR (Infant mortality rate)
IMR = (Number of deaths under one year of age/ Number of live births) × 1000
= (160/1856) × 1000
= 0.0862 × 1000
∴ IMR = 86.2

7. The census population of a district in 1981 and 1991 was 20,00,000 and 26,00,000 respectively calculate:
Mid Year population of 1989
What is the present growth rate of India

Sol:

Using arithmetical progression method
Population of a district in 1981 = 20,00,000
Population of a district in 1991 = 26,00,000
Increase in 10 years = 26,00,000 – 20,00,000 = 600,000
∴ Average increase per year = 60,000
∴ Mid year population in 1989 = Pt = Po+rt (from AP)
= 20,00,000 + 60000 × 8 + 60000 × 1/3
(1/3 Means 1st March to June 30th)
= 20,00,000 + 480,000 + 20,000
= 25,00,000

8. *In an estimated MYP of 100,000 there were 1500 live births and 850 deaths in 1995.*

No. of abortions reported	: 300
No. of fetal deaths (1000 gm)	: 50
Deaths 0-7 days	: 50
Deaths 8 day to 1 month	: 25
Deaths 1 month to 1 year	: 50

Woman in the child bearing age group constituted 20 percent of the population 400 deaths occurred in the age group of 45 years and above. These were:

Heart disease	: 200
Chronic lung disease	: 50
Neoplasms	: 80
Suicides	: 20
Others	: 50

Calculate
a. General fertility rate
b. IMR
c. PMR
d. Proportional mortality of deaths overs 45 years due to heart disease.

Sol. a. General fertility rate :

GFR = (No. of live births in one year/ No. of women aged 15-49 years) × 1000

GFR = (1500/20000) × 1000 = 75

(∵ 20% of the population are women in the child bearing age group).

b. IMR = (Number of deaths under one year of age/No. of live births) × 1000

∴ IMR = (50 + 25 + 50/1500) × 1000
= (125/1500) × 1000
= 0.0833 × 1000

∴ IMR = 83.3

c. PMR = (Late fetal deaths (after 28 weeks or more) + deaths under one week/Total births) × 1000
= (50 + 50/1500) × 1000

∴ PMR = (100/1500) × 1000 = 66.66

d. Proportional mortality of deaths over 45 years due to heart disease. Proportional mortality rate
= (No. of deaths due to specific cause/Total deaths) × 100

PMR = (200/400) × 100

(Deaths, due to heart disease = 200)

PMR = 50%

9. *Estimate the midyear population in the year 1985 given 1971 census population 548.1 million and 1981 census population 685.2 million.*

Sol. Population in the year 1981 = 685.2 million
Population in year 1971 = 548.1 million
Population growth in 10 years = 137.1 million
Annual rate of growth $= (P_t - P_0)/P_0 \times 1/10$
= (137.1/548.1) × 1/10
= 0.025

It is assumed that 'r' remains contant approximately.
Then by geometric growth model

$$P_t = P_0 (1 + r)^t$$

$$\text{Log } P_t = \text{Log}P_0 + t\log (1+ r)$$
$$= \log 685.2 + (4 + 1/3) \log (1 + 2.5/100)$$
$$= \log 685.2 + 13/3 \log 1.025$$
$$= 2.8358 + 4.33 \times 0.0107$$

$= 2.8358 + 0.0463$

$\therefore \quad \log P_t = 2.8821$

$\therefore \quad P_t = \text{Antilog}\ (2.8821)$

$= 762.3$ million.

EPIDEMIOLOGICAL AND NUTRITIONAL EXERCISES

1. *In a boarding house inhabited by 100 children all below 10 years, on 1/3/88, 10 cases of measles occurred. On the 11th a second batch of 35 cases were detected. Interrogation of those who had not contracted the disease revealed that 15 of them were previously immunized against measles. Determine the serial interval and the secondary attack rate of measles.*

Sol. Serial interval

= Gap between the onset of primary and secondary case.

= Gap between 1st and 11th March = 10 days.

Secondary attack rate

= No. of exposed persons developing diseases/Total no. of exposed/susceptible contacts × 100

Total no. exposed are 100 – 10 = 90

Out of these 15 who were immunized are not susceptible.

So no. susceptible are 90 – 15 = 75

∴ Secondary attack rate = 35/75 × 100

= 46.66%

2. *The 1994 MYP of a place was 5,000. There were 750 children below 5 years, and 500 from 5 to 10 years.*

   A lameness survey revealed that 4 of the children 5 to 10 years were lame. Determine the annual incidence of:

   a. Paralytic and

   b. All cases of poliomyelities in the total population.

Sol. Prevalence of polio in children of 5 to 10 years:

= Polio cases in 5-10 age group/Population of 5-10 age group × 1000

= 4/500 × 1000 = 8 per 1000

Correction for those cases not involving lower extremities:

= Prevalence of polio in 5-10 years group × 1.25

= 8 × 1.25 = 10 per 1000

Average annual incidence rate of 0-4 years:

= Corrected prevalence/No. of years of risk = 10/5 = 2 per 1000

a. Annual paralytic incidence for whole population:

= Average incidence of 0-4 years × proportion of 0-4 population

= 2 × 750/5000 = 0.3 per 1000

b. Incidence of all cases of poliomyelitis:

= Annual incidence × 1.33

= 0.3 × 1.33 = 0.399 per 1000

3. *The average daily calorie consumption of a weighing 60 kg person is 2770, and the protein intake 60 G. Determine his percent protein calories and comment.*

He is currently taking 100 G. Eggs daily and no groundnuts. He wishes to replace eggs with groundnuts. How much of the latter he must eat so that it furnishes him the same amount of absorbed protein as 100 G of eggs ? If the cost of egg is 2.50 per 100 G and of groundnuts, 25 per kg, how much less/ more he have to spend ?

Sol. a. Percent protein calories

= Energy given by protein/Total energy × 100

= 60 × 4.1/2770 × 100 = 8.88%

This is within the required range of 7 to 12 percent

b. Net protein utilization of egg is 96 percent

100 G of eggs have 13.3 G of Protein

of this 96/100 × 13.3 or 12.77 G is net protein utilization

Net protein utilization of groundnut is 55 percent

To get 55 G of protein utilization in this body 100 G of nut protein have to be consumed.

So to get 12.77———?

(12.77/55) × 100 = 23.22 G of Groundnut protein.

The percentage of protein is 25 percent so 23.22 G of Groundnut protein will be obtained from 23.22 × 100/1000 = 93 G

So, 100 G of egg costing 2.50 rupees should be replaced by 93 G of groundnut costing 93 × 25/1000 = 2.33 rupees.

Therefore, he will be saving 2.50 – 2.33 = 0.17 rupees.

4. *The estimated MYP of place for 1994 was 9,000. Its CBR was 30/1000 population IMR, 80/1000 live births and under 1 to 3 mortality 10/1000 children below three years.*

a. How many packets of ORS and how many tablets of septran with 20 mg. Methoprim and 100 mg, Sulphamethoxazole will be required for the treatment of episodes of acute diarrheal and respiratory diseases, respectively ? No change in the incidence is expected.

b. A mass polio-immunization camp is planned for January and another for February 1995 in which all children below three years would be given polio vaccine irrespective of previous history of vaccination. Determine the vials of oral polio vaccine that will be required. How many vaccine carriers will be needed to carry the vaccine to different immunization centers?

c. The place is being brought under CSSM Program in 1995. How many bottles of vitamin A concentrate will be required for carrying out vitamin A prophylaxis among infant during 1995?

Sol. a. i. Under 5 population is 15 percent

∴ Under 5 population = 15 percent of 9000 = 1,350

Average incidence of diarrhea is 2.5/epiosde/year/child.

∴ Total episodes of diarrhea in under fives:

$= 1{,}350 \times 2.5 = 3{,}375$

Only 10 percent require ORS packets.

That is 337.5 or 338 children require ORS packets.

Two packets per episodes with wastage of 30 percent

∴ ORS packets required = 338 × 2 + 30 wastage

= 676 + 203

= 879 packets of ORS.

ii. Incidence of respiratory diseases under 5 is 3 episodes/year/child.

∴ No. of episodes in 1350 children = 1350 × 3 = 4,050

Fifteen percent episodes or moderate or severe which need drug.

∴ 15% of 4050 = 608 episode need drug.

Each episode needs 2 tablets bd for 5 days, that is 20 Tablets per episodes.

∴ Total No. of Tablets = 608 × 20 = 12,160

b. To find the estimated population of Under 3, the following formula is used.

Estimated under 3 population:

= 3 MYP × Birth rate as decimal × (1-3 Death rate under 3 as decimal)

= 3 × 900 × 0.03 × (1-3 × 0.01) = 785.7 or 786

∴ Total doses of OPV required to immunize 786 under 3 children for second rounds:

2 × no. of children × WMF = 2 × 786 × 2 = 3144

1 OPV vial has 20 doses.

∴ OPV vials required = 3144/20 = 157.2 or 158

So, for 1st round 79 vials and second round also 79 and each vaccine carrier accommodates 15 vials.

∴ Vaccine carriers need = 79/15 = 5.2 or 6

Six vaccine carriers will sufficient for both round.

c. Estimated infants under one year:

= MYP × Birth rate as decimal × (1-IMR as decimal)

= 9000 × 0.03 × 0.92 = 248.4 or 249.

One lakh IU of vitamin A for 1 baby Under 1 years is required:

So, for 249 babies 249 lakh IU of vitamin A is required:

One bottle of vitamin A = 100 Ml

Each 1 ml = 1 lakh IU of vitamin A

Therefore, for 1 lakh IU we require 1 ml

For 249 lakh IU we require 249 ml, bottles are therefore – 3

5. *a.* *50,000 liters of water with fluorine concentration of 0.4 mg/L have to be fluoridated so as to bring the concentration to 1 mg/L determine the quantity of sodium fluoride required.*

   b. *During 1994, in an industry employing 1,000 workers, 200 remained absent. Of the later 10 were absent each for one day only; 20 for 2 days each; 30 for 4 days each, 40 for 6 days each; 60 for 12 days each and the remaining for 14 days each. Calculate the absenteeism rate of this industry for 1994.*

Sol. a. Fluorine concentration is 0.4 mg/liter.

Therefore, to get concentration of 1 PPM add 0.6 mg of fluorine per liters water.

Sodium fluoride contains 45 percent fluorine ions.

That is 1 mg Sodium fluorine gives 0.45 mg of fluorine.

Therefore, to get 0.6 mg fluorine sodium fluoride added is:

= 0.6/0.45 = 1.33 mg

Therefore, to get 1 PPM fluorine level, add 1.33 mg/liter of Sodium fluoride.

Required Sodium fluoride for 50,000 liters of water:

= 1.33 × 50,000 mg

= 66,500 mg = 66.5 gm.

No. of days absent	*No. of workers*	*Total no. of days of absenteeism*
10	1	10
20	2	40
30	4	120
40	6	240
60	12	720
40	14	560
		Total 1690

b. Absenteeism rate

= Total no. of days of absenteeism/Total no. of workers

= 1690/1000 = 1.69 days/head/year

6. *In June 1989, an epidemic of acute gastroenteritis occurred in a village. There were 160 cases of which 20 died. There are two wells in the village. Well 'A' is in the north which is used by 600 persons; 120 cases were noted among them. Well 'B' in the south is the source of water for the remaining 1000 persons among whom 40 cases were recorded.*

   The age and sex-distribution of the population of the village along with the cases and deaths in each age sex group is shown below.

Age group	*Males*			*Females*		
	Pop.	*Cases*	*Deaths*	*Pop.*	*Cases*	*Deaths*
0	130	30	12	120	20	8
5	200	40	0	180	20	0
15	270	25	0	300	15	0
35	150	10	0	100	0	0
55 and above	70	0	0	80	0	0
Total	820	105	12	780	55	8

a. *Analyze and interpret the above data.*
b. *What further information is necessary to elucidate the epidemiology of the epidemic?*

Sol. a. Analysis and interpretation:

i. Attach rate = 160/1600 × 1000 = 100/1000 population.

ii. Case fatality rate = Deaths/Cases × 100

$$= \frac{20}{100} \times 100 = 12.5\%$$

iii. CFR under 5 = Deaths < 5/Cases < 5 × 100
= 20/50 × 100 = 40%

Comment: All the deaths under five years. None in older children. This may be due to complicity of malnutrition in under fives.

iv. Attack rate in males = 105/820 × 1000 = 128/1000 males.
Attack rate in Females = 55/780 × 1000 = 70.5/1000 females

Comment: The disease is 128/70.5 or 1.8 time more in males.

v. Attack rate in different age groups:
Cases in that age group/Total persons in that age group × 1000

a. 50/250 × 1000 = 200/1000, children below 5
b. 60/380 × 1000 = 157.9/1000 children 5 -< 15
c. 40/570 × 1000 = 70.2/1000 persons 15 - < 35
d. 10/250 × 1000 = 40/1000 adults 35 - < 55
e. 0/150 × 1000 = Zero after 55 years age group

Comment: There is steady decline in the attack rate with rise in age up to 54 years. After 55 there are no cases. 'A'

vi. Well 'A'/Attack rate = 120/600 × 100 = 20%
Well 'B' attack rate = 40/1000 × 100 = 4%
Is this difference statistically significant.
H_o: There is no difference in the attack rates.

$$\text{Test criteria is Z} = \frac{|P_1 - P_2|}{SE_{(P_1 - P_2)}}$$

$$= SE_{(P_1 - P_2)} = \sqrt{\frac{p_1q_1}{n_1} + \frac{p_2q_2}{n_2}}$$

$$\therefore \quad SE_{(P_1 - P_2)} = \sqrt{\frac{20 \times 80}{600} + \frac{4 \times 96}{1000}} = 1.75$$

$$\therefore \quad Z = \frac{20 - 4}{1.75} = 9.14$$

Here Z = 9.14 > 1.96 $\therefore$ reject H_o

Therefore p.001

Therefore, rejected null hypothesis = 1.75

Comment: This epidemic is due to contamination of the water of well 'A'.

Miscellaneous Problems

1. *2000 smokers and 1000 matched non-smokers were followed-up. Lung cancer developed in 120 smokers and 20 nonsmokers. Find the absolute risk, relatives risk, attributable risk of lung cancer in smokers and comment on them.*

	Persons with lung cancer	*Persons without lung cancer*	*Total*
Smokers	120(a)	1880 (b)	2000 (a+b)
Non-smokers	20 (c)	980 (d)	1000 (c+ d)

Sol. Absolute Risk = Incidence of disease among smokers.

= a/a + b = 120/2000 = 0.06 or 6%

Relative risk

= Ratio of incidence of lung cancer between smokers and nonsmokers

$$= \frac{a/a+b}{c/c+d} = \frac{a\,(c+d)}{c\,(a+b)} = \frac{120 \times 1000}{20 \times 2000} = 3$$

Attributable risk

= incidence (risk) of disease that is attributed to smoking

$$= \frac{\frac{a}{a+b} - \frac{c}{c+d}}{\frac{a}{a+b}} \times 100$$

$$= \frac{0.06 - 0.02}{0.06} \times 100$$

$$= \frac{0.04}{0.06} \times 100 = 66.6\%$$

Comments:

- Lung cancer is three times commoner in smokers than non-smokers.
- Lung cancer among 66.6 percent smoker is due to smoking, the rest due to background effect.
- Results of other studies in other part of world should be considering before concluding there is casual relationship between smoking and lung cancer.

2. *According to past records the hookworm prevalence rate in a community is 25/1000 population. It is decided to conduct a fresh hookworm survey. Determine the size of the sample for this survey, allowing an error of 10 percent with a confidence limit of 95 percent.*
The formula to calculate the sample size with 95 percent confidence limit with d percent error is true prevalence 'p' of disease is:

$$n = \frac{4pq}{d^2}, \text{ where } q = 1 - p$$

Sol. Given information:

Prevalence of hookworm = p = 25/1000 = 0.025

q = 1 – p = 0.975

Error allowed = d = 10% of p = 10% of 0.025 = 0.0025

4 pq 4 × 0.025 × 0.975

$$\text{Required sample size } n = \frac{4pq}{d^2} = \frac{4 \times 0.025 \times 0.975}{(0.0025)^2}$$

$$= \frac{0.0975}{0.000000625} = 15600$$

3. *The 1993 estimated mid-year population of a town was 200,000. The numbers of registered vehicles during the year were 5,000. Of these 100 were not driven during 1993 at all. The average number of KMS per day run by the remaining vehicles is given below:*

1,900 vehicles	10
2,500 vehicles	50
500 vehicles	100

The numbers of persons killed in motor vehicular accident in 1993 were 500, of which 400 were the occupants of vehicles. Calculate all possible accident fatality rates.

Sol. 1. Accident death rate per 100,000 population

$$= \frac{\text{Deaths due to accidents}}{\text{Mid-year population}} \times 100000$$

= (500 × 100,000)/200000= 250/100000 population.

2. Death rate per 1000 registered vehicles = 500 × 1000/5000
= 100/1000 registered vehicles.

3. Total vehicle kilometers are
= (1900 × 10) + (2500 × 50) + (500 × 100) × 365
= (19000 + 125000 + 50000) × 365
= 70,810,000

Death rate per 100,000 Vehicle kilometers
= 500 × 100,000/70,810,000
= 0.7/100,000 vehicle kilometer

Death rate of vehicle occupants per 1000 vehicles per year
= 400 × 1000/5000 = 80/1000 vehicle occupants.

4. *A new screening test for a certain disease was administered to 490 persons, 60 of whom are known to have the disease. The test was positive in 50 of the persons with the disease, as well as in 20 persons without the disease. Calculate the following:*
a. Sensitivity of the test
b. Specificity of the test.
c. Percentage of false positive
d. Percentage of false negatives
e. Prevalence of disease
f. Predictive value of a positive test
g. Predictive value of a negative test.

Screening test results	*Diagnosis*		*Total*
	Diseased	*Non-diseased*	
Positive	50 (a)	20 (b)	70 (a + b)
Negative	10 (c)	400 (d)	410 (c + d)
Total	60 (a + c)	420 (b + d)	480

Sol. a. Sensitivity of screening test = a/(a + c) × 100
= 50/60 × 100 = 83.33%

b. Specificity of screening test = d/(b + d) × 100
= 400/420 × 100 = 95.24%

c. Percentage of false positives = b/(b + d) × 100
= 20/420 × 100 = 4.76%

d. Percentage of false negatives = c/(a + c) × 100
= 10/60 × 100 =17.67%

e. Prevalence of disease = a + c/(a+ b+ c+ d) × 100
= 60/480 × 100 =12.5%

f. Predictive value of positive test = a/(a+b) × 100
= 50/70 × 100 = 71.43%

g. Predictive value of negative test = d/(c + d) × 100
= 400/410 × 100 = 97.56%

5. *In a clinical trial, 240 patients suffering from depression were included. These matched groups were made. The first was put on drug 'A' second on drug 'B' and third on a placebo. The results of the trial are shown below:*

Drug/ placebo	*No. felt better*	*No. felt worse*	*No. unchanged*	*Total*
'A'	47	6	29	82
'B'	52	3	22	77
Placebo	32	16	33	81

Determine if drug 'A' is statistically more effective than 'B'

Sol. To compare efficacy of drug A with B, exclude placebo results from analysis. Also club the results 'not felt worse' and 'number unchanged' as 'not felt better'. The results can be tabulated as:

Drug	*No. felt better*	*No. felt worse*	*Total*
'A'	47 (a)	35 (b)	82 (a+ b)
'B'	52 (c)	25 (d)	77 (c+ d)
Total	99 (a+ c)	60 (b+ d)	159 (N)

Null hypothesis: Drug 'A' and 'B' are equally effective

Use Chi-Square test. χ^2 for 2 × 2 table is:

$\chi^2 = (ad - bc)^2 \times N/(a+b)\,(c + d)\,(a + c)\,(b + d)$

$= (645)^2 \times 159/99 \times 60 \times 82 \times 77$

$= 66147975/37505160 = 1.763$

Degree of freedom = (r – 1) (c – 1) = (2 – 1) (2 – 1) = 1

For one degree of freedom, χ^2 value at 0.05 level of significance is 3.84. The calculated χ^2 is less than critical value of χ^2. Therefore, accept null hypothesis. Therefore, drug 'A' is not more effective than drug 'B'.

Chapter 30 Visits

CHAPTER OUTLINE

- INTEGRATED COUNSELING AND TESTING CENTER (ICTC)
- VISIT TO BLIND SCHOOL
- A VISIT TO DEAF AND DUMB SCHOOL
- VISIT TO DISTRICT HEALTH LABORATORY
- VISIT TO PRIMARY HEALTH CENTER (PHC)
- POSTPARTUM CENTER
- DELIVERY OF INTEGRATED SERVICES FOR MATERNAL AND CHILD HEALTH, FAMILY PLANNING, NUTRITION AND IMMUNIZATION
- THE BABY FRIENDLY HOSPITAL INITIATIVE
- WORLD BREASTFEEDING WEEK
- ANGANWADI
- INTEGRATED CHILD DEVELOPMENT SCHEME
- VISIT TO DISTRICT TUBERCULOSIS CENTER
- VISIT TO DISTRICT REHABILITATION CENTER
- VISIT TO PLACES OF NATURAL CALAMITIES
- SCHOOL HEALTH SERVICE
- VISIT TO DISTRICT LEPROSY CENTER

INTEGRATED COUNSELING AND TESTING CENTER (ICTC)

An Integrated Counseling and Testing Center (ICTC) is a place where person is counseled and tested for HIV, on his own or advised by a medical provider. This common facility will remove fear, stigma and discrimination among the clients. The ICTCs have common televise and video-based health education material that are screened continuous in the waiting area. The main functions of ICTC include:

1. Early diction of HIV
2. Provision of basic information on modes of transmission and prevention of HIV/AIDS for promoting behavioral change and reducing vulnerability.
3. Link people with other HIV prevention, care and treatment services.

Strategies adopted in ICTCs for HIV testing:

- "Opt out" and "opt in" strategy
- "Opt out" strategy.

Provider-initiated counseling and testing—"opt out": There are three varieties of patients who are offered provider counseling and testing:

a. Patients who present at a health facility with symptoms suggestive of HIV infection (pneumonia, TB and persistent diarrhea).
b. Patients with STI/RTI.
c. Pregnant women who register at antenatal clinic.

In such cases the client in given basic information on HIV, and educated about testing for HIV. The counselor will ask each client, "Do you wish to test for HIV or not?" The client can "opt out" or choose not to test for HIV. If a client does not "opt out" then he/she is tested for HIV.

Client initiated counseling and testing "opt in " or Direct walk in client. These clients who present themselves at the ICTC of their own free will based on their individual risk behavior or information and advice received from a friend, sexual partner, or outreach worker or peer educator. Here the client is counseled for HIV and then "opts in" or actively aggress to be tested for HIV. Written consent has to be obtained from such clients before testing.

ICTC can be located in the Obstetric and Gynecology Department for pregnant women, or with tuberculosis microscopy center for TB patients at work place, on national highways and on universities.

There are two typed of ICTCs:

1. Fixed facility ICTC
2. Mobile ICTCs.

A fixed facility ICTC can be two types:

- "Stand alone" ICTC having full time counselor and a laboratory technician located in medical colleges and district and in some sub-district hospitals. It is envisaged under NACP-III to have such ICTCs established up to the level of CHC.
- "Facility-integrated" ICTC which does not have full time staff and provides HIV counseling and testing as a service along with other services. Such center canters to small number of clients.

VISIT TO BLIND SCHOOL

In India, there are 140 blind schools of which 4 are in Karnataka in Hubli, Davangere, Mysore and Gulbarga; Blind School at Davangere is exclusively for girls.

Admission Criteria

Students are admitted in the month of June-July every year the students should be blind and should produce a certificate from an ophthalmologist. He should also produce an age certificate, a caste certificate in case of a SC, ST student, also three passport size photos. Age group for admission into 1st Std is 6 to 10 years. In case of an orphan a certificate from the magistrate is needed. There is no admission fees.

Government Authority

The school is government school under the directorate of disabled welfare which looks after the blind, physically handicapped, deaf and dumb, mentally handicapped and those suffering from cerebral palsy.

Everything is provided free of cost. Besides education the other facilities for blind are:

1. KSRTC has completely exempted the travelling charges for blind people in ordinary buses.
2. In the Indian Railways, the blind persons has to pay only 25 percent of the fare. For travel of the person needs an escort, the escort also has to pay only 25 percent of the fare.
3. They are given Rs 125/- month as disabling allowance.
4. The blind students get a reader's allowance of Rs 50 per month.

Syllabus for the Blind

There is no exemption in the syllabus for the blind up to VII Std but after VII Std instead of mathematics and science, they can study economics, political science, music and history (choose any two subjects). The special script for blind is called Braille script. Invented by Louis Braille (divine life for blind).

Staffing Pattern

Consists of 24 members. In which are included the superintendent, teachers with physical director to look after the affairs of the school. There is also one visiting medical officer.

Specific Program for Prevention of Blindness

1. Vitamin A prophylaxis program
2. Trachoma control program
3. School age health services.

National and International Agencies

1. National Association for Blind (NAB) established in 1962.
2. Royal Common Wealth Society for Blind (1950).
3. International Agency for Prevention of Blindness.
4. Danish International Development Association (DANIDA).

A VISIT TO DEAF AND DUMB SCHOOL

There are four government schools in Karnataka:

1. Mysore upto SSLC
2. Gulbarga upto 7th Standard
3. Bellary upto 7th Standard
4. Belgaum upto 7th Standard

The Belgaum school is only for girls, rest all are only for boys.

Staffing Pattern

1. Gazetted post—Superintendent.
2. Two FDA (1st division assistant).
3. Two SDA (2nd division assistant). They look after the administration and other problems individually.
4. Matron: Food, clothing, bedding are provided by him.
   To assist them more in cooking staff two cooking posts.
5. Four graduate assistants who teach upto high school.
6. One primary school teacher undergraduate.
7. One tailoring instructor.
8. Two weaving assistants.
9. Night watchman.

Rules and Regulations

Boys and girls 6 to 10 years are admitted along with their records.
1. Birth certificate from municipality corporation, panchayat.
2. Income certificate and caste certificate from Tahsildar.
3. Photographs—four.

The capacity of student accommodation is 100 in each school. The government is providing training facilities to all teachers. Teachers training institute are formed for this purpose now it is at Bangalore.

There are two categories:
1. Institute for oral training
2. Institute for sign training.

VISIT TO DISTRICT HEALTH LABORATORY

In each district there is one district health laboratory.

Staffing Pattern

1. Medical Officer	1
2. Senior Laboratory Technician	4
3. Attender	4
4. Peon	2
5. Sweeper	1

Functions

1. Preparation of stain for all PHCs.
2. Conducting malaria clinics.
3. Surveillance: (a) Active surveillance, (b) Passive surveillance.
4. Training for paramedical staff.
5. Examination of malaria slides from all PHCs and rural sub-centers.
6. Routine laboratory work: Total count, differential count, ESR, Hb%, VDRL, pregnancy test.

Urine Test: Bile salts, bile pigment, sugar, albumin and microscopic examination. Stool examination for ova and cyst.

Staining Procedure for Malarial Smear

The stain used for this is JSB stain (Jaswant Singh Bhattacharya). Two solutions of JSB are used—JSB_1 solution and JSB_2 solution. After dehemoglobinization of the smear, dip the smear in JSB_2 solution for 30 to 40 seconds which contains eosin. Wash it with buffer water containing KPO_4 and disodium hydrogen phosphate. Then dip in JSB_1 solution for 30 to 40 seconds and again wash with buffer water. Dry it and examine under oil immersion lens using liquid paraffin. JSB_1 solution contain methylene blue, water, etc.

VISIT TO PRIMARY HEALTH CENTER (PHC)

The National Health Plan (1983) proposed reorganization of primary health centers on the basis of one PHC for every 30,000 rural population in the plains, and one PHC for every 20,000 population in hilly, tribal and backward areas for more effective coverage. As on 30th June 1999, 22807 primary health centers have been established in the country against the total requirement of about 23,000.

Functions of the PHC

1. Medical care
2. MCH including family planning
3. Safe water supply and basic sanitation
4. Prevention and control of locally endemic diseases
5. Collection and reporting of vital statistics
6. Education about health
7. National Health Programs—as relevant
8. Referral services
9. Training of health guides, health workers, local dais and health assistants
10. Basic laboratory services.

Staffing Pattern

At present in each community development block, there are one or more PHCs each of which covers 30,000 rural population. In the new set-up each PHC will have the following staff:

At the PHC Level

Medical Officer	1
Pharmacist	1
Nurse midwife	1

Health worker (Female) ANM	1
Block extension educator	1
Health assistant (Male)	1
Health assistant (Female)/LHV	1
UDC	1
LDC	1
Laboratory technician	1
Driver (subject to availability of vehicle)	1
Class IV	4
	15

At the Sub-center Level

Health worker (female)/ANH	1
Health worker (male)	1
Voluntary worker (Paid Rs 50 per month as honorarium)	1
	3

POSTPARTUM CENTER

Introduction

The history of postpartum concept dates back to the year 1966 when the Population Council, New York, developed an International Program to test the idea that the post delivery (or postpartum) period is the point of highest motivation for family planning and therefore the best occasion for providing information and service. Government of India launched the All India Hospitals Postpartum Program in 1969.

The postpartum program has been defined as "A maternity centered hospital based approach to Family Welfare Program to motivate women with in the reproductive age group (15-44 years) or their husbands for adopting small family norms through education and motivation particularly during prenatal and postnatal period".

Over a period of years the concept of postpartum program has undergone a change. The service of the postpartum center now include MCH and Family Planning Services. The postpartum centers function as referral centres for peripheral institution.

It ensures effective Obstetric Services leading to decline in maternal and infant mortality and better acceptance of family planning methods (Table 30.1).

Table 30.1: Staff pattern of the postpartum center attached to medical college

1.	Assistant Professor in OBG	1
2.	Lecturer in Health Education and FP	1
3.	Lecturer in Statistics and Demography/ Lecturer in Social Preventive Medicine	1
4.	Lecturer in Pediatrics	1
5.	Anesthetist (Asst. Surgeon Gr.I)	1
6.	Projectionist-cum-Mechanic	1
7.	Medical Officer (1 Male and 1 female)	2
8.	Public Health Nurse/LHV	1
9.	Auxilliary Nurse Mid-wife	2
10.	Family Welfare Worker (M)	1
11.	Store Keeper cum/Clerk	1
12.	Steno-typist	1
13.	LDC	1
14.	Driver	1
15.	Attendant	1
16.	Cytotechnician	1

Functions of Postpartum Unit

The Postpartum Unit as a whole is responsible for carrying out the following functions.

A. To provide contraceptive advice and services primarily to obstetric and abortion cases attending the Department of Obstetrics and Gynecology and various other Departments, knowledge regarding available methods and follow-up of acceptors, in addition to this, advice/service treatment of infertility for both male and female recanalization.

B. To provide out reach services and extend material and Child Health Family Welfare Hospital. This all should cover at least a population of 50,000 or the whole town if the population is less than 50,000.

C. Immunization of all children delivered at the Postpartum Center and those attending hospital Outpatient Department. To provide nutritional education to women during antenatal, correct methodology of weaning of the child. Health education on prevention of anemia, protein malnutrition and vitamin 'A' deficiency in addition to other diseases also needs to be imparted. The above services shall also be provided to the community of the field area.

D. To involve all the departments and staff of the hospital in addition to the Department of Obstetrics and Gynecology in the Family Welfare Program.

E. To detect early cases of cervical cancer among users and not-users of family welfare methods through Postpartum Pap Smear test facilities wherever such facility is provided under the Postpartum Program.

F. To conduct teaching and training program in family welfare for under graduate and postgraduate medical and paramedical students.

G. To develop an over all plan for distribution of conventional contraceptives and identify depot holders to meet the demand of the people in the area served by the Center.
H. To participate in the State Level Seminar and suggest methods for improving the Program and removing the bottleneck if any.

Department of Obstetrics and Gynecology

Shares the major responsibility of implementing the program while the other departments viz. Pediatrics, Surgery and Preventive and Social Medicine supplement the efforts of the Department of Obstetrics and Gynecology.

In the case of non-teaching hospitals, the Medical Superintendent or Civil Surgeon acts as Program Director and Senior Medical Officer as Project Officer.

Monitoring and Evaluation Aspects

Program monitoring is considered as one of the most essential tools for the successful implementing of the program. It helps in studying day-to-day developments to the program.

Institutional Level Monitoring and Evaluation

At institutional Level the program is monitored by way of maintaining proper records like eligible couple survey register of field area population served, acceptors motivated at various intervals of time, etc. and evaluated by Coordination Committee constituted in every Institution as per the norms suggested by Government of India.

Guidelines for Constitution of Coordination Committee

In order to evaluate and review the working of the program and to bring about further improvement in effective functioning of the program, Coordination Committees are formed in all the Medical Institutions Hospital/covered under the program. The composition of the Co-ordination Committee may be as follows (Table 30.2).

Table 30.2: Composition of the coordination committee

1.	Program Director—Principal/Dean in case of Medical College/Teaching Institution Medical Superintendent/Civil Surgeon in case of nonteaching Hospital/Institution	Chairman
2.	Project Director—Head of the Department of Obstetrics of Gynecology	Member
3.	Head of the Department of Pediatrics	Member
4.	Head of the Department of Preventive and Social Medicine	Member
5.	Head of the Department of Surgery	Member
6.	Regional Director (H and FW, Government of India) if available	Member
7.	State Family Welfare Officer/District, Family Welfare Officer or any person outside the Medical College May be co-opted as Member at the discretion of the Chairman if necessary	Member

In those Postpartum Units where Pap Smear Test Facility has been sanctioned, Professor of Pathology/Cytopathologist may be co-opted as member of coordination Committee.

Broad Functions

The broad functions of the committee in an institution are:

I. To evaluate and review the progress of the postpartum program.
II. To adopt corrective measures for improvement of the program.
III. To meet at least once in three months.
IV. To apprise State Government of the development taking place in the field.

DELIVERY OF INTEGRATED SERVICES FOR MATERNAL AND CHILD HEALTH, FAMILY PLANNING, NUTRITION AND IMMUNIZATION

The health of the mother and child are interviewed so that the services of maternal and child health, family planning, nutrition and immunization are closely and required to be delivered as an integrated package of family health care. This is indicated in Figure 30.1.

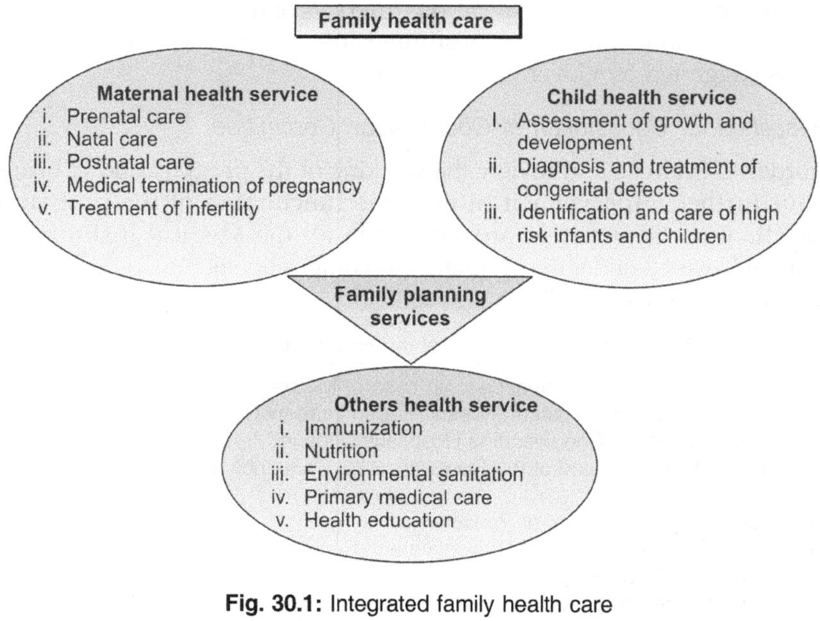

Fig. 30.1: Integrated family health care

THE BABY FRIENDLY HOSPITAL INITIATIVE

What is BFHI?

This is global program aimed at giving quality care to mothers and children and to ensure that every newborn baby gets the best start in its life. The program commits itself to protecting, supporting, and promoting breastfeeding.

Why this Program?

It is generally felt that all mothers in this part of the world breastfeed their babies anyway. So why worry about such a program?

If we think for a moment and apply our mind to this situation, we all know that there are many mothers who deliver a baby for the first time, many more mothers are delivered by cesarean section (this figure is on the increase especially among urban mothers), one-third of the babies born in our state are low-birth weight and nearly 12 to 15 percent are preterm babies Mothers delivering with episiotomy wound and forceps extraction are also quite a few. These are situations found by each one of us wherein newborn babies and mothers have breastfeeding difficulties.

Studies conducted from 222 villages of Central Karnataka has shown that rural mothers delay the first feed, administer prelacteal feeds, quite a few discard colostrum considering that it is unsuitable to the child and exclusive breastfeeding is not optimally practised. Quite a few mothers bottle-feed their babies.

Taking all these points into consideration, we have to conclude that where ever there is a maternity service and where ever there are lactating mothers there must be high level of expertise available among MCH care staff to deal appropriately with any lactation management difficulty. Hence, this program is very relevant to us.

What is New About it?

- Lactation management focuses its attention on understanding the physiology of the newborn and parturient mothers and critically looks at factors that govern initation and establishment of lactation.
- The dynamics of breast milk transfer is now understood in proper perspective. We now know that baby should attach in a good position and its tongue should remove all the milk from the lactiferous sinuses (the reservoirs of milk). Complete emptying results in more production of breast milk.

- Early initiation results in practical disappearance of breast engorgement
- Sore nipples, fissures, cracks and pain experienced by the mother while breastfeeding are the result of nipple feeding.
- The art of manual expression of breast milk tries to mimic the action of baby at the mothers breast.

What is this Program All About? Can it be Simply Described in a Few Words?

Yes, the program comprises of:

A. Ten simple steps that should be implemented in a maternity service.

B. Learning five basic skills by all the MCH care staff.

The Ten Steps

1. Have a written breastfeeding policy that is routinely communicated to all health care staff.
2. Train all health care staff in skills necessary to implement this policy.
3. Inform all pregnant women about the benefits and management of breastfeeding.
4. Help mothers initiate breastfeeding within half an hour of birth.
5. Show mothers how to breastfeed and how to maintain lactation even if they should be separated from their infants.
6. Give newborn infants no food or drink other than breast milk unless medically indicated.
7. Practice "rooming-in" allowing mothers and infants to remain together 24 hours a day.
8. Encourage breast-feeding on demand.
9. Give no artificial teats or pacifiers to breastfeeding infants.
10. Foster the establishment of breastfeeding support groups.

The Five Basic Skills

1. To learn the skill of initiating breastfeeding and to assure that baby is placed in a good position at the mothers breast.
2. To learn the skill of manual expression of breast milk.
3. To learn how to prevent and treat insufficient milk supply.
4. To learn how to prevent and treat sore nipples.
5. To learn how to prevent and treat breast engorgement.

What are the Benefits of Making My Hospital Baby Friendly?

There are many benefits of making my hospital baby friendly:

1. Firstly you will have the satisfaction of providing scientific and updated information and technical help to lactating mothers.
2. Infant mortality will come down.

3. Your hospital staff will work as a cohesive team and will derive pride in their work.
4. Your hospital will get National and International recognition.
5. This program will place us on a global forefront.

What are the Investments Needed and What is the Cost Involved?

Nothing. There is no financial involvement. However, you will have to spend lots of time training your MCH care staff.

What should I do to get My Hospital Recognized as Baby Friendly Hospital?

The steps are three folds:

1. Obtain self-assessment form.
2. Complete the form, Xerox two copies and send to coordinator baby friendly hospital initiative for Karnataka State (Retain one copy with you).
3. Train your health care staff and await inspection.

WORLD BREASTFEEDING WEEK

Each year we have been observing " World Breastfeeding Week" from 1st to 7th August every year. We all know that exclusive breastfeeding for the first six months and continued breastfeeding for two years along with home made semi solids, is the best way of bringing up a child.

- Most mothers in our country want to breastfeed their children.
- Though 90 percent of mothers are successful in breastfeeding their children, primi mothers, mothers delivering by LSCS and mothers having preterm and low-birth weight children more often have breastfeeding difficulties.

What are Our Problems?

Delayed Start

Mothers usually delay the first feed for three days and offer cows milk, honey, sugar water using cloth or cotton wisp. These pre-lacteal feeds are unnecessary and can introduce infection in the baby. They also interfere with the physiology of lactation and delay establishment of breast milk, They can cause breast engorgement by 4th or 5th postnatal day.

Hence, we have to spread an important message that " babies should be put to breast in first half an hour of birth". During this period, the neonate is awake, alert and all his neonatal reflexes such as rooting, sucking and swallowing are very sharp. This is the right time when we should initiate breastfeeding.

Mothers delivering by LSCS: Such mothers have lot of pain and difficulty looking after themselves. Such mothers need the help of trained nursing staff who are able to support and assist them with breastfeeding. The number of LSCS deliveries are increasing. Hence, we have to create adequate expertise in all maternity facilities.

Primi mothers: For these mothers, all said and done, it is their first experience. Mothers have many doubts and fears about breastfeeding and carrying for their young ones. They need to be adequately supported and helped. Most difficulties are in the first few days after birth.

Working mothers: Mothers who have to return to work are constantly under stress as to how to manage feeding once they return to work. Usually such mothers end up bottle feeding their young ones inviting risks and hazards of artificial feeding. There is explosion in knowledge and technical expertise in helping such mothers.

Common breastfeeding problems: Sore nipples, mastitis, engorgement, difficulty in positioning and breast refusal are some of the common problems seen. These problems can be easily prevented by simple measures because of better understanding of physiology of lactation and breast milk transfer.

What can We do for the World Breastfeeding Week (WBW)?

There is tremendous amount of responsibility with each one of us to ensure that no mothers will have any difficulty with breastfeeding their young ones.

At individual level:

1. Every newborn baby that you come across, please make sure that the baby is sucking in proper position.
2. Ensure that breastfeeding is initiated early and baby fed on demand as frequently as needed.
3. Train Nurses to assist mothers delivering by LSCS with breastfeeding.
4. Help mothers in manual expression of breast milk in situation like-baby very small or preterm, mother who has to return to work.
5. Create supporting environment for the mother.
6. Congratulate every mother who is doing well with breastfeeding.
7. Encourage every mother to exclusive breastfeed for six months.
8. Each one of us involved in neonatal care can contribute to better lactation management in our day to day work, involving nurses and mothers.

At community level:

1. Organize talks and meetings with Pediatricians, Obstetricians, IMA members and Medical Practitioners. Include all nursing staff in such meetings.

2. Hold public meetings with Lions Club, Rotary Club and other such Voluntary Organizations.
3. Organize meetings with Mahila Mandals and Womens organizations.
4. Give radio talks and TV talks.
5. Write in daily newspapers, magazines and other print media.

Promote BFHI Concept

The Baby Friendly Hospital Initiative aims at promoting, protecting and supporting breastfeeding in the community.

Let us rededicate our efforts to help all mothers in attaining their best in their role of child rearing. Please note that these activities are not limited to just the week alone but should become a part and way of life.

Please plan your activities along with your District Branch President and Secretary.

ANGANWADI

The focal point for the operation of the ICDS at the village level, is an Anganwadi. It covers a population of about 1000 in urban and rural areas and 700 in tribal areas. The worker who coordinates and offers the services is the Anganwadi Worker (AWW).

Some of the important tasks to be performed by the AWW are as follows:

1. To survey the community and identify child and mother beneficiaries.
2. To monitor the growth of children using weight for age and identify children suffering from malnourishment.
3. To maintain growth charts and records of attendance, immunisation, births, deaths, etc. at the Anganwadi.
4. To provide supplementary feeding to children.
5. Assist the LHV in distributing Vitamin A to children and iron and folic acid supplements to pregnant and lactating women; and refer patients to local health services.
6. To teach nonformal preschool education to three to six years old children and functional literacy classes for adult women.
7. To make home visits in order to enlist community and beneficiary to supports various activities.
8. To organize women's clubs (Mahila Mandals) for health and nutrition education and centers for income-generating activities.

INTEGRATED CHILD DEVELOPMENT SCHEME

A majority of India's children live in impoverished economic, social and environmental conditions which impede their physical and mental development. As a response to the unmet needs of this vast and vulnerable population, the Government of India introduced in 1975 its most ambitious and comprehensive plan to increase child survival rates among the poorest and enhance the health, nutrition and learning opportunities of pre-school children and their mothers. Drawing upon experience called from twenty years of planned social development, the Integrated Child Development Scheme (ICDS) is designed both as a preventive and developmental effort. If extends beyond the existing health and education systems to reach children and their mothers in villages and slums and delivers to them an integrated package of services.

Objectives

Its major objectives are to:

i. Reduce malnutrition, morbidity and mortality of children in the age group 0 to 6 years
ii. Improve their health and nutritional status
iii. Provide the environmental conditions necessary for their psychological social and physical development
iv. Enhance the ability of mothers to provide proper care to their children
v. Achieve effective coordination among various departments providing developmental services to children.

Package of Services

To achieve these goals a package of services consisting of the following was introduced:

a. Supplementary feeding (Details given in Table 30.3).
b. Immunization
c. Health check-up
d. Referral services
e. Nutrition and health education
f. Pre-school education and
g. Non-formal education for women.

Table 30.3: Nutritional supplements

Recipients	*Calories*	*Grams of protein*
1. Child up to 6 years	300	8-10
2. Adolescent girls	500	20-25
3. Pregnant and nursing mothers	500	20-25
4 Malnourished children	Double the daily supplement provided to the other children (600) and/or special on medical recommendation	

Organizational Set-up

The Ministry of Social Welfare is responsible for the budgetary control and administration of the scheme forms the center and coordinates activities with the Ministries of Education, Health Family Welfare and Rural Development.

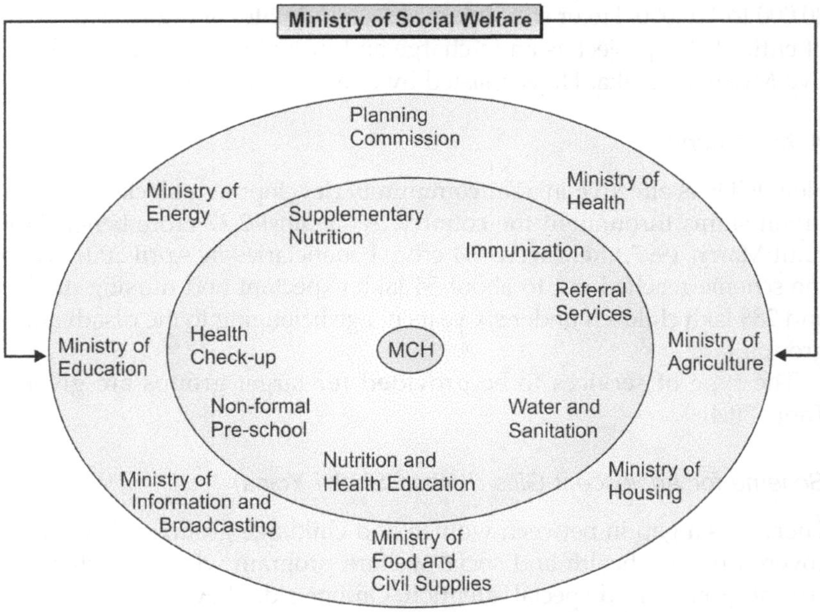

Fig. 30.2: Convergence of ICDS services

At the State level, the Department of Social Welfare is mainly responsible, although in some states, other Departments (e.g. Tribal Welfare, Women and Child Welfare, Health or Rural Development) may take primary responsibility for implementation.

At the block level, the Block Development Officer (BDO) exercises overall responsibility for the project, co-ordinating activities with the main ICDS functionary, the Child Development Officer (CDPO) (Fig. 30.2).

Anganwadi Worker

Anganwadi worker is a part-time trained voluntary worker and receives an honorarium of Rs. 700 per month. She is assisted by a helper who is also a local women and paid an honorarium.

Mukhya Sevika (MS)

Mukhya Sevika is a full-time worker who supervises the work of 20, 25 and 17 Anganwadi workers in urban, rural and tribal projects respectively. She visits each Anganwadi at least once a month, and liaise with lady health visitor in nutritional and health activities.

Child Development Project Officer

For one project there is one Child Development Project Officer (CDPO) who cover one community development block having a population of

80,000 to 120,000. He or she supervises, co-ordinates and guides the work of entire ICDS project as an in-charge and provide supervision to four to five Mukhya Sevika. He is assisted by one assistant CDPO.

Achievements

New ICDS is effective in 5171 community development blocks and major urban slums throughout the country. As against 2.27 crore beneficiaries until March 1997, there were 3.4 crore beneficiaries in April 2001. Today the scheme reached out to about 54 lakh expectant and nursing mothers and 288 lakh children under six years of age belonging to the disadvantage groups.

The type of services to be provided for target groups are given in Table 30.4.

Scheme for Adolescent Girls (Kishori Shakti Yojna)

There was a gap in between women and child age group which was not covered by any health and social welfare program whereas girls in this crucial groups need special attention. On one side they need appropriate nutrition, education, health education, training for adulthood, training for acquiring skills as the base for earning an independent livelihood, training for motherhood, etc. Similarly on the other side their potential to be a good community leader has to be realized. A scheme for adolescent girls in ICDS was launched by the Department of Women and Child Development, Ministry of Human Resource Development in 1991.

Table 30.4: Type of services to be provided for target groups

Beneficiary	*Service*
1. Expectant and nursing mothers	i. Health check-up ii. Immunization of expectant mothers against tetanus iii. Supplementary nutrition iv. Functional literacy
2.Other women 25-45 years	i. Nutrition and health education ii. Functional literacy
3. Children less than 3 years	i. Supplementary nutrition ii. Immunization iii. Health check-up iv. Referral services
4. Children between 3-6 years	i. Supplementary nutrition ii. Immunization iii. Health check-up iv. Referral services v. Nonformal preschool education

Common services: All adolescents girls in the age group of 11 to 18 years (70%) receive the following common services:

1. Watch over menarche
2. Immunization
3. General health check-ups once in every six months
4. Training for minor ailments
5. Deworming
6. Prophylactic measures against anemia, goiter, vitamin deficiency, etc. and
7. Referral to PHC/District hospital in case of acute need.

This scheme for adolescent is extended to 3.51 lakh adolescent girls in 507 ICDS blocks covering all states and union territories. It is proposed to extend the scheme in 2000 community development blocks during ninth plan covering 12.8 lakh adolescent girls.

VISIT TO DISTRICT TUBERCULOSIS CENTER

National Tuberculosis Program (NTP)

National Tuberculosis Program (NTP) has been in operation since 1962 NTP operates through the District Tuberculosis Program (DTP) which is the backbone of the NTP. Over 600 TB clinics have been set up in the country, of which 390 have been upgraded todate as District TB Centres (DTC) to undertake districtwise TB control in association with general health and medical institutions.

Organization

A District Tuberculosis Program consists of one District Tuberculosis Center (DTC) and on an average 50 peripheral health institutions comprising of PHCs, general hospitals, rural dispensaries, etc.

To implement the program, a specially trained team of key program personnel (Trained at the National Tuberculosis Institute, Bangalore for a period of 13 weeks) is posted at each DTC. The team consists of:

- One District Tuberculosis Officer (DTO)
- One Second Medical Officer
- Two Laboratory Technicians
- Two Treatment Organzer/Health Visitor
- One X-ray Technician
- One Non-medical Team Leader
- One Statistical Assistant
- One Pharmacist.

The program is integrated with primary health care system (general health services) and is brought within the ambit of the District Health Organization. The District Health Officer is made directly responsible for the DTP, with the DTO as a specialized staff officer to assist him in the management of DTP. Not only the peripheral health institutions, but also the caders of health workers and MPWs are all involved in the program of case detection and treatment.

VISIT TO DISTRICT REHABILITATION CENTER

The Government of India launched District Rehabilitation Center (DRC) scheme in early 1985, for providing a package of model comprehensive rehabilitation services to the rural disabled. The scheme, at present is operated in 11 different places of the country. The scheme covered: (1) Locomotor handicap, (2) Speech and hearing impaired, (3) Visually impaired, (4) Mentally handicapped, and (5) Multiple handicaps.

Services Provided

1. Preventive and early detection
2. Medical intervention and surgical correction
3. Fitment of artificial aids and appliances
4. Therapeutic services such as physiotherapy, speech therapy, and occupational therapy
5. Provision of educational services in special and integrated school
6. Provision of training, for acquisition of skills through vocational training, job placement in local industries and trade with proper linkages with on going training and employment programs
7. Provision of self employment opportunities and bank loans
8. Establishing a meaningful linkage with existing government scheme such as disability/old age pension, scholarship, etc.
9. Creating of awareness movement of community and family counseling.

At Village Level

Anganwadi worker, teacher, health workers, etc. undertake the work of prevention, detection, and referral to PHC/CHC/District Hospital or voluntary organizations.

At PHC/CHC Level

Medical officers and paramedical staff are trained and oriented to prevent, detect, and appropriate intervention at their level and timely referral to highest centers.

DRC Level

District unit:

1. Provide service to handicaps
2. Act as referral center to PHC/CHC and for village level staff
3. Organizing camps

4. Education, vocational training, coordinating work with voluntary agencies and other departments.

Regional Rehabilitation Training Center were set up in Lucknow, Chennai, Cuttack, Mumbai to provide technical support to the DRCs.

National Program for Rehabilitation of Persons with Disabilities

National Sample Survey Organization of 1991 indicated 1.8 percent of the population in the country as disabled which is now 1.9 percent and 2-2.5 percent has mental retardation. The prevalence rate of disability is 22.7 per 1000 males and 16.9 per 1000 females. Disability was more in rural than urban areas and above national average in states of AP, HP, MP, Karnataka, Orissa, Punjab, and Tamil Nadu.

Objectives

1. To create services delivery system at state/district block/gram panchayat level so as to provide comprehensive based rehabilitation services.
2. Prevention, early intervention and information dissemination.

VISIT TO PLACES OF NATURAL CALAMITIES

WHO defines disaster as "Any occurrence that causes damage, ecological disruption, loss of human life, deterioration of health and health services, on a scale sufficient to warrant an extraordinary response from outside the affected community or area."

Disasters

Disasters are classified in various ways, e.g. natural versus manmade disasters or sudden versus slow-onset disasters.

Phases of a Disaster (Fig. 30.3)

Predisaster phase: The phase before a disaster strikes is the pre-disaster phase.

Alert phase: This phase refers to the period when a disaster is developing and when it has not yet hit the community.

Impact phase: There is no well-defined impact phase for gradual onset disasters, and sudden onset disasters are unpredictable in every way.

Post impact phase: This is the phase following the actual impact of the disaster.

Reconstruction and rehabilitation phase: This is a long-term phase. It aims at getting the community back to where it was before the emergency and to strengthen its ability to prevent and/or mitigate other diseases.

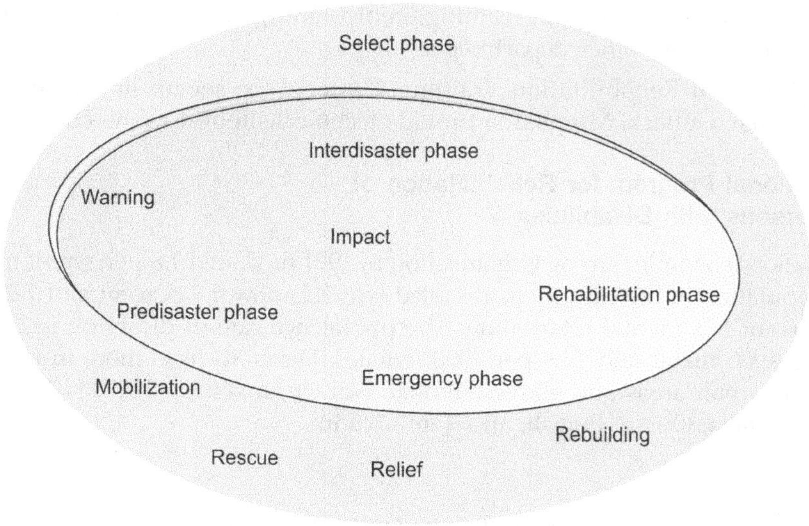

Fig. 30.3: Prototype acute disaster cycle

Effect of Disasters on Health (Table 30.5)

Objectives of health disaster preparedness:
The objectives of disaster preparedness and response activities in the health sector may be expressed as follows:

a. To prevent excess mortality due to the disaster, which may be caused by the direct impact of the disaster, by delays in rescue and relief activities, by lack of appropriate and timely health care, by the disruption of the normal health care and breakdown of preventive measures, and sometimes by malnutrition.
b. To provide appropriate and timely care for casualties due to the disaster. These include injuries, trauma and burns in natural disasters; malnutrition in situations of food shortage; acute cases of communicable disease in epidemic outbreaks, etc.
c. To prevent exposure to adverse climatic and environmental conditions including lack of food, water, sanitation, shelter, clothing, chemical or nuclear exposure, etc.
d. To prevent short-term and long-term disaster related morbidity:
Outbreaks of communicable disease usually due to changes in the local ecological conditions, disruption of health services, interruption of control measures, lack of sanitation, overcrowding;
Increase in morbidity and mortality due to destruction of health infrastructure and to the provision of basic health services;
Introduction of new diseases due to resettlement or imported by external relief workers;
Occurrence of wide-spread malnutrition/under-nutrition.

Table 30.5: Effect of disasters on health

Effect	*Earthquake*	*High wind (without floodings)*	*Tidal waves/ flash flood*	*Flood*	*Drought*
Deaths	Many	Few	Many	Few	Moderate
Severe injuries requiring extensive care	Overwhelming	Moderate	Few	Few	Moderate
Increase risk of communicable diseases		Potential risk following all major natural disasters (Probability rising with overcrowding and deteriorating sanitation)			
Food scarcity	Rare (May occur due to factors other than food shortage)	Rare	Common	Common	Common
Major population move-ments	Rare (May occur in heavily damaged urban areas)	Rare	Common	Common	Common
Under-nutrition/ Famine	Occasional	Rare	Occasional	Moderate	Common

e. To re-establish health services to or above pre-disaster levels, with special attention to:
   - Reconstruction and repair of damaged health facilities;
   - Renovation of health facilities to adequate and appropriate level;
   - Reorganization of health services based on Primary Health Care.

Examples of Some Disasters

A few examples of disasters which are still fresh in the memory of living generations are as under:

Atom bombing of Hiroshima (6 August 1945) and Nagasaki (9 August 1945): During the second world war is regarded as the worst manmade disaster of the century with estimated casualties of 120,000 and 75,000 respectively.

Guatemala earthquake (1976): In which 92 percent lost their homes, about 76,000 sustained injuries and some 23,000 got killed. A sample survey of victims of this disaster brought out such startling findings as:

- Eighty-four percent of the victims had no social security in the form of insurance.
- Forty-six percent were dissatisfied with the medical care received by them.
- Thirteen percent could not return to their former employment because of their injury, i.e. they needed vocational rehabilitation.

- Twelve percent had to wait 2-3 days and 16 percent for one week before admission into a hospital.
- Even for first-aid, 13 percent had to wait for 2-4 hours, 12 percent for four to eight hours and 21 percent for two to three days.

Bhopal gas tragedy (1984): It is regarded as the worst air pollution disaster so far and was due to accidental leakage of methylisocynate (MIC) from its plant. It affected about two lakh people and claimed 1,754 lives, according to one published report.

SCHOOL HEALTH SERVICE

School health is an important branch of community health. According to modern concepts, school health service is an economical and powerful means of raising community health.

Benefits of School Health Programs

School health programs have a beneficial impact on students, family, nation and all people at large:

1. Investment in school health programs is the most efficient and cost effective way to improve students health, and consequently their academic performance. Beside the students, teachers and other staff also get health benefits.
2. It has been estimated that 1.3 years of schooling to the mother reduces child mortality by about 15 percent. More years of education a female receives, the more likely it is that her children will survive the first 5 years of life (World Development Report, 1993).
3. School food programs also have a marked effect on attendance and school performance.
4. Carefully designed and implemented comprehensive health education curricula can prevent certain adverse behaviors, including tobacco use, illicit drug use, unhealthy dietary practices, unsafe sexual behavior, and physical inactivity.
5. Schools setting provides an efficient means of improving young people's health, self-esteem, life skills (abilities related to effective decision-making, communication, understanding emotions, critical thinking, coping with stress, etc.) and behavior. School can also provide the setting to introduce health information and technologies to the community and can lead the community by advocating policies and services that promote health.
6. Schools can reach about one billion students worldwide everyday and, through them, their families and communities that is the world broadest and deepest channel for putting information at the disposal of its citizens (UNICEF 1988).

Objectives of School Health Service

The objectives of the program of a school health service are as follows:
1. The promotion of positive health
2. The prevention of diseases
3. Early diagnosis, treatment and follow-up of defects
4. Awakening health consciousness in children
5. The provision of healthful environment.

School Health Program in India

Formal school health program is nonexistence in India. However, school medical inspection was started first in Baroda city in 1909. In the succeeding years practically every province in British India introduced some form of school health program particularly in middle and high schools. But after independence there was not much progress made in school health program. At the government level, a School Health Committee was set up in 1960 to review the program at national level. The committee recommended that in the first phase (1962-66) school health services should be developed in an area close to primary health unit to cover 40 primary schools and in cities all primary school children in slums must be covered. In the second phase (1966-71) these services should be extended to all primary schools in both rural and urban area (GOI 1960-61). Again the progress in this direction has been rather very slow (Lal 1998).

It is suggested by the School Health Committee that primary health centers should also cover schools in their jurisdiction for health care delivery including inspection. One PHC is responsible for more than 5000 students per year. In urban area school health service schemes are run by corporation or nongovernmental organization.

Aspects of School Health Service

The tasks of a school health service are manifold, and vary according to local priorities. Where resources are plentiful, special school health services may be developed. Some aspects of a school health service are as follows:
1. Health appraisal of school children and school personnel
2. Remedial measures and follow-up
3. Prevention of communicable diseases
4. Health school environment
5. Nutritional services
6. First aid and emergency care
7. Mental health
8. Dental health
9. Eye health
10. Health education

11. Education of handicapped children
12. Proper maintenance and use of school health records.

VISIT TO DISTRICT LEPROSY CENTER

The distribution of leprosy within districts is quite uneven and equally the services available in the districts for leprosy control vary considerably. There are many reasons for this including the availability of number of staff, difficult terrain, lack of logistic support and limited participation of general health staff and community in program activities.

A district level leprosy elimination cell under the chairmanship of CDMO with ADMO (PH), skin and orthopedic specialists of HQ hospital, one LCU medical officer, MO incharge and one PHC medical officer as members of the district leprosy cell could do the planning and monitoring of leprosy elimination activities in the district. The district leprosy elimination plan to be comprehensive should include all core activities for leprosy elimination and take care to see that leprosy services reach every patient in every village. The plan should be placed before the DLES and sent to JDHS (Lep) for their information and approval.

District Infrastructure (Table 30.6)

Main Activities

The main activities are to be focused at the district level are:
- To expand MDT services to all health facilities.
- To treat all leprosy patients with MDT given free of cost.
- To detect all leprosy cases undetected in the district and treat them with MDT.
- Capacity building at local level.
- To inform and impart health education to community on leprosy and seek their support.
- Referral services for leprosy patients.
- The prevention of disability (POD).
- Monitoring, supervision and evaluation.
- To promote health system research (HSR).

Table 30.6: District infrastructure according to endemicity level

District classification	Infrastructure sanctioned
by prevalence levels at the start of phase-1-218 high endemic districts (PR>50/10000)	• Leprosy Control Units (LCU): 1 per 4.5 lakh rural population A LCU is manned by one Medical Officer (MO) 4 Non-medical Supervisors (NMS) and 20 paramedical workers • Modified LCUs: Rural areas • Urban Leprosy Centers (ULCs):1 per 50,000 population 1 PMW/NMS (reporting to the MO of a dispensary or a hospital)

Contd...

Contd...

	• Temporary Hospitalization Wards (THWs): To provide specialized services to leprosy patients with complications/problems. The THWs were supplemented by limited number of centers identified that doing restructured surgery
79 Moderately endemic districts	2 Mobile Leprosy Treatment Units (MLTU) for each moderately endemic 1 MLTU for each low endemic district
193 Low-endemic districts	• MLTU for leprosy patients at drug delivery with the help of general health staff. Each MLTU consists of following staff appointed on contract basic: MO-1, NMS-1, PMS-2, Driver-1, Total 350 MLTUs sanctioned in the country • SET Centers: Survey Education and Treatment Centers attached to PHCs/hospitals in rural endemic pockets. One SET covers 25,000 population. Staff one PMW under the guidance of PHC medical officer • ULCs in urban endemic pockets

Goal of National Health Policy 2002
"Elimination of Leprosy by 2005"

Project Phase II 2000 Onward

The Project Implementation Plan (PIP) for the NLEP Phase II.

- *Part A:* National plan setting out the project design for the country.
- *Part B:* Plan for eight high endemic states (Madhya Pradesh, Orissa, Bihar,Uttar Pradesh and West Bengal, Uttaranchal, Chhattisgarh, Jharkhand)
- *Part C:* Plan for the remaining 27 states and Union Territories

Project Phase II Objectives

1. To achieve elimination of leprosy at national level by the end of the project.
2. To accomplish integration of leprosy services with the general health care system in the 27 low endemic states/UTs—union territories.
3. To proceed with integration of services as rapidly as possible in the eight high endemic states.

Project Phase II Components

1. Decentralization and institutional development
2. Strengthening and integration of service delivery
3. Disability care and prevention
4. Information, education and communication
5. Training.

BIBLIOGRAPHY

1. J Kishore, National Health Programmes of India, 4th edn, 2002.
2. Karnataka Paediatric Journal. April-Sept 2000;14:243
3. Park's Textbook of Preventive and Social Medicine, 16th edn, Nov, 2000.
4. Should disaster strike—Be prepared—Central Health Bureau Directorate, General of Health Services, Government of India.
5. Swasth Hind, Annual Report 1999-2000.

Appendix

GOALS TO BE ACHIEVED BY 2000-2015

Year	*Goals to be achieved*
2003	: Enactment of legislation for regulating minimum standard in Clinical Establishment/Medical Institutions
2005	: Eradicate poliomyelitis and yaws
	: Eliminate leprosy
	: Establish an integrated system of surveillance, National Health Accounts and Health Statistics
	: Increase State Sector Health spending from 5.5 to 7 percent of the budget
	: One percent of the total health budget for Medical Research
	: Decentralization of implementation of public health programs.
2007	: Achieve zero level growth of HIV/AIDS
2010	: Eliminate kala-azar
	: Reduce Mortality by 50 percent on account of TB, Malaria and other Vector and Water-borne diseases
	: Reduce prevalence of blindness to 0.5 percent
	: Reduce IMR to 30/1000 And MMR to 100/Lakh
	: Increase utilization of public health facilities from current level of <20 to >75 percent
	: Increase health expenditure by government from the existing 0.9 to 2.0 percent of GDP.
	: Two percent of the total health budget for Medical Research
	: Increase share of Central grants to constitute at least 25 percent of total health spending
	: Further increase of State Sector Health spending to eight percent
2015	: Eliminate lymphatic filariasis

THEMES OF THE WORLD NO TOBACCO DAYS

- "A World No Smoking Day", April 7, 1988
- World No Tobacco Day, May 31

On 31 May of each year, WHO celebrates World No Tobacco Day, highlighting the health risks associated with tobacco use and advocating for effective policies to reduce consumption. Tobacco use is the second cause of death globally (after Hypertension) and is currently responsible for killing one in 10 adults worldwide.

The World Health Assembly created World No Tobacco Day in 1987 to draw global attention to the tobacco epidemic and its lethal effects. It provides an opportunity to highlight specific tobacco control messages and to promote adherence to the WHO framework convention on tobacco control. Tobacco use is the number one preventable epidemic the health community faces.

Year	*Themes*
1988	: Tobacco or Health—choose health
1989	: Women and tobacco—the female smoker—at added risk
1990	: Childhood and youth without tobacco—growing up without tobacco
1991	: Public places and transport—better be tobacco free
1992	: Tobacco free workplaces—safer and healthier
1993	: Health services—our windows to a tobacco-free world
1994	: Media and tobacco—get the message across
1995	: Tobacco costs more than you think
1996	: Sport and art without tobacco—play it tobacco free
1997	: United for a tobacco-free world
1998	: Growing up without tobacco
1999	: Leave the pack behind
2000	: Tobacco kills, don't be duped
2001	: Second-hand smoke kills
2002	: Tobacco-free sports
2003	: Tobacco-free film, tobacco free fashion
2004	: Tobacco and poverty, a vicious circle
2005	: Health professionals against tobacco
2006	: Tobacco—deadly in any form or disguise
2007	: Smoke free inside
2008	: Tobacco-free youth
2009	: Tobacco health warnings
2010	: Gender and tobacco with an emphasis on marketing to women

World Diabetes Day

In recent years, World Diabetes Day has focused particularly on raising awareness of the complications of diabetes affecting the heart, eyes, kidneys, and feet.

The following themes have been addressed since World Diabetes Day began in 1991:

1991 : Diabetes Goes Public
1992 : Diabetes—A Problem of All Ages in All Countries
1993 : Growing up with Diabetes
1994 : Diabetes and Growing Older
1995 : The Price of Ignorance
1996 : Insulin for Life!
1997 : Global Awareness—Our Key to a Better Life
1998 : Diabetes and Human Rights
1999 : The Costs of Diabetes
2000 : Diabetes and Lifestyle in the New Millennium
2001 : Diabetes and Cardiovascular Disease
2002 : Your Eyes and Diabetes
2003 : Diabetes and Kidneys
2004 : Diabetes and Obesity
2005 : Diabetes and Foot Care
2006 : Diabetes and the Disadvantaged and Vulnerable
2007 : Diabetes in Children and Adolescents
2009–2013 : Diabetes Education and Prevention

INTERNATIONAL DECADES

2011–2020 : Decade of Action for Road Safety.
2008–2017 : Second United Nations Decade for the Eradication of Poverty.
2006–2016 : Decade of Recovery and Sustainable Development of the Affected Regions (third decade after the Chernobyl disaster).
2005–2015 : International Decade for Action, "Water for Life".
2005–2014 : United Nations Decade of Education for Sustainable Development.
Second International Decade of the World's Indigenous People.
2003–2012 : United Nations Literacy Decade—Education for All.
2001–2010 : International Decade for a Culture of Peace and Non-violence for the Children of the World.
Decade to Roll Back Malaria in Developing Countries, Particularly in Africa.

Second International Decade for the Eradication of Colonialism.
1997–2006 : Decade for the Eradication for Poverty.
1995–2004 : Decade for Human Rights Education.
1994–2004 : Decade of the World's Indigenous People.
1993–2003 : Third Decade to Combat Racism and Racial Discrimination.
1991–2000 : Second Industrial Development Decade for Africa.
Second Transport and Communications Decade in Africa.
United Nations Decade Against Drug Abuse.
Fourth United Nations Development Decade.
1990–2000 : International Decade for the Eradification of Colonialism.
1990–1999 : United Nations Decade of International Law.
: International Decade for Natural Disaster Reduction.
1990s : Third Disarmament Decade.
1988–1997 : World Decade for Cultural Development.
1983–1993 : Second Decade to Combat Racism and Racial Discrimination.
1983–1992 : United Nations Decade for Disabled Persons.
1981–1990 : International Drinking Water Supply and Sanitation Decade.
Third United Nations Development Decade.
1980–1990 : Second Disarmament Decade.
1980S : Industrial Development Decade for Africa.
1978–1988 : Transport and Communications Decade for Africa.
1976–1985 : United Nations Decade for Women—Equality, Development and Peace.
1973–1983 : Decade to Combat Racism and Racial Discrimination.
1971–1980 : Second United Nations Development Decade.
1970s : Disarmament Decade.
1960–1970 : United Nations Development Decade.

IMPORTANT ACTS RELATED TO HEALTH

Acts

- The Indian Medical Council Act, 1956 and Regulations, 2002
- The Indian Nursing Council Act, 1947
- The Dentists Act, 1948
- The Pharmacy Act, 1948
- The Rehabilitation Council of India Act, 1992
- The Indian Medicine Central Council Act, 1970
- The Homeopathy Central Council Act, 1973
- The Consumer Protection Act (CPA), 1986
- The Registration of Births and Deaths Act, 1969
- The Epidemic Diseases Act, 1897
- The Transplantation of Human Organ Act, 1994

- The Prevention of Food Adulteration Act, 1954
- The International Health Regulation
- The Medical Termination of Pregnancy (MTP) Act, 1971
- The Maternity Benefit Act, 1961
- The Dowry Probihition Act, 1961
- The Immoral Traffic (Prevention) Act, 1956
- The Prenatal Diagnostic Techniques (Regulation and Prevention of Misuse) Act, 1994
- The Infant Milk Substitutes, Feeding Bottlers and Infant Foods (Regulation of Production, Supply and Distribution) Act, 1992
- The Juvenile Justice (Care and Prevention of Children) Act, 2001
- The Child Labor (Prohibition and Regulation) Act, 1986
- The Child Marriage Restraint Act, 1929
- The Persons with Disabilities (Equal Opportunity, Protection of Rights and Full Participation) Act, 1995
- The Mental Health Act, 1987
- The SCs and the STs (Prevention of Atrocities) Act, 1989
- The Narcotic Drugs and Psychotropic Substances Act, 1985
- The Drugs and Cosmetics Act, 1940
- The Drugs (Control) Act, 1948
- The Drugs and Magic Remedies (Objectionable Adverstiments) Act, 1954
- The Minimum Wages Act, 1948
- The Dangerous Machine (Regulation) Act, 1983
- The Plantation Labor, Act, 1951
- The Factories Act, 1948
- The Mines Act, 1952
- The Employees State Insurance (ESI) Act, 1948
- The Workmen's Compensation Act, 1923
- The Bonded Labor System (Abolition Act)
- The Environment (Protection) Act, 1986
- The Biomedical Waste (Management and Handling) Rules, 1998
- The Municipal Solid Waste (Management and Handling) Rules, 2000
- The Hazardous Waste (Management and Handling) Rules,1989
- The National Environmental Tribunal Act, 1995
- The Air (Prevention and Control of Pollution) Act, 1981
- The Water (Prevention and Control of Pollution) Act, 1974
- The Insecticides Act, 1988
- The Motor Vehicles Act, 1988
- Red Cross Society Act, 1936

YEARS OF LAUNCHING NATIONAL HEALTH PROGRAMS

National program	*Year*
Sexual Transmitted Diseases Program	1949
BCG Vaccination Program	1951
Community Development Program	1952
National Malaria Control Program	1953
National Family Planning Program	1953
Contributory Health Service Scheme	1954
National Water Supply and Sanitation Program	1954
National Leprosy Control Program	1955
National Filaria Control Program	1955
National Malaria Eradication Program	1958
National Small Pox Eradication Program	1962
School Health Program	1962
National Goiter Control Program	1962
District Tuberculosis Program	1962
Applied Nutritional Program	1963
National Trachoma Control Program	1963
Contributory Health Services renamed as Central Government Health Scheme	1963
Expanded Family Planning Program	1963
National Trachoma Control Program	1968
All India Hospital (Postpartum) PP Program	1969
Accelerated Rural Water Supply Program	1972
National Program of Minimum Needs	1973
National Program for Prevention of Visual Impairment and Control of Blindness	1976
Rural Health Scheme	1977
Re-oriented Medical Education (ROME)	1977
Modified Plan of Operation (MPO)	1977
Expanded Program on Immunization (EPI)	1978
National Guineaworm Eradication Program	1979
National Mental Health Program	1982
National Leprosy Eradication Program	1983
National Health Policy	1983
Universal Immunization Program (UIP)	1985
New 20 Point Program	1987
National Diabetes Control Program	1987
National AIDS Control Program	1987
Blood Safety Program	1989
Child Survival and Safe Motherhood Program	1992
Reproductive and Child Health Program	1994
Integrated Disease Surveillance Project (IDSP)	2004

Contd...

Contd...

National program	*Year*
Reproductive and Child Health Program II (RCH II)	2005
Integrated Management of Childhood Illness (IMCI)	2007-2010
Integrated Management of Neonatal and Childhood Illness	2010
National Rural Health Mission	2005-2012
National Urban Health Mission	2008-2012

WORLD HEALTH DAY

What is the World Health Day?

The seventh of April each year is celebrated as the World Health Day and it marks the date 1948 when sufficient countries had ratified their signature to bring the Constitution of the World Health Organization into force. Ever since 1950, a theme related to international public health has been chosen for the World Health Day, with an appropriate slogan. Thus in 1955, the slogan was "Clean Water Means Better Health". In 1962, "Preserve Sight—Prevent Blindness" and in 1980, "Smoking Health—the Choice is Yours".

All over the world, governments, WHO national commities, United Nations association and Nongovernmental Organizations help to arrange events related to the theme. Over the years, the World Health Day events have attracted more and more coverage by media—whether newspapers or radio and television. And the impetus does cease when the day is over—the them is regarded as valid for the rest of the year.

LIST OF WORLD HEALTH DAY THEMES

1950 : Know Your Own Health Services
1951 : Healthy for Your Child and the World's Children
1952 : Healthy Surrounding Make Healthy people
1953 : Health is Wealth
1954 : The Nurse, Pioneer of Health
1955 : Clean Water Means Better Health
1956 : Destroy, Disease Carrying Insects
1957 : Food for Health
1958 : Ten Years of Health Progress
1959 : Mental Illness and Mental Health in the World Today
1960 : Malaria Eradication—A Word Challenge
1961 : Accidents need not Happen
1962 : Preserve Sight—Prevent Blindness
1963 : Hunger, Disease of Millions
1964 : No Truce for Tuberculosis

1965 : Smallpox—Constant Alert
1966 : Man and His Cities
1967 : Partners in Health
1968 : Health in the World of Tomorrow
1969 : Health, Labor and Productivity
1970 : Early Detection of Cancer Saves Lives
1971 : A Full Life Despite Diabetes
1972 : Your Heart is Your Health
1973 : Health Begins at Home
1974 : Better Food for a Healthier World
1975 : Smallpox—Point of No Return
1976 : Foresight Prevent Blindness
1977 : Immunize and Protect your Child
1978 : Down with High Blood Pressure
1979 : A Healthy Child, A Sure Future
1980 : Smoking or Health—The Choice is Yours
1981 : Health for All by the Year 2000
1982 : Add Life to Years
1983 : Health for All by the Year 2000—The Count down has Begun
1984 : Children's Health—Tomorrow's Wealth
1985 : Healthy Youth—Our Best Resource
1986 : Healthy Living—Everyone a Winner
1987 : Immunization—A Change for Every Child
1988 : Health for All—All for Health
1989 : Let Us Talk Health
1990 : Our planet, our health—think globally act locally
1991 : Should disaster strike—Be prepared
1992 : Heart beat—The rhythm of health
1993 : Handle Life with Care—Prevent Violence and Negligence.
1994 : Oral Health for a Healthy Living
1995 : Target 2000—A World without Polio
1996 : Healthy City for Better Living
1997 : Emerging Diseases—Global alert, Global response
1998 : Pregnancy is Precious "Let us make it safe"
1999 : Active Ageing Makes Difference
2000 : Safe blood starts with me, blood saves life.
2001 : STOP Exclusion dare to care
2002 : Move for Health
2003 : Shape the Future of Life—Healthy Environments for Children.
2004 : Road Safety.
2005 : Make every mother and child count.
2006 : Working together for health.

2007 : International Health Security.
2008 : Protecting health from the adverse effects of climate change.
2009 : Save lives, Make Hospitals Safe in Emergencies.
2010 : 1000 cities, 1000 lives.

IMPORTANT INTERNATIONAL EVENTS AND DAYS

9th January	Cancer Day
30th January	Anti-Leprosy Day
1st February	Deaf and Dumb Day
8th March	International Women's Day
15th March	World Consumer Rights Day + World Disabled Day
16th March	Measles Day
20th March	World Forestry Day
24th March	World TB Day
7th April	World Health Day
26th April	Anniversary of Chernobyl disaster
30th April	Child Labor Day
1st May	World Labor Day
8th May	World Red Cross Day
12th May	Red Cross Day
13th May	Mothers Day
24th May	Dr Olle Hansson Day
31st May	World No Tobacco Day
5th June	World Environment Day
26th June	International Day against Drug Abuse and Illicit Trafficking
1st July	Doctors Day (India)
1st August	World Breastfeeding Day World breastfeeding week
5th August	World Breastfeeding Practice Day
6th August	Hiroshima Day
9th August	Nagasaki Day
20th August	World Mosquito Day
1st October	World Voluntary Blood Donation Day
1-7th September	National Nutrition Week
8th September	International Literacy Day
20th September	International Peace Day
3rd October	Habitat Day
10th October	World Mental Health Day
11th October	National No Tobacco Day
13th October	Anti-National Disaster Day
14th October	World Standards Day
16th October	World Food Day

24th October	United Nations Day
15th November	World Diabetes Day
18th November	World Epilepsy Day
1st December	International Pollution and Prevention Day + World AIDS Day
2nd December	National Pollution and Prevention Day
3rd December	Bhopal Gas Tragedy Day
8th December	National Day for the Mentally Retarded
10th December	World Human Rights Day
11th December	UNICEF Day.

POLICIES

National Policies Related to Health

1. National Health Policy 2002
2. National Population Policy 2000
3. National AIDS Prevention and Control Policy 2002
4. National Blood Policy 2002
5. National Policy for the Empowerment of Women (2001)
6. National Policiy and Charter for Children Draft
7. National Policy for Old Person 1999
8. National Nutrition Policy 1993
9. National Health Research Policy Draft
10. National Policy on Education
11. National Water Policy
12. National Conservation Strategy and Policy Statement on Environment and Development 1992
13. Census of India 2001.

ACRONYMS

AFP	Acute Flaccid Paralysis
AIDS	Acquired Immunodeficiency Syndrome
ANM	Auxiliary Nurse-Midwife
ARI	Acute Respiratory Infection
BFHI	Baby Friendly Hospital Initiatives
CBO	Community Based Organization
CBR	Crude Birth Rate
CHC	Community Health Center
CIDA	Canadian International Development Agency
CMO	Chief Medical Officer
CPA	Consumer Protection Act
CPR	Couple Protection Rate
CSSM	Child Survival and Safe Motherhood
DALY	Disability Adjusted Life Year Lost

DGHS	Director General of Health Services
DHO/DMO	District Health/Medical Officer
DHS	Directorate of Health Services
DOTS	Directly Observed Therapy Short-course
DPT	Diphtheria, Pertussis, and Tetanus Vaccine
EPI	Expanded Program on Immunization
FAO	Food and Agriculture Organization
FWP	Family Welfare Program
GBD	Global Burden of Disease
GDP	Gross Domestic Product
GNP	Gross Net Product
GOI	Government of India
HIV	Human Immunodeficiency Virus
ICCIDD	International Council for Control of Iodine Deficiency Disorders
ICDS	Integrated Child Development Service
IEC	Information, Education and Communication
IFA	Iron and Folic Acid
ILO	International Labor Organization
IMA	Indian Medical Association
IMR	Infant Mortality Rate
ISM	Indian System of Medicine
IUD	Intrauterine Device
LHV	Lady Health Visitor
MCH	Maternal and Child Health
MDR	Multi-Drugs Resistance Tuberculosis
MDT	Mutli-Drugs Therapy of Leprosy
MMR	Maternal Mortality Rate
MOHFW	Ministry of Health and Family Welfare
MPW	Multipurpose Worker
MS	Medical Superintendent

Index

Page numbers followed by *f* refer to figure and *t* refer to table